PROFESSIONALISM IN MEDICINE

A Case-Based Guide for Medical Students

Medical professionalism is a challenging, evolving, and lifelong endeavor. *Professionalism in Medicine: A Case-Based Guide for Medical Students* helps begin this process by engaging students and their teachers in reflection on cases that resonate with the experiences of life in medicine. Through the book's seventy-two cases, commentaries, videos, and literature-based reviews, students explore the many challenging areas of medical professionalism. Readers will appreciate the provocative professionalism dilemmas encountered by students in the pre-clinical years and clinical rotations and by physicians of various specialties. Each case is followed by two commentaries by writers who are involved in health care decisions related to that case, and who represent a wide variety of perspectives. Authors represent forty-six medical schools and other organizations and include physicians, medical students, medical ethicists, lawyers, psychologists, nurses, social workers, pharmacists, health care administrators, and patient advocates.

John Spandorfer, M.D., is an Associate Professor of Medicine and an Associate Dean for Education at Jefferson Medical College, and a Fellow in the American College of Physicians.

Charles A. Pohl, M.D., is a Professor of Pediatrics and an Associate Dean for Student Affairs at Jefferson Medical College, and a Fellow in the American Academy of Pediatrics.

Susan L. Rattner, M.D., is a Professor of Medicine and Family and Community Medicine and Senior Associate Dean for Academic Affairs and Undergraduate Medical Education at Jefferson Medical College, and a Fellow in the American College of Physicians.

Thomas J. Nasca, M.D., is Chief Executive Officer of the Accreditation Council for Graduate Medicine, a Professor of Medicine and formerly the Gertrude M. and Anthony F. DePalma Dean (2001–2007) at Jefferson Medical College, and a Master in the American College of Physicians.

To my son Adam, he is always with me. *JS*

To my friend and colleague Philip Wolfson, M.D., whose passion and commitment inspire this work. *SLR*

To Janice, Emma, and Annie, who serve as my role models and give us hope for a better tomorrow. *CAP*

To Jean and our sons, whose sacrifices made all we do possible. *TJN*

And to our patients, whose gift of trust is the reward of professionalism. *The Editors*

CAMBRIDGE UNIVERSITY PRESS
Cambridge, New York, Melbourne, Madrid, Cape Town,
Singapore, São Paulo, Delhi, Tokyo, Mexico City

Cambridge University Press
32 Avenue of the Americas, New York, NY 10013-2473, USA

www.cambridge.org
Information on this title: www.cambridge.org/9780521704922

First published 2010
Reprinted 2010, 2011

A catalog record for this publication is available from the British Library.

Library of Congress Cataloging in Publication Data

Professionalism in medicine : a case-based guide for medical students /
edited by John Spandorfer . . . [et al.].
    p. ; cm.
Includes bibliographical references and index.
ISBN 978-0-521-87932-3 (hardback) – ISBN 978-0-521-70492-2 (pbk.)
1. Medicine–Vocational guidance–Case studies. 2. Medical ethics–Case
studies. 3. Clinical competence–Case studies. I. Spandorfer, John. II.
Title.
[DNLM: 1. Clinical Competence. 2. Physician's Role. 3. Professional
Autonomy. W 21 P9645 2009]
R690.P763 2009
610.69–dc22   2009027844

ISBN 978-0-521-87932-3 Hardback
ISBN 978-0-521-70492-2 Paperback

Professionalism in Medicine

A Case-Based Guide for Medical Students

Edited by

John Spandorfer, M.D.

Associate Professor of Medicine
Associate Dean for Education
Jefferson Medical College

Charles A. Pohl, M.D.

Professor of Pediatrics
Associate Dean for Student Affairs and Career Counseling
Jefferson Medical College

Susan L. Rattner, M.D., M.S.

Professor of Medicine
Professor of Family and Community Medicine
Senior Associate Dean for Academic Affairs and Undergraduate Medical Education
Jefferson Medical College

Thomas J. Nasca, M.D.

Chief Executive Officer
Accreditation Council for Graduate Medical Education
Professor of Medicine
Jefferson Medical College

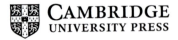

CAMBRIDGE
UNIVERSITY PRESS

Contents

Contributors

David Abraham, Ph.D.
Professor of Microbiology and Immunology
Jefferson Medical college

Salman Akhtar, M.D.
Professor of Psychiatry and Human
 Behavior
Jefferson Medical College

Josephine Albritton, M.D.
Assistant Professor, Department of Psychiatry
 and Health Behavior
Medical College of Georgia

Irene Alexandraki, M.D.
Assistant Professor of Medicine
University of Florida College of Medicine-
 Jacksonville

Kiona Allen, M.D.
Former student, University of Pennsylvania
 School of Medicine

Armand Antommaria, M.D., Ph.D.
Assistant Professor of Pediatrics
University of Utah School of Medicine

Louise Arnold, Ph.D.
Professor and Associate Dean
Office of Medical Education and Research
University of Missouri–Kansas City
 School of Medicine

David Axelrod, M.D., J.D.
Assistant Professor of Medicine
Jefferson Medical College

Phil Barbosa, M.D.
Former student, University of Minnesota
 Medical School

Catherine Belling, Ph.D.
Assistant Professor of Medical Humanities
 and Bioethics
Northwestern University Feinberg
 School of Medicine

Paul J. Bellino III, M.D.
Residency Program Director, Pediatrics
Geisinger Medical Center

Sarah Bergman Lewis, M.D.
Former student, University of Washington
 School of Medicine

Kim Best, M.D.
Director of the Division of Psychiatric
 Education
Albert Einstein Medical Center

Linda Blank
Vice President, The Culliton Group
Robert G. Petersdorf Scholar (2006–2007)
Association of American Medical
 Colleges

Justin Brandt, M.D.
Former student, Jefferson Medical College

Monica Branigan, M.D., M.H.Sc.
Family Physician in Palliative Care
St Joseph's Health Center

E. Ray Dorsey, M.D., M.B.A.
Assistant Professor of Neurology
University of Rochester Medical Center

David J. Doukas, M.D.
William Ray Moore Endowed Chair of
   Family Medicine and Medical
   Humanism
University of Louisville

Patrick Duff, M.D.
Associate Dean for Student Affairs
University of Florida College of
   Medicine

Kevin Eanes, M.D.
Former student, Jefferson Medical College

JoAnne Earp, Sc.D.
Professor and Interim Chair
Department of Health Behavior and Health
   Education
Gillings School of Global Public Health
University of North Carolina

Molly Eaton, M.D.
Former student, Jefferson Medical College

Jeffrey Ecker, M.D.
Associate Professor of Obstetrics,
   Gynecology, and Reproductive
   Biology
Harvard Medical School

Karen Edwards, M.D.
Associate Dean for Primary Care
New York Medical College

Henry C. Fader, Esq.
Health Care Services Group of Pepper
   Hamilton LLP

Anthony Farah
Student, Jefferson Medical College

Arthur Feldman, M.D.
Magee Professor and Chairman
Department of Medicine
Jefferson Medical College

Anna Filip, M.D.
Student editor
Former student, Jefferson Medical College

Faith Fitzgerald, M.D.
Professor of Internal Medicine
University of California, Davis School of
   Medicine

Laura J. Fochtmann, M.D.
Professor of Psychiatry and Behavioral
   Sciences
Stony Brook University School of
   Medicine

Julia Puebla Fortier
Director, Resources for Cross Cultural Health
   Care

Parry Frew, M.D.
Former student, Oregon Health and Science
   University

Kelly Fryer-Edwards, Ph.D.
Associate Professor
Department of Bioethics and Humanities
University of Washington School of
   Medicine

Jorge Galante, M.D., DMSc
Professor
Department of Orthopedic Surgery
Rush University Medical Center

Thomas H. Gallagher, M.D.
Associate Professor of Medicine
Department of Medical History & Ethics
University of Washington

David Garcia, M.D.
Associate Professor of Medicine
Department of Internal Medicine
University of New Mexico School of
   Medicine

Karen Glaser, Ph.D.
Associate Professor of Family and
   Community Medicine
Associate Professor of Psychiatry and Human
   Behavior
Associate Dean, Academic Affairs
Jefferson Medical College

Michael Golinkoff, Ph.D.
Bala Cynwyd, PA

Kenneth W. Goodman, Ph.D.
Professor of Medicine
Miller School of Medicine
Director, Bioethics Program
University of Miami

Stephen Gordin, M.D.
Director, Clinical Affairs
Horizon Health Care of New Jersey

Bridget K. Gorman, Ph.D.
Associate Professor, Department of Sociology
Rice University

Meghan Gould, M.D.
Former student, University of California,
    San Francisco School of Medicine

Neerav Goyal, M.D., M.P.H.
Former student, Jefferson Medical College

Michael Green, M.D., M.S.
Professor, Departments of Humanities and
    Medicine
Penn State College of Medicine

Amy M. Haddad, Ph.D.
Dr. C.C. and Mabel L. Criss Endowed
    Chair in the Health Sciences
Creighton University Medical Center

Frederic W. Hafferty, Ph.D.
Professor of Behavioral Sciences
University of Minnesota Medical School

Chris Henry, M.D.
Former student, Jefferson Medical College

Steven K. Herrine, M.D.
Professor of Medicine
Assistant Dean for Academic Affairs
Jefferson Medical College

Gerald B. Hickson, M.D.
Professor of Pediatrics
Vanderbilt University School of Medicine

Peter J. Hoffman, Esq.
Eckert, Seamans, Cherin and Mellott, LLC,
    Philadelphia, PA

Eric Holmboe, M.D.
American Board of Internal Medicine

Paul Indman, M.D.
Private Practice, Gynecology
Los Gatos, California

Gerry Isenberg, M.D.
Surgery section editor
Associate Professor of Surgery
Jefferson Medical College

Kathy Jensen
Salt Lake City, UT

John C. Kairys, M.D.
Assistant Dean for Graduate Medical
    Education and Affiliations
Vice Chairman for Education
Department of Surgery
Jefferson Medical College

Adina Kalet, M.D., M.P.H.
Associate Professor of Medicine and
    Surgery
New York University School of Medicine

Gregory C. Kane, M.D.
Professor of Medicine, Vice Chair for Education
Jefferson Medical College

Dylan Kann, M.D.
Former student, University of California,
    Davis School of Medicine

Lawrence Kaplan, M.D.
Professor of Medicine
Assistant Dean for Clinical Education
Temple University School of Medicine

David J. Karras, M.D.
Professor of Emergency Medicine
Temple University School of Medicine

Michael G. Kavan, M.D.
Professor of Family Medicine
Associate Dean for Student Affairs
Creighton University School of Medicine

Peter King, M.D.
Former student, Medical University of
    South Carolina

Elizabeth Kramer
Bala Cynwyd, PA

Daniel Kremens, M.D., J.D.
Neurology section editor
Assistant Professor of Neurology
Jefferson Medical College

Shanu Kohli Kurd, M.D.
Student editor
Former student, Jefferson Medical College

Thomas Lagrelius, M.D.
President, Society for Innovative Medical
  Practice Design
University of Southern California Keck
  School of Medicine

Christine Laine, M.D., M.P.H.
Editor
Annals of Internal Medicine

David Lambert, M.D.
Senior Associate Dean for Medical Student
  Education
University of Rochester School of Medicine
  and Dentistry

J. Lindsey Lane, M.D.
Pediatrics section editor
Associate Professor of Pediatrics
Jefferson Medical College

Stephen Latham, J.D., Ph.D.
Deputy Director, Interdisciplinary
  Center for Bioethics
Yale University

Jeremy Lazarus, M.D.
Clinical Professor of Psychiatry
University of Colorado Denver School of
  Medicine

Amanda Lerman, M.D.
Former student, Jefferson Medical College

Bernard Lopez, M.D.
Assistant Dean for Student Affairs and
  Career Counseling
Professor of Emergency Medicine
Jefferson Medical College

Beth A. Lown, M.D.
Assistant Professor of Medicine
Harvard Medical School

Kenneth M. Ludmerer, M.D.
Professor of Medicine
Washington University School of
  Medicine

Anne Drapkin Lyerly, M.D., MA
Associate Professor, Obstetrics and
  Gynecology
Duke University School of Medicine

Dianne MacRae
Department of Surgery
Jefferson Medical College

Barry D. Mann, M.D.
Professor of Surgery
Program Director, Lankenau Surgical
  Residency Program
Jefferson Medical College

Peter Mattoon, Esq.
Ballard, Spahr Andrews and
  Ingersoll, LLP

Andrew Matuskowitz
Student editor
Student, Jefferson Medical College

Robert McFadden, M.D.
Director, Student Personal Counseling
  Center
Jefferson Medical College

William McNett, M.D.
Division Chief, General Pediatrics
Jefferson Medical College

Brad Meier, Ph.D.
Delaware Psychiatric Center

Kenneth Mendel, M.D.
Clinical Associate Professor of Medicine
Temple University School of Medicine
Crozer Chester Medical Center

Elaine C. Meyer, Ph.D., R.N.
Associate Professor of Psychology
Harvard Medical School

Robin Miller, M.D.
Division of Hematology-Oncology
Alfred I. duPont Hospital for Children

Sohail K. Mirza, M.D., M.P.H.
Vice Chair and Professor
Department of Orthopedics
Dartmouth Medical School
The Dartmouth Institute for Health Policy and
   Clinical Practice

Stephen Ray Mitchell, M.D.
Dean for Medical Education
Georgetown School of Medicine

John A. Morris, M.S.W.
Director, Human Services Practice
The Technical Assistance Collaborative, Inc.
Professor, Department of Neuropsychiatry
   and Behavior Science
University of South Carolina School of
   Medicine

Jock Murray, M.D., M.A.C.P.
Professor Emeritus
Dalhousie University

Maryann Napoli
Associate Director
Center for Medical Consumers

David Nash, M.D., M.B.A.
Dr. Raymond C. and Doris N. Grandon
   Professor of Health Policy
Dean, Jefferson School of Health Policy and
   Population Health

Alvita Nathaniel, Ph.D., FNP-BC, FAANP
Associate Professor
Coordinator, Nurse Practitioner Track
West Virginia University School of
   Nursing

Elizabeth Norheim, M.D.
Former student, Jefferson Medical
   College

Karen Novielli, M.D.
Professor of Family and Community
   Medicine
Senior Associate Dean, Faculty Affairs
Jefferson Medical College

Sarah O'Brien
National Alliance on Mental Illness

Molly Osborne, M.D., Ph.D.
Professor of Medicine
Associate Dean, Student Affairs
Oregon Health and Science University

Kayhan Parsi, J.D., Ph.D.
Associate Professor of Bioethics and Health
   Policy
Neiswanger Institute for Bioethics and
   Health Policy
Stritch School of Medicine
Loyola University

Kathleen Flynn Peterson, R.N., J.D.
Past President of the American Association
   for Justice
Robins, Kaplan, Miller and Ciresi

James W. Pichert, Ph.D.
Professor of Medical Education and
   Administration
Vanderbilt University School of
   Medicine

James Plumb, M.D.
Professor, Department of Family
   and Community Medicine
Jefferson Medical College

Danielle Ku'ulei Potter, M.D.
Former student, Creighton University School
   of Medicine

Kimmie Pringle, M.D.
Former student, Jefferson Medical College

Carolyn D. Prouty, D.V.M.
Department of Medical History & Ethics
University of Washington

Howard Rabinowitz, M.D.
Ellen M. and Dale W. Garber Professor of
   Family Medicine
Director, Physician Shortage Area
   Program
Jefferson Medical College

Lee Rabinowitz, M.D.
Former student, Jefferson Medical College

Andrew Radu, M.D.
Former student, Jefferson Medical College

Susan Reichwein, B.A.S.W.
Program Coordinator
Parkinson's Disease and Movement Disorder
    Center
University of Pennsylvania

Carol Reife, M.D.
Clinical Associate Professor of Medicine
Jefferson Medical College

Caroline Rhoads, M.D.
Associate Professor of Medicine
University of Washington

J. Adam Rindfleisch, M.D., M.Phil.
Assistant Professor, Department of Family
    Medicine
University of Wisconsin School of
    Medicine

Christine Lee Ruehl, M.D.
Former student, Penn State College of
    Medicine

Robert Sade, M.D.
Professor of Surgery
Director, Institute of Human Values in
    Health Care
Medical University of South Carolina

Pamela Sankar, Ph.D.
Associate Professor, Department of Medical
    Ethics
Center for Bioethics
University of Pennsylvania School of
    Medicine

Ira Schwartz, M.D.
Associate Professor of Family and Preventive
    Medicine
Associate Professor of Pediatrics
Associate Dean of Medical Education and
    Student Affairs
Director of Admissions
Emory University School of Medicine

H. Edward Seibert, M.D.
Assistant Residency Director
Department of Emergency Medicine
Jefferson Medical College

Steven R. Simon, M.D., M.P.H.
Associate Professor
Department of Ambulatory Care and
    Prevention
Harvard Medical School

Thomas G. Sinas, J.D.
Robins, Kaplan, Miller and Ciresi

Lois Snyder, J.D.
Director, Center for Ethics and
    Professionalism
American College of Physicians

Richard Sobel, Ph.D.
Program in Psychiatry and
    the Law
Harvard Medical School

Paul Sorum, M.D.
Professor of Internal Medicine and
    Pediatrics
Albany Medical College

Jeffrey Spike, Ph.D.
Professor and Director, Campus-Wide Ethics
    Program
McGovern Center for Health, Humanities
    and the Human Spirit
University of Texas Health Science Center

Beth Ann Swan, Ph.D., C.R.N.P.
Associate Professor and Associate Dean of
    the Graduate Program
Jefferson School of Nursing

Mark Sylvester, M.D.
Former student, University of Miami

George Thompson, M.D.
Associate Professor
Office of Medical Education and
    Research
University of Missouri–Kansas City School of
    Medicine

Thomas Tomlinson, Ph.D.
Professor and Director
Center for Ethics and Humanities in the Life
    Sciences
Michigan State University

Griffin Trotter, M.D., Ph.D.
Associate Professor
Department of Health Care Ethics
Department of Surgery, Emergency Medical
    Division
St. Louis University School of Medicine

Walter Tsou, M.D., M.P.H.
Past President American Public Health
    Association
Center for Public Health Initiatives
University of Pennsylvania

Jon Veloski, M.S.
Center for Research in Medical Education and
    Health Care
Jefferson Medical College

Neil Vidmar, Ph.D.
Russell M. Robinson II Professor of Law
Duke Law School
Professor of Psychology
Duke University

Stanley F. Wainapel, M.D., M.P.H.
Professor of Clinical Physical Medicine and
    Rehabilitation
Albert Einstein College of Medicine

Delese Wear, Ph.D.
Professor of Behavioral Sciences
Northeastern Ohio Universities College of
    Medicine

Howard Weitz, M.D.
Vice Chair, Department of Medicine
Professor of Medicine
Jefferson Medical College

Ben Wilfond, M.D.
Professor and Head, Division of
    Bioethics
Department of Pediatrics
University of Washington School of
    Medicine

Paul Wolpe, Ph.D.
Asa Griggs Candler Professor of Bioethics
Director of the Center for Bioethics
Emory University

Erin Wright, M.D.
Cooper University Hospital

James Wu, M.D., M.P.H.
Former student, University of Wisconsin
    School of Medicine

Charles Yeo, M.D.
Samuel D. Gross Professor and Chair of
    Surgery
Jefferson Medical College

Chris Yingling, M.D.
Former student, Jefferson Medical
    College

Acknowledgments

Through the process of creating and editing this book, we have benefited from the collaboration of many people. First, we are deeply indebted to the 161 authors who diligently contributed commentaries and reviews. We have tried to ensure that this book represents their thoughtful and varied perspectives.

We would like to thank our editors at Cambridge University Press. We especially want to acknowledge Beth Barry's initial work, Angela Turnbull's editing, and Marc Strauss', Allan Ross', and Shelby Peak's help in shepherding this book through its completion. Since the inception of this project many colleagues, friends, and family have given us important counsel, feedback, and support. We are particularly grateful for the assistance of Rachel Adams, Kate Berg, John Caruso, Susan Coffin, Mitchell Cohen, Richard Cruess, Sylvia Cruess, Chris Jerpbak, Sal Mangione, Jen Mendel, Judy Mendel, Ken Mendel, Jared Meshekow, Anne Morganti, Janice Nevin, David Paskin, Carol Reife, David Spandorfer, Julia Spandorfer, Lester Spandorfer, Merle Spandorfer, John Veloski, Abigail Wolf, and the late Philip Wolfson. Also, the guidance, insight, and support of Dale Berg, Paul Brucker, Jonathan Zimmerman, and our section editors, Gerry Isenberg, Dan Kremens, Lindsey Lane, and Bernie Lopez, have been enormously helpful throughout the planning and editing of the vignettes and commentaries.

We feel fortunate to have worked with three exceptional medical student–editors. Anna Filip, Shanu Kurd, and Andrew Matuskowitz were invaluable in their feedback as they made time in their busy medical student schedules to add their perspectives to the vignettes and commentaries. In appreciation of our students, we will direct all royalties from this book toward funding professionalism projects in medical education.

Finally, our deepest gratitude goes to Amy Jordan, whose persistent support, constructive critique, and editorial expertise have helped turn the concept of this text into a reality.

Introduction

Concerns have been raised, both within and outside medicine, that physicians and the medical education system have lost their commitment to medical professionalism. One senses that in the perennial struggle between self-interest and altruism self-interest may be winning out. The realities of today's medicine, including commercialism, conflicts of interest, decreased autonomy, and increased oversight, have led to the erosion of the idealistic values expected of physicians since the conception of the Hippocratic Oath. This attrition of professionalism has, in turn, led to renewed calls to refine how professionalism is taught in medical schools. Many organizations, including the Association of American Medical College, the Accreditation Council for Graduate Medical Education, and the American College of Physicians have advocated initiatives to emphasize professionalism in medicine and medical education.

Despite the calls for change, challenges remain about how an ethos of professionalism should be inculcated in doctors-in-training. Professionalism is taught in the explicit and the implicit curriculum in most medical schools. Early in their education, students are first taught professionalism through the explicit curriculum. This occurs mainly during lectures, small group discussion and isolated events, including the "white coat ceremony." The challenge with learning professionalism in these settings is manifold. The explicit curriculum (1) may not be consistently and readily integrated with the four-year curriculum; (2) may be overly simplistic; (3) tends to focus more on the negative aspects of professionalism (such as using lists of rules and behaviors and describing the negative consequences of bad actions); and (4) lacks a single resource or text used for teaching students about medical professionalism. Perhaps the greatest challenge of learning professionalism is that the behavior stressed in the classroom setting is only partially corroborated by the students' experience in the clinical setting. As students advance in their training, learning professionalism skills increasingly occurs through the implicit, or hidden, curriculum. Values that were learned in lecture, small groups, and ceremonies become less memorable as students are more influenced by what they observe first-hand. Unfortunately, many of these first-hand observations are not ideal. Students often complain that a significant number of their educators display unprofessional conduct. The adage "do as I say, not what I do" well describes the conflict students have as they consider both their lessons learned in the classroom and in real-world settings. The cognitive dissonance generated through exposure to unprofessional behaviors in the hospital and outpatient setting frustrates and confuses students, and the behaviors observed trump those of the explicit curriculum every time!

Another challenge to teaching about this subject is gaining a common understanding of what the term *professionalism* means. Many physicians claim to "know it when they see it," yet when pressed have difficulty defining it. Each profession – the clergy, law, engineering, architecture, and the multiple professions of medicine – has at its foundation a social contract between that profession and society. From this perspective, professionalism may be defined as the means by which members of that group fulfill the obligations of that profession's social contract. In the case of medicine, several benefits may follow from the contract. One benefit is that the profession is permitted to autonomously set expectations and guidelines for the field, while it regulates and disciplines physicians when deviation from standard practices occur. The returned benefit for society from the social contract is that it can then trust that physicians will be capable, moral, accountable, and will act in the best interest of those whom they are serving.

Our primary goal in the creation of *Professionalism in Medicine: A Case-Based Guide for Medical Students* is to give medical educators and medical students a resource that can be useful throughout the four years of the medical school experience. We aim to facilitate discussion and further understanding of a wide range of topics within the domain of medical professionalism. Following a review in **Part I** on how professionalism has been defined, the book is organized around a collection of cases, commentaries, and literature reviews. The seventy-two cases portray real life medical challenges that are relevant to the experiences of medical students. Many of the cases focus on ethical dilemmas where there is no clear resolution. Some are dilemmas encountered where solutions may be easier, but other issues arise that demand deliberation. And still other cases broach topics where students and physicians struggle with the friction between the patient's welfare and the practitioner's own self-interest. Through applying clinical judgment and fundamental ethical and professionalism principles, the commentators explore reasoning behind and potential approaches to the case dilemmas.

The organization of this book is based on a view of professionalism described in the publication *Medical Professionalism in the New Millennium: A Physician Charter* (Ann Intern Med 2002:136:243–246). Developed by the American Board of Internal Medicine, the American College of Physicians, and the European Federation of Internal Medicine, the Charter has been endorsed by specialties throughout the world and in all fields of medicine. The Charter recognizes a set of three principles and ten professional responsibilities that must be practiced by the medical profession and understood by society (see Table). Such an expansive set of ideals, avowed by each physician, allows the public to place their trust in an ideal or virtuous physician.

The Physician Charter

Fundamental Principles
Principle of primacy of patient welfare
Principle of patient autonomy
Principle of social justice

Set of Professional Responsibilities
Commitment to professional competence
Commitment to honesty with patients
Commitment to patient confidentiality
Commitment to maintaining appropriate relations
Commitment to improving quality of care
Commitment to improving access to care
Commitment to a just distribution of finite resources
Commitment to scientific knowledge
Commitment to maintaining trust by managing conflicts of interest
Commitment to professional responsibilities

Very early in their medical education – with the start of anatomy dissection or with the first patient interview in front of the class – students realize that even this stage in their education presents encounters with ethical meaning. In **Part II** of the book, medical students are the central characters in cases. Each of the thirteen areas of the Physician Charter is explored by two cases, one in which the student is at an earlier stage in his or her medical education, and one later. Following each case, two commentaries are written, one authored by a faculty member and another by a medical student. Many of the cases raise issues asking students to balance their own health and welfare, their own expectations, or their own educational needs with the needs of their patients and with their vulnerable status in the academic educational hierarchy.

Students aspire to learn from situations in which doctors have the leading role. The cases in **Part III**, the main section of this text, shift to vignettes based on situations that physicians across medical specialties encounter. This section comprises forty-two cases, each followed by two commentaries that explore eight of the thirteen areas of professionalism in the Physician Charter: the three principles (patient welfare, patient autonomy, and social justice) and five of the professional responsibilities (honesty with patients, patient confidentiality, improving quality of care, managing conflicts of interest, and professional responsibilities). Following each case, two commentaries are authored. The first, a physician commentary, is written by specialists from family medicine, internal medicine, obstetrics-gynecology, pediatrics, psychiatry, surgery, neurology, and emergency medicine. The physician-commentator briefly describes the clinical issues that are relevant to render a judgment, explains the salient professional issues to be considered, and offers an opinion about how they would proceed with resolving the dilemma.

A second commentary is included because it is important to understand that perspectives and approaches to the cases will differ. The authors of these commentaries represent a wide variety of voices, each with a stake in health care decisions. These authors include ethicists, lawyers, psychologists, nurses, social workers, pharmacists, health administrators, health service researchers, patient advocates, and other medical educators. Family members of patients also comment on several of the cases. A unique format for learning about medical professionalism has been created with the video production of eight of the cases. These cases are brought to life by specially trained standardized patients from the Rector Clinical Skills and Simulation Center at Jefferson Medical College of Thomas Jefferson University. For access to the videos and more information on medical professionalism, see http://professionalism.jefferson.edu/.

Professionalism requires not only allegiance to the qualities discussed in the Physician Charter, but also an understanding of the medical literature and an awareness of where opinions originate. With this in mind, each of the eight areas of medical professionalism in **Part III** includes a comprehensive literature-based review of that topic. The authors also reflect on the commentaries and connect these writings with current literature.

Learning medical professionalism is a challenging, evolving, lifelong endeavor. *Professionalism in Medicine: A Case-Based Guide for Medical Students* will help this process by engaging students and their teachers in reflection on and discussion of cases that will resonate with life experiences. If this text, reinforced by appropriate clinical role models, fortifies the aspirations of future physicians to practice medicine guided by the precepts of professionalism, we will have achieved our purpose.

PART ONE

Defining Medical Professionalism

1 Defining, Teaching, and Learning Professionalism

Professionalism is frequently described as the fundamental core of medicine. This chapter discusses the importance of professionalism, its historical contexts, the current challenges, and the Physician Charter[1] as a worldwide medical response to these challenges. The chapter also examines and elaborates on other definitions of professionalism, explores how professionalism is acquired and strengthened, and summarizes current medical education approaches to promoting professionalism.

PROFESSIONALISM TODAY

Why Is Professionalism Important?

The Physician Charter avers in its preamble that "professionalism is the basis of medicine's contract with society."[1] This pact or agreement denotes a reciprocal, though tacit, relationship between the public and the medical profession. The public gives physicians rights and privileges in return for their adherence to values that enable them to protect the public health, which is vital to the very existence of society itself. That is, in exchange for authority to control key aspects of their working conditions, the public expects physicians to maintain high standards of competence and moral responsibility. According to the Charter, trust is essential to this contract.[1] Public trust depends on whether the actions of physicians and their leaders demonstrate the values of medical professionalism.

The authors would like to acknowledge the University of Missouri-Kansas City School of Medicine, the Arnold P. Gold Foundation, Harry Palmer, the Avatar course, Peter Senge and his collaborators.

Why Is Professionalism Increasingly Important?

Healers across time and cultures have embraced the values of professionalism. Derived from the need to care for the sick, professionalism in Western societies expanded in Hellenic Greece to include service and in medieval England to include obligations to society and individual patients. In the early 1900s William Osler reminded physicians in North America and Britain that medicine is a calling, not a business. He also stressed the role of empathy in doctoring. Later, leading the charge to reform medical education in the United States, Abraham Flexner added excellence and self-regulation to the notion of medical professionalism. As medicine increasingly relied upon science, expertise became an ever greater part of professionalism. In the last two decades of the twentieth century, the American Board of Internal Medicine (ABIM) reintroduced the notions of service and caring, and triggered a growing movement to reaffirm the importance of professionalism in medicine in both the United States and abroad.[2]

Why has this groundswell for professionalism emerged among physicians and the public alike? Authors of the Physician Charter note that physicians everywhere face unprecedented challenges that endanger the existence of medical practice as a profession.[1] These challenges involve the changing nature not only of medicine, but also of health care systems, resources for health care, physicians, and even patients.

Advances in medical technology and our increased reliance on it in patient care, for example, have diminished physicians' expression of humanism.[1,3] With the enormous advances in medical science have come significant progress in helping the sick, as well as heightened anxiety about the efficacy and safety of procedures and powerful drugs.[4] Technology has outpaced our ability to use it wisely.

Importantly, health care has become a business where commercial values clash with those of the profession.[1,5–9] Health is a commodity to be bought and sold to customers where market forces dictate health care delivery. Consumer and physician media marketing have influenced and perhaps corrupted medical decision making. Other highly skilled health care professionals compete with physicians for the health care dollar. Bureaucracy, at times, trumps patient care. Limited resources fail to meet patient needs, and result in unequal access to and coverage for health care.[1,6] These colliding forces have led to rising health care costs with an added pressure to contain costs.[1,7]

The intentional and unintentional acts of physicians themselves have markedly contributed to the interest in medical professionalism among physicians and the public.[7,10,11] Faced with the above changes in medicine, health care delivery, and resources, physicians have found it increasingly difficult to meet their responsibilities to patients and society.[1] They did not anticipate and adapt to the changing context of medical practice.[6] They were reluctant to become socially engaged[12] and address the injustices in health care,[13] and they placed undue emphasis on income and power to the detriment of patient welfare and the primacy of the patient's interest.[1,13] They failed to regulate themselves and allowed incompetent and unethical physicians to continue to practice medicine.[10,12–14] In addition, a younger generation of physicians favors a more balanced lifestyle.[4] In these ways, physicians themselves have contributed to the rising interest in professionalism within and without the profession.

For their part, patients have heightened expectations for the efficacy of medicine, while disparities among the legitimate needs of patients grow.[1] With greater access to medical information[4,8] and the rise of patient choice and empowerment,[7,8] patients have become dissatisfied with physicians and medical care. Moreover, there is a generalized mistrust in society today. This mistrust not only transcends the profession of medicine, but targets it as well.[6]

As a consequence of all these factors, external oversight and other outside influences have become more dominant in health care. This, in turn, has made it more difficult, yet more important, to maintain a commitment to medical professionalism.[12,15]

What Is the Physician Charter?

In response to the challenges facing the medical profession, authors from the United States, Canada, and Europe developed and propagated the Physician Charter, which enunciates three principles of medical professionalism and specifies ten professional responsibilities.[1]

The *primacy of patient welfare, patient autonomy, and social justice* constitute the Charter's principles. The principle of patient primacy contributes to patient and societal trust by ensuring that "the interest of the patient" will not be compromised by "market forces, societal pressures, and administrative exigencies…"[1] The principle of patient autonomy requires physicians to be honest with their patients and to empower them so they can make informed and appropriate decisions about their own care. The principle of social justice demands that the profession promotes the fair distribution of health care resources and works to eliminate discrimination in health care.

Among physicians' professional responsibilities are those that focus directly on their *commitments to patients: to be honest with them, safeguard*

patient confidentiality, and maintain appropriate relations with patients.
Honesty requires that patients understand their condition and treatment.
It involves telling patients about medical mistakes, should they occur, and
reporting and analyzing mistakes to prevent them in the future. Patient confidentiality extends to persons acting on a patient's behalf when the patient
cannot give consent. Commitment to confidentiality is more important than
ever because of electronic information systems. However, physicians must
recognize that considerations in the public interest must occasionally override confidentiality.

Several other principles in the Physician Charter refer to broad social
issues such as *commitment to improved access to care and just distribution
of finite resources.* Physicians must strive to eliminate barriers to health care,
so that uniform and adequate care is available. Commitment to equity in
care entails promotion of public health, preventive medicine, and public
advocacy without concern for self-interest of the physician or the profession.
A just distribution of finite resources requires physicians to develop guidelines for cost-effective care and scrupulous avoidance of unnecessary tests
and procedures.

The remaining principles relate to the collective responsibilities of the
profession. These include the *commitment to professional competence,
improvement of the quality of care, and scientific knowledge.* They also
include *commitment to the management of conflicts of interest and discharge of professional responsibilities to the profession and its members.*
Regarding professional competence, physicians themselves must engage
in lifelong learning; the profession as a whole must ensure that the means
exist for all of its members to achieve professional competence. In addition,
physicians must be dedicated to improving quality of care by working with
other professionals to increase patient safety and optimize outcomes of
care, by developing and using better measures of quality, and by creating
better mechanisms to encourage continuous quality improvement of care.
The commitment to scientific knowledge entails the duty to uphold scientific standards, promote research, create new knowledge, ensure its appropriate use, and guard the integrity of medical knowledge. To maintain
public trust, physicians and their organizations must recognize, disclose,
and deal with conflicts of interest that arise in the course of their multiple
activities. Professional responsibilities include collaboration to maximize
patient care and respect for one another. Other responsibilities address
standard setting for current and future members of the professions and
self-regulation, including remediation and discipline of members who have
failed to meet professional standards. A final aspect of professional

responsibility is the acceptance of internal assessment and external scrutiny of all aspects of professional performance.

How Have Others Explained Medical Professionalism?

Teachers, clinicians, and learners have struggled with the meaning of professionalism because it is a complex multidimensional concept.[16] Frequently they say they cannot define it but know it when they see it. However, scholarship in the social sciences and medicine has produced more systematic explanations of medical professionalism that can enable medical faculty, practitioners, and physicians-in-training to better understand its meaning.

In the social sciences, early theoretical analyses of occupations distinguished the professions from other types of work and identified medicine as the prototype profession. The features of a profession were: a specialized body of knowledge, the altruistic service to patients and society, the right to establish practice standards for its members who maintain them through self regulation, and the responsibility to guard the integrity of the profession's knowledge and its use.[16] The nature of the relationship between client and professional was key. In the specific case of medicine, the placement of the welfare of the patient above self-interest was a central and positive feature of the profession.[11,17]

In medicine, the American Board of Internal Medicine (ABIM) contributed to delineating professionalism through its project on humanism.[18,19] The Board identified three humanistic qualities that a physician should bring to the profession of medicine: integrity, respect, and compassion.[18,19] In the mid-1990s, it defined professionalism per se in terms of aspiration to altruism, accountability, excellence, duty, service, honor, integrity, and respect for others.[20] It noted that altruism – serving the best interests of patients, not self-interest – is the essence of professionalism. It also listed challenges to professionalism such as greed, arrogance, and impairment.

By the end of the 1990s, the Accreditation Council on Graduate Medical Education (ACGME) designated professionalism as one of six core competencies for resident physicians to demonstrate. It specified professionalism as "a commitment to carrying out professional responsibilities, adherence to ethical principles, and sensitivity to a diverse patient population."[21] About the same time, the Association of American Medical Colleges (AAMC) published a normative definition of professionalism to assist medical schools with understanding and assessing professionalism.[22,23] It listed nine behaviors necessary for physicians to exhibit in order to meet their obligations to patients, communities, and their profession.

Physicians subordinate their own interests to the interests of others; adhere to high ethical and moral standards; respond to societal needs and their behaviors reflect a social contract with the communities served; evince core humanistic values including honesty and integrity, caring and compassion, altruism and empathy, respect for others, and trustworthiness; exercise accountability for themselves and for their colleagues; demonstrate a continuing commitment to excellence; exhibit a commitment to scholarship and to advancing their field; deal with high levels of complexity and uncertainty; and reflect upon their actions and decisions.[22]

Next, the AAMC and the National Board of Medical Examiners (NBME) joined forces to embed professionalism in medical education more thoroughly through assessment. Toward that end, an invitational conference reviewed and organized principles of professionalism derived from the literature and produced a catalog of professionalism behaviors.[7] Subsequently, a task force at the Center for Innovation of the NBME developed a set of sixty professional behaviors for use in an assessment tool, which emphasized altruism, followed by responsibility and accountability, leadership, caring, compassion and communication, excellence and scholarship, respect, and honor and integrity.[24]

Having declared that the literature lacked an inclusive yet concise definition, Cruess, Cruess, and Johnston proposed a working definition of professionalism in 2004.[15] Previously, professionalism was circumscribed as a series of qualities or behaviors. Their efforts resulted in a definition of profession serving as the etymological root of the frequently used words professional and professionalism. The definition efficiently combined the major elements of a profession as outlined by key sociologists and by scholars in medicine and offered a comprehensive guide for teaching professionalism. But it was not a definition of medical professionalism per se.

A "new professionalism" movement attempted to redefine professionalism in terms of greater physician engagement in the public arena while retaining the commitment to the care of individual patients. New professionalism assigns physicians public roles for advocacy and for participation in improving community conditions that affect the health of individuals, especially access to care and socioeconomic factors directly influencing health, such as poor housing conditions.[25] More pointedly, civic professionalism equates fulfilling the social contract between the public and the profession with physicians' improving the quality of care for individual patients and for the health care system through policy activism.[26] Reflective practice organizations[27] and the medical profession itself have been assigned major roles in spearheading policy initiatives.[28–30] A similar movement also appeared in the United Kingdom.[31,32]

Still searching for a crisp, clear definition of professionalism that would cover the meaning of preceding definitions and identify observable behaviors for assessment purposes, Arnold and Stern equated professionalism to "the aspiration to and wise application of the principles of excellence, humanism, accountability, and altruism that rest upon a foundation of clinical competence, communication skills, and ethical and legal understanding."[16]

The definition points to the necessary but not sufficient elements of professionalism – clinical competence, ethical understanding, and communication – which the authors depict as the foundational steps to a Greek temple. It thereby recognizes the attitudes, knowledge, and skills that underpin the application of the principles of professionalism. It refers to the additional necessary and sufficient elements of professionalism – excellence, humanism, accountability, and altruism – as aspirational principles, depicted by the columns of the temple. The definition thus views professionalism as a set of virtues toward which physicians continually strive. Further, it highlights the application of those principles in observable behaviors, which is the crux of the definition that supports assessment of professionalism. The definition implies that the principles may conflict and leads to the assertion that those who can wisely resolve the conflicts may be considered truly professional.[16] It is through application of these principles that physicians meet the health care needs of not only patients but also communities and society.

Common themes can be found among the definitions of professionalism.[2,16] These include the importance of physicians' knowledge, skill, learning, and the process of safeguarding the validity of medical knowledge. The definitions also typically mention the primacy of patient welfare over self-interest or altruism, a concept critical to patients' trust in physicians and to healing. If patients are not able to believe that the advice they receive from physicians is in their best interests, then the bond between patient and doctor dissolves. The Charter itself opens with the statement "[Professionalism] demands placing the interests of patients above those of the physician."[1] Historically, the definitions often describe professionalism in terms of a list of physician qualities or behaviors such as responsibility, reliability, and accountability; honesty and integrity; respect and other interpersonal skills; and self-improvement. Compassion and empathy are commonly included too, but they are notably missing in the Physician Charter. Their absence turns our attention to exploring differences in the definitions.

One striking difference turns on whether a definition treats professionalism as duty or virtue-based and envisions it as a contract or covenant relationship. Swick and colleagues[33] argue that the Charter envisions professionalism as a competent, timely service; well-defined, circumscribed tasks characteristic of an occupation; and a duty-based ethical framework. They maintain, however, that duty is not enough. They advocate for a definition of professionalism that transcends duty and competence and subscribes to the ideals of a higher professionalism, namely, exceptional service that transcends the provider's self-interest, work as a calling with often open-ended tasks, and a virtue-based ethical framework. The importance of the difference between duty and virtue-based can best be illustrated by contrasting the pursuit of competence with excellence. Embracing competence equals a commitment to meeting minimal standards, whereas embracing excellence equals a continual conscientious effort to exceed ordinary expectations.[16,20] Examples of pursuing the values of excellence and exceptional service can be found in the successful quest for better means to treat patients with cystic fibrosis,[34] and in the conscious choice of the physician who identified severe acute respiratory syndrome (SARS) and subsequently died after contracting the illness.

Related to the distinction between duty and virtue-based professionalism is whether a contract or a covenant shapes the relationship between the public and the medical profession. According to Swick and colleagues, the language of contract conveys a formal agreement explicitly codified and enforceable by law.[33] In turn, that legalistic language supports an interpretation of professionalism as mere rules to be followed. It also suggests that the relationship between the public and the profession is grounded in mistrust leading to " 'ethical minimalism,' in which physicians limit themselves to the 'precise letter of agreement.' "[33] Swick and colleagues claim that the Charter advances a duty or rule-based approach to professionalism.

An alternative approach to professionalism posits a covenant as the basis of the relationship between the public and the profession. A covenant is a solemn promise or pledge, exemplified by the oath that physicians take upon entering the profession. When recited, the oath represents a publicly binding promise that involves something beyond self-interest. It is a first step toward securing trust between the public and medicine, and providing a moral framework within which to consider the dilemmas that physicians and patients encounter.

Another striking difference in definitions is who the primary constituents are (i.e., individual physicians in service to individual patients or the profession as a collectivity with responsibility to society). Some definitions of professionalism, for example, largely describe the elements of professionalism in terms of qualities, behaviors, or values of individuals. Others implicate the responsiveness of individual physicians as well as the profession and its leaders in delineating professionalism.

Other variations across definitions reflect distinct physician qualities, commitments, and/or behaviors; different emphases on these elements;

and alternative interpretations of their meanings. Several of the definitions, for example, are distinctive because they include autonomy and self-
regulation as elements of professionalism.[10,13,15,35] Another definition adds
the ability to deal with uncertainty as a critical element of professionalism.[22]
One focuses on reflection and mindful practice[36] while another introduces
the obligation to express regret, apologize, and make amends for patient
errors.[37] Authoritative organizations and scholars assign varying degrees of
importance to the elements. Altruism, for example, is central to professionalism in some definitions,[20] while its explicit use is absent in the Charter and
other definitions.[1,38] Duty, advocacy, service, and/or social responsiveness,
on the other hand, are central to other definitions.[12,15,27–32] One definition
places knowledge as foundational to professionalism while highlighting
excellence, humanism, accountability, and altruism.[16] As for differences in
the interpretations of the elements' meanings in defining professionalism,
accountability is variously defined across authors.[20,39,40] The Charter shifts
respect for patients as persons to respect for patient autonomy, and one
scholar claims that this lexical change has impoverished how physicians treat
patients.[41]

The differences just identified among definitions stem from several factors:
the academic disciplines that inform the definition, the purpose of the definition, and the health care delivery systems and cultural traditions in which
those systems reside. For example, the Charter's notion of professionalism is
anchored in the bioethics movement with a heavy emphasis on patient
autonomy,[33] while the Cruesses' definition of profession reflects sociological
traditions.[15] The Arnold and Stern definition of professionalism was tailored
to meet specifications of effective assessment,[16] whereas Inui's definition,
which has the qualities of the virtuous person at its core, serves as inspiration
and a guide to instruction and understanding.[42] The absence of explicit reference to altruism in a definition from the Netherlands results, in part, from
the difficult fit between altruism and clinical practice there.[38]

Knowing the contents of the Physician Charter, identifying the elements of
professionalism, and being able to discuss the similarities and differences
among the various definitions of professionalism alone are not tantamount
to being a virtuous physician. We therefore turn our attention to the question
of how professionalism is acquired and strengthened.

HOW PROFESSIONALISM IS ACQUIRED AND STRENGTHENED

Cruess and Cruess provide an excellent outline to guide the teaching and
learning of medical professionalism.[43] They emphasize that students indeed
must learn the "cognitive base" of professionalism at the outset of their

careers (i.e., what professionalism is, where it came from, and the context in which it exists). Once students intellectually acquire the principles of professionalism, they must have access to opportunities to apply these principles in authentic learning activities in order to bridge the gap between "knowing what" and "knowing how."[43] By reflecting upon these experiences, students can then begin to build mindfulness[36] about the principles and engage in reflection-in-action.[44] The environment must support students as they learn, apply the professionalism principles, and come to adopt them as their own because they are the values of the profession they wish to join. This process, technically termed "socialization," is therefore a process of value transmission that occurs through meaningful experiences reflected upon within supportive communities.

How Do Medical Schools Currently Teach Professionalism?

To facilitate the socialization process, medical schools and residencies are designing programs that will eventually lead to comprehensive, evidence-based education for professionalism. Medical schools' curricula now include the cognitive information on professionalism through readings and didactic lectures. Small group discussions, standardized patient interactions, and self-reflection papers further refine, highlight, and clarify aspects of professionalism and its application. In addition, respected role models provide live examples of professionalism and discuss their actions in order to give students first-hand experience of professionalism.

In short, educational programs need to include a combination of explicit didactic and experiential approaches in authentic contexts in order to support a learner's socialization to the profession. This book itself is an example of such an approach. Cases about professionalism and professional lapses are a starting point for discussions grounded in "authentic activities" where learners can explore the application of principles without the risk of adverse outcomes. Another example is a web-based education workbook that includes stories about highly professional behavior.[45] It also describes experiential activities to undertake such as brainstorming solutions to professionalism conflicts, rehearsing what to do in professionally challenging situations, and practicing respectful interactions with challenging patients.

These approaches require the assumption that professionalism is developmental and can be taught, nurtured, and learned. There is increasing recognition that human capacities related to professionalism do develop, that their development can be deliberately accelerated, and that there are useful models to inform the process.

How Is Professionalism Developed and Nurtured?

Medical educators describe the development of professionalism as dependent upon career stage[16] and involving acquisition of practical wisdom through a prolonged period of experience and reflection on experience.[46] Likewise, the psychologist Lawrence Kohlberg points out that development of morality, a specific human quality related to professionalism, unfolds in a predictable sequence of stages[47] and is accelerated through challenging social experiences such as directed student discussions about thorny issues.[48]

The real challenge of professionalism is learning to resolve tensions and conflicts in medicine with wisdom and compassion.[16] A key reason that professionalism issues are thorny is that conflicts between principles remain invisible. In the authors' work collecting narratives about professionalism,[49] we saw situations in which it would be difficult, for example, to be both humanistic and accountable or to be both compassionate and excellent. Yet there was often little awareness of the existence of, implications for, and solutions to the tension. This problem can be addressed by using cases in this book to learn to recognize, name, and discuss unresolved issues in professionalism. These discussions will contribute to new reflective experiences and, in turn, foster growth in professionalism of learners and faculty alike.

Didactic descriptions of professionalism principles may disguise the fact that it is easy to act professionally when well rested and well provisioned and when the compassionate route is clearly marked. Yet the value of professionalism is most visible when the stakes are high, information is incomplete, and no predictable solution to the situation exists.[50] Such events, as depicted by the cases in this book, are familiar to the individual practitioner, to leaders of medical institutions, and to the profession as a whole. These circumstances can be associated with harmful reactions and emotions and unhelpful thought patterns that diminish one's ability to act professionally. Professionalism thus involves the art of deliberately choosing one's actions according to principles.[51] Self-control, emotional control, and cognitive self-reflection support students' and physicians' ability to act on principle and avoid destructive responses. The self-control literature provides strategies to limit instinctive reactions like anger.[52] Literature on emotional regulation and character development[53,54] describe how to develop positive emotions and thereby increase helping behaviors,[48] inspire further virtuous action,[47] and support expressions of empathy and altruism.[55] Achieving critical self-reflection entails cognitive self-regulation that leads to an awareness of the thoughts and emotions of oneself and others, along with a decrease in thinking patterns that lead to unpleasant emotions.[56] When not controlled, these damaging human tendencies not only threaten a physician's interactions with patients, but also put our survival as a species at risk. Indeed, Fawcett cautions that violence and vulnerability may lead humanity to self-annihilation within five to ten generations.[57]

In this context, development of professionalism brings an unexpected benefit. This chapter has outlined significant challenges now threatening physicians' ability to practice healing. Despite these challenges, a global network of physicians has endorsed a code of professional behavior, attitudes, values, and ideals.[16] As physicians adopt and embrace these professional ideals, they undergo a personal evolution toward noticing suffering, feeling its impact, and doing what they can to provide relief. These ideals call for physicians to treat their patients with respect, compassion, and integrity, regardless of their origins, beliefs, attitudes, or behavior. A code of humanism must not waver in the face of difference, difficulty, or hostility. Accepting these ideals provides a worldwide model for reducing intolerance, cruelty, and violence and expressing a humanism that encompasses all of us. An unintended benefit of openly practicing professionalism is that physicians do their part to shift the planet toward a saner time. That is a fundamental importance of practicing professionalism with as much heart as one can.

Louise Arnold, Ph.D.
Professor, Associate Dean
Office of Medical Education and Research
University of Missouri-Kansas City School of Medicine

George Thompson, M.D.
Associate Professor
Office of Medical Education and Research
University of Missouri-Kansas City School of Medicine

REFERENCES

1. ABIM Foundation. American Board of Internal Medicine, ACP-ASIM Foundation. American College of Physicians-American Society of Internal Medicine, European Federation of Internal Medicine. Medical professionalism in the new millennium: A physician charter. *Ann Intern Med.* 2002;**136**(3):243–246.
2. Arnold L. Assessing professional behavior: Yesterday, today, and tomorrow. *Acad Med.* 2002;**77**(6):502–515.
3. Brody H. Professionalism, ethics, or both? Does it matter? *Med Hum Rep.* 2003;**24**:1–4.

4. Working Party of the Royal College of Physicians. Doctors in society. medical professionalism in a changing world. *Clin Med.* 2005;**5**(6 Suppl. 1): S5–40.

5. Swick HM. Academic medicine must deal with the clash of business and professional values. *Acad Med.* 1998;**73**(7):751–755.

6. Bruhn JG. Being good and doing good: The culture of professionalism in the health professions. *Health Care Manag (Frederick).* 2001;**19**(4):47–58.

7. Association of American Medical Colleges, The National Board of Medical Examiners. Embedding professionalism in medical education: Assessment as a tool for implementation.

8. Bligh J. Professionalism. *Med Educ.* 2005;**39**(1):4.

9. Hafferty F. Viewpoint: The elephant in medical professionalism's kitchen. *Acad Med.* 2006;**81**(10):906–914.

10. Cruess RL, Cruess SR, Johnston SE. Professionalism: An ideal to be sustained. *Lancet.* 2000;**356**(9224):156–159.

11. Cruess SR, Cruess RL. Professionalism must be taught. *BMJ.* 1997;**315**(7123): 1674–1677.

12. Rothman DJ. Medical professionalism – focusing on the real issues. *N Engl J Med.* 2000;**342**(17):1284–1286.

13. Cruess RL, Cruess SR. Teaching medicine as a profession in the service of healing. *Acad Med.* 1997;**72**(11):941–952.

14. Cruess SR. Professionalism and medicine's social contract with society. *Clin Orthop Relat Res.* 2006;**449**:170–176.

15. Cruess SR, Johnston S, Cruess RL. "Profession": A working definition for medical educators. *Teach Learn Med.* 2004;**16**(1):74–76.

16. Arnold L, Stern DT. What is medical professionalism. In: Stern DT, ed. *Measuring Medical Professionalism.* Oxford, England: Oxford University Press; 2006: 15–37.

17. Parsons T. *The Social System.* Glencoe, IL: The Free Press; 1951.

18. Evaluation of humanistic qualities in the internist. *Ann Intern Med.* 1983;**99**(5): 720–724.

19. American Board of Internal Medicine. *Guide to Awareness and Evaluation of Humanistic Qualities in the Internist.* Philadelphia, PA: American Board of Internal Medicine; 1992.

20. American Board of Internal Medicine. *Project Professionalism.* Philadelphia, PA: American Board of Internal Medicine; 1994.

21. ACGME Outcome Project. Enhancing Residency Education through Outcomes Assessment, General Competencies, Version 1.2. ACGME Web site. http://www.acgme.org/outcome/comp/compFull.asp. Updated 1999. Accessed October 26, 2007.

22. Swick HM. Toward a normative definition of medical professionalism. *Acad Med.* 2000;**75**(6):612–616.

23. Association of American Medical Colleges Group on Educational Affairs. Assessment of Professionalism Project. www.aamc.org/members/gea/professionalism.pdf. Updated 2002. Accessed October 26, 2007.

24. National Board of Medical Examiners. Professional Behaviors. Assessment of Professional Behaviors Web site. http://professionalbehaviors.nbme.org/current-work.html. Accessed June 22, 2007.

25. Gruen RL, Pearson SD, Brennan TA. Physician-citizens – public roles and professional obligations. *JAMA*. 2004;**291**(1):94–98.

26. Brennan TA. Physicians' professional responsibility to improve the quality of care. *Acad Med*. 2002;**77**(10):973–980.

27. Frankford DM, Patterson MA, Konrad TR. Transforming practice organizations to foster lifelong learning and commitment to medical professionalism. *Acad Med*. 2000;**75**(7):708–717.

28. Sullivan WM. What is left of professionalism after managed care? *Hastings Cent Rep*. 1999;**29**(2):7–13.

29. Sullivan WM. Medicine under threat: Professionalism and professional identity. *CMAJ*. 2000;**162**(5):673–675.

30. Sullivan WM. Can professionalism still be a viable ethic? *The Good Society*. 2004;**13**:15–20.

31. Irvine D. The performance of doctors: The new professionalism. *Lancet*. 1999;**353**(9159):1174–1177.

32. Irvine D. Patients, professionalism, and revalidation. *BMJ*. 2005;**330**(7502):1265–1268.

33. Swick HM, Bryan CS, Longo LD. Beyond the physician charter: Reflections on medical professionalism. *Perspect Biol Med*. 2006;**49**(2):263–275.

34. Gawande A. The bell curve: What happens when patients find out how good their doctors really are. *The New Yorker*. December 6, 2004.

35. Cruess RL, Cruess SR, Johnston SE. Renewing professionalism: An opportunity for medicine. *Acad Med*. 1999;**74**(8):878–884.

36. Epstein RM. Mindful practice. *JAMA*. 1999;**282**(9):833–839.

37. Fiester A. Viewpoint: Why the clinical ethics we teach fails patients. *Acad Med*. 2007;**82**(7):684–689.

38. van de Camp K, Vernooij-Dassen M, Grol R, Bottema B. Professionalism in general practice: Development of an instrument to assess professional behaviour in general practitioner trainees. *Med Educ*. 2006;**40**(1):43–50.

39. Emanuel EJ, Emanuel LL. What is accountability in health care? *Ann Intern Med*. 1996;**124**(2):229–239.

40. Evetts J. The sociological analysis of professionalism: Occupational change in the modern world. *Int Sociol*. 2003;**18**:395–415.

41. Ross LF. What is wrong with the physician charter on professionalism. *Hastings Cent Rep*. 2006;**36**(4):17–19.

42. Inui T. A Flag in the Wind. https://services.aamc.org/Publications. Updated 2003. Accessed October 26, 2007.

43. Cruess RL, Cruess SR. Teaching professionalism: General principles. *Med Teach*. 2006;**28**(3):205–208.

44. Schon DA. *The Reflective Practitioner: How Professionals Think in Action*. New York, NY: Basic Books; 1983.

45. Thompson GS, Arnold L. Strengthening Professionalism through Humanistic Narratives. www.umkc.edu/profstories. Accessed October 26, 2007.

46. Hilton SR, Slotnick HB. Proto-professionalism: How professionalisation occurs across the continuum of medical education. *Med Educ.* 2005;**39**(1):58–65.

47. Crain WC. *Theories of Development.* New York: Prentice-Hall; 1985.

48. Peterson C, Seligman MEP. *Character Strengths and Virtues: A Handbook and Classification.* Oxford and New York: Oxford University Press; 2004.

49. Quaintance JL, Arnold L, Thompson G. Promoting medical professionalism through narratives: The students' perspective. poster presentation, research in medical education session, central group on educational affairs, Indianapolis, IN, 2007.

50. Patterson K, Grenny J, McMillan R, Switzler A, Covey SR. *Crucial Conversations: Tools for Talking When the Stakes Are High.* New York: McGraw Hill; 2002.

51. Palmer H. *Living Deliberately.* Altamonte Springs, FL: Star's Edge International; 1994.

52. Strayhorn JM Jr. Self-control: Toward systematic training programs. *J Am Acad Child Adolesc Psychiatry.* 2002;**41**(1):17–27.

53. Seligman ME, Steen TA, Park N, Peterson C. Positive psychology progress: Empirical validation of interventions. *Am Psychol.* 2005;**60**(5):410–421.

54. Seligman ME, Csikszentmihalyi M. Positive psychology: An introduction. *Am Psychol.* 2000;**55**(1):5–14.

55. Eisenberg N, Fabes RA, Murphy B, Karbon M, Smith M, Maszk P. The relations of children's dispositional empathy-related responding to their emotionality, regulation and social functioning. *Dev Psychol.* 1996;**32**:195–209.

56. Goleman D. *Emotional Intelligence.* New York: Bantam Books; 1995.

57. Fawcett J. It's a wonder that we make it. *Psychiatric Annals.* 2007;**376**:385.

PART TWO

Cases Involving Medical Students

2 Student and Faculty Cases

PATIENT WELFARE 1

A student, a few months into the winter of his first year of medical school, is increasingly anxious. He also has had frequent episodes of insomnia and abdominal pain. He is now struggling academically. Prior to medical school, he had no medical or mental health problems. Despite his ill health, he does not seek medical attention.

A Medical Student Perspective

When I place myself in this student's shoes, part of me is inclined to think, "I'm an adult. I can treat or ignore my health problems as I wish. My health is my business." Do you agree? Can physicians' failure to care for themselves negatively impact their patients? Does caring for others introduce an ethical obligation to care for oneself?

As a medical student, my basic responsibilities for self-care expand when I assume the role of caregiver. I think my patient care responsibilities begin with a responsibility for my own health. A number of studies document an effect of physician health and health practices on patient care. For example, in an article on depression among medical students, Rosenthal and Okie report that failing to seek treatment for depression can have a negative impact on patient care.[1] In a discussion of when it is appropriate for physicians to call in sick, Swinker acknowledges the dangers to patients when physicians continue to practice despite suffering from communicable illnesses such as TB or gastroenteritis. However, she also acknowledges a strong motivation to continue working despite illness because of a perceived "wimp factor," as well as the inconvenience of rescheduling a day's worth of appointments.[2] In an article examining physicians' preventive health practices, Frank and colleagues report that physicians' personal health habits may influence the health counseling they give to their patients.[2] Collectively, these studies point to a real ethical responsibility for self-care on the part of physicians in order to provide quality patient care.

Stress management is one aspect of self-care significant to students. The stress response, while important for memory formation, is known to impair learning and memory in the chronic phase.[3] Moreover, chronic stress makes us susceptible to illness. When a student is suffering from stress and illness, what happens to his ability to learn and retain the information he will need to care for his patients? From my own experiences studying the basic sciences during medical school, the information I learned during times of effective stress management was certainly better retained than the material I studied during stressful times or times of distraction. This underscores the importance of effective stress management in the early years of medical training for long-term retention of essential information.

Medical school, while certainly a time for clocking long hours with our textbooks, is also a time for establishing healthy stress-management behaviors such as regular exercise and formal relaxation (yoga, meditation, getting outdoors). In fact, in an article on physician impairment, Miller and McGowen reason that maintaining healthy lifestyles as well as setting professional limits and pursuing leisure activities outside of work are necessary to establish a buffer against the stresses of medical practice.[4] I interpret this as an endorsement of having fun during medical school or at least achieving a balance.

In many ways, the stressors of medical education can be seen as positive stressors. Entering a new hospital with a new team and new patients at the start of each clinical block presents challenging but positive experiences for many medical students. As we experience these stressors our bodies respond through release of substances such as cortisol and β-endorphin.[5] For the student in the vignette, managing stress may include seeking formal medical attention, following good sleep hygiene, getting adequate nutrition and adhering to a daily exercise regimen. Well-managed stress means that we experience the benefits of the body's stress responses, including a sense of accomplishment in meeting our challenges and the support of learning and memory.

Molly Eaton
Medical Student, Jefferson Medical College

A Faculty Perspective

Medical student and physician distress is a serious, pervasive problem. About half of physicians rate their morale as "five or lower" (on a scale of one to ten). Two-thirds report emotional burnout. About one in twenty report job-stress-associated suicidal ideation. However, only about one in four seeks personal counseling.[6] A similar fraction of medical students report burnout, with the percentage increasing as their training progresses.[7]

As I read the vignette, I considered the student's differential diagnosis. But there was so little information! I took the problem to my wife, who listened calmly, then stated, "Well, I think you'd have to rule out pheochromocytoma. Can you find out if the patient is having diarrhea or any other symptoms?" Before speaking with her, I'd only considered anxiety and depression. I was unsure what to do next.

I took time later to reflect on my thoughts and responses. It occurred to me that some sort of identification with the student in the vignette had happened. Perhaps I could understand my reactions apropos of the student and his situation. Specifically,

1. The confusion of roles – Am I supposed to diagnose this myself or seek help?
2. The uncertainty of how to proceed – Should I keep asking friends who are in medicine for help (analogous to *curbsiding*)?
3. The pressure of time – Do I have the time to deal with this right now, or can it be put off?

There is a correlation between some obstacles I was experiencing and obstacles medical students encounter in dealing with illness. The difficulties most frequently reported by medical students seeking care are financial concerns, concerns about confidentiality, not having access to care, and that they are "too busy to take time off." In fact, more than six in ten students report seeking informal consultation, stating reasons of convenience, decreased expense, and speed.[8]

In their quest for consensual validation, students will ask others students about their experiences as patients. The stories they hear may be further incentive to avoid getting treatment, or to circumvent the "usual" channels. In a poignant story written by a first-year medical student being treated for an AVM, the student did not report difficulty with accessing care. However, she was left wanting for more communication, recognition of her distress, and recognition of the inappropriateness of her being a "teaching case" during her treatment.[9]

During their pre-clinical years, medical students will learn about different learning theories. They will learn that modeling is the most effective way to learn new, complex behaviors. Caring for one's own illness is an intricate problem, and modeling will be a very important means by which students will adapt solutions. In a paper on medical student distress, Dyrbye et al.

proposed some ideas for promoting well-being during medical training. Their ideas fell under four headlines: creating a nurturing learning environment, identifying and assisting struggling students, teaching skills for stress management/promoting self-awareness, and helping students promote personal health.[10] Although these four headlines represent a well-considered strategy, I think the authors of the paper stop just short of a comprehensive approach. If modeling is a means of skills acquisition for the students, then having workshops for residents and attendings on managing stress and illness is an overlooked necessity.

Clearly medical students are:

1. very vulnerable to illness, and
2. at risk to experience difficulties accessing appropriate care.

Any efforts by educators to model healthy care-seeking behaviors would be a high-yield investment. What would you do if you needed to deal with an illness? Concerning the student from our vignette – how should he move forward? His most pressing needs are recognizing that there is a problem, and seeking help. Ideally, the services at his school system (student health, student personal counseling, academic affairs) could work together. The goals are to assure that he receives support, examines his options, and knows how to begin appropriate treatment.

Robert F. McFadden, M.D.
Director, Student Personal Counseling Center
Jefferson Medical College

PATIENT WELFARE 2

A third year student has just finished a very busy day and overnight call on her pediatrics rotation. She has had only an hour of sleep. Although the clerkship syllabus states that it is appropriate to leave at noon after a night on call, her resident has not sent her home. She is feeling the lack of sleep and is concerned about her twenty-minute drive home. She is also concerned that asking to leave will reflect poorly on her and affect her evaluation.

For a video of the vignette, see http://professionalism.jefferson.edu/.

A Medical Student Perspective

As a medical student, my quality of life depends on finding balance between work responsibilities and personal needs. However, my professional standing seems to depend on my work ethic and the sacrifices I'm willing to make for my training.

What might be the negative repercussions of a student choosing to leave her shift when she feels too tired or stressed out? Students often know the most about a patient's social and emotional state, so leaving without adequately signing out psychosocial issues could compromise patient care. Some patients may prefer to have a student present for support during procedures or in family meetings. The student's absence may affect the patients' perception of their care. Less time spent with patients could also result in missed learning opportunities. The grueling environment of clinical rotations may be a requisite "initiation" for the life-or-death decisions that will come in the years ahead.

When faced with a difficult decision on the wards, perhaps the most salient consequence for students is a poor evaluation. Medical students confronting ethical dilemmas often make decisions based on how their residents will evaluate them.[11] Most strive to be a "team player" and are reluctant to speak up about moral conflicts fearing it will reflect poorly on performance.[12] Even when work obligations are complete, leaving a shift without offering additional help risks being perceived as uncommitted and lazy. Nevertheless, students making every effort to be a team player may find themselves compelled to doing things they feel are unethical and counter-productive to their learning.[11] The first time a student is asked to do a difficult procedure can result in failed attempts and suffering for the patient.[11] Working extra hours while sleep deprived can compromise learning and health. Sleep loss from a night on call has been shown to impair cognitive performance[13] and increase the risk of motor vehicle accidents,[14] and may be contributing to the high rates of depression and anxiety among medical students.[15] Psychological distress can lead to poor academic performance and decreased empathy towards patients.[15] Sleep loss and subsequent poor quality of life, therefore, can interfere with the very reason we train to be doctors – to provide the best possible care for our patients.

Perhaps finding the courage to address the dilemmas we face is a step in the right direction? The fear of being poorly judged for simple decisions, like eating lunch or asking to leave, is real. However, the assumption that drives that fear is often irrational. Most of my residents and attendings are reasonable people who understand my need to eat and sleep. One of my greatest epiphanies was realizing this obvious fact: the only way my residents can know that I'm done with my work and ready to leave is to tell them! So, when I'm exhausted on post-call days, I have found what often works is simply asking my resident if there's anything else I can do before I leave. This can be an effective and sensitive approach to finding balance between supporting my team and advocating for my personal health.

Meghan Gould
Medical Student, University of California, San Francisco
School of Medicine

A Faculty Perspective

The tension between service to patients and attention to personal concerns is pervasive in medicine and can be especially poignant for students because of the importance of meeting supervisors' expectations. Altruism, the commitment to put the interests of others before one's own, is a core value of medicine but making it a living value, that can be both aspired to and enacted daily, is challenging. This challenge has increased over the past generation as medicine has become substantially feminized, obviating the division of labor that allowed physician-fathers to devote themselves to their patients while stay-at-home mothers managed the household.

The third year medical student in the vignette is faced with a discrepancy between her understanding of the expectations for her post-call responsibilities and what she believes her resident requires. Her perceptions of her resident's standards for a third year student may be inaccurate, but perhaps not. Unfortunately, residents too commonly say, "Where I went to medical school, the students stayed all night with their teams," or "Students carried as many patients as the interns." Once the resident has even intimated such expectations it is difficult for a conscientious student to choose to fall short of them. And, while students overestimate the importance of "putting in the hours," the resident's opinion of her diligence and commitment to patients will certainly color her evaluation.

The impact of duty hour reduction (DHR), mandated for residents in 2003, has been complex and controversial. There are five outcomes of particular interest: the quality of patient care;[16,17] resident personal life and safety; fostering of altruism; accomplishment of work previously done by residents; and teaching and learning by all trainees.[18–20] Although directed at house staff, DHR has implications for medical students. Better-rested residents might be more willing to teach or, given the obligation to be out of the hospital within thirty hours of the beginning of a shift, residents may prioritize patient care over teaching. Faculty and students may feel that they are filling in for residents who are mandated to be out of the hospital. Predictably, the specific strategies used to reduce resident duty hours influence whether the impact is regarded as beneficial or deleterious.[21]

Medical schools must ensure that student patient-care responsibilities conform to school policy and that student learning is not compromised by policy changes intended to address other issues. Medical students already evaluate resident teaching and the learning opportunities afforded by their clerkships. Perhaps evaluations should contain additional items encouraging students to reflect on the balance between service to patients and their own personal needs and addressing the clerkship's conformance to school policy. The student might be asked to respond to items such as: "This clerkship supported my continued learning about altruism and balancing my service to patients with my other roles and responsibilities," and "The resident's expectations of my performance were consistent with school policy (night call, patient load, scut, etc.)." Medicine in the twenty-first century requires a "new professionalism";[22] there is more to devotion to patients than working to exhaustion.

Molly Cooke, M.D.
Professor of Medicine
Director, the Haile T. Debas Academy of Medical Educators
University of California, San Francisco School of Medicine

PATIENT AUTONOMY 1

A second year student is assigned to obtain a history and perform a physical exam on an elderly patient who was hospitalized for treatment of pneumonia. After thirty minutes, the patient appears tired and politely asks if the student can return the next day to finish the history and examination. The student is expected to present to her attending and to hand in her H&P at the end of the session that day.

A Medical Student Perspective

From the day we first put on the white coat, we take on a responsibility to hold our patients' health above our own interests. Faced with this situation, the student in the vignette might choose to explain to the patient the importance of the assignment and beseech her to keep going. After all, what harm would be done with just a couple more questions?

I think this rationalization uses dangerously selfish logic. While the proper completion of the assignment may be a very real concern to the medical student, it is far less important than the wishes of the patient lying in bed in front of her. The medical student must recognize that while this assignment is a valuable learning experience, it probably has no therapeutic benefit for the patient. I would argue that the only ethically sound choice is for the student to respect the patient's wishes and leave to find another patient.

The medical student has a responsibility towards the patient, but I don't believe that the patient has any such responsibility towards the student. I fondly remember the time during my Family Medicine rotation when I entered the room to see an elderly woman with chronic sinusitis. As I was introducing myself she interrupted: "No, No, I'm here to see the doctor, not just anybody," she said, shooing me away. I smiled and told her the doctor would be in shortly. I was taken aback by her rudeness but I begrudgingly accepted her choice not to contribute to my medical education.

I am not "just anybody." I am a future doctor who has studied countless hours and has overcome many hardships to get here. Yet it is a common mistake made by medical students to summarize our worth based on academic achievement. Our grades and test scores as undergraduates got us here and our performance in medical school will determine entrance into residency. However, the ongoing drive for personal achievement can sometimes compromise our ability to act courteously towards others. The second year student in the vignette may feel indignant at the patient's request. She may think to herself: "My grade in this course, my entire future, is at stake and you're too tired to give me your stupid history? I'm tired too!" What is really at stake is the patient's autonomy, which is of greater value than any one assignment or grade. Although a treating physician may be justified in trying to change a patient's mind to accomplish an important intervention, the medical student must be mindful that is not the case here.

It can be quite easy for an enthusiastic medical student in a shiny white coat to coerce the seriously ill patient. It is far more difficult for the student to look the attending physician in the eye and explain that by respecting the patient's wishes she was not able to complete the assignment. Further, it is critical that the educators of medical students be flexible in these situations and consistently reinforce the need to handle difficult situations with grace and good communication.

Andrew Radu
Medical Student, Jefferson Medical College

A Faculty Perspective

At first blush, this scenario seems very simple. The student should thank the patient for his time and leave. But that's easy for an attending to make that determination. In fact, the reality of medical education dictates that the student must get this assignment done. This reality includes completing an assignment within a relatively short amount of time, writing up the medical history, researching the patient's diagnosis in order to discuss it with the instructor (in case asked), and all with a quick turn-around time. The bottom line is the patient's non-participation creates a problem.

If this was a third year medical student on an inpatient rotation at a hospital where all patients had a student assigned to participate on their care teams, one might have a stronger argument for participation, since the student might positively impact the patient's medical care. Or if the learner was a resident, then it would be almost mandatory that they be involved in the patient's care. (I have made rare exceptions on my inpatient service under extraordinary circumstances to allow a patient not to have resident contact.)

The bigger consideration is whether the patient is obligated to participate in a student's educational pursuits. One can give convincing arguments that both support and refute this premise but ultimately it comes back to respecting a patient's autonomy.

In this scenario, the student has three choices, all fraught with a potentially poor outcome:

1. The student can gently urge the patient to continue, although at the risk of having the quality of the information obtained in the history impacted by the patient's fatigue, and, more importantly, agitating the patient and exacerbating the illness.

2. The student can offer to come back later that day after the patient has rested. If the student comes back later, he risks not being able to finish the assignment in a timely manner.

3. The student can find another patient to help them complete the assignment. This allows the patient to be autonomous. The student does have to spend extra time interviewing a second patient but hopefully something is learned from the first patient encounter.

I believe the third option is best. And communication with the clinical instructor is important.

This scenario reminds us that flexibility is necessary when interacting with patients and completing clinical assignments. The nature of the healing arts and taking care of ill people includes many variables, some which are unpredictable and uncontrollable. Because patient care is a fluid and dynamic venture, the instructor should understand that a patient's cooperation is part of this process. The instructor should be flexible enough to either give an extension to the student's assignment so the interview can be completed with the initial patient or help find another patient in order to complete the interview.

William G. McNett, M.D.
Division Chief, General Pediatrics
Jefferson Medical College

PATIENT AUTONOMY 2

A surgical resident and fourth year medical student on rounds see a patient scheduled for an elective femoral-popliteal bypass. The patient looks at them anxiously and says "I hope that Dr. White is doing the entire operation. I know you are both here to learn, but I came to this hospital because Dr. White is the best and I only want him to operate on me." The resident explains that Dr. White will be doing the entire procedure and he will be assisting and the student will be watching. Near the completion of the operation, Dr. White turns to the student and asks her to help close the incision.

For a video of the vignette, see http://professionalism.jefferson.edu/.

A Medical Student Perspective

It is not hard to imagine that helping close the incision would be the easiest choice for the student, as such participation is expected of a fourth year student and would be done at the request of the attending. Closing incisions also gives a student the opportunity to make a more personal contribution to the case while practicing a useful skill. However, if she did so, the student would knowingly break the agreement formed with the patient during rounds. The fact that the student's action would have little impact on the outcome of the operation is not sufficient reason to ignore the patient's preferences. Doing so would place the trust of the patient at risk as well as the patient–surgeon and patient–student relationships.

An appropriate first step is to make Dr. White aware of the conversation from rounds. The student is thus showing respect for the patient and acknowledging his right to make autonomous decisions regarding his care. These are fundamental principles of the informed consent process. Informed consent is considered an ongoing dialogue between patient and surgeon,[23] and the resident and student are participants in this process. They have a mutual understanding with the patient regarding their roles in the operation and should honor those expectations. Additionally, the patient's expression of personal preferences before a procedure should be a foremost consideration when making decisions regarding an anesthetized patient.

As medical students on clinical rotations, we see the look of hesitancy some patients express when we ask permission to participate in their care. Most patients are willing to interact with students, but this willingness varies with the clinical setting.[24] One survey in an outpatient clinic noted that only 2 percent of patients would not allow students to watch surgery but 59 percent said they would probably or definitely not allow students to suture incisions.[24] As in this case, the appropriate response to patients' concerns is to err on the side of giving more information regarding trainees' roles rather than less. If open discussions do not resolve concerns over student involvement, patients ultimately have the right to choose from whom they receive treatment.[25]

Because of their willingness to interact with students, we come to expect patients' consent, even though our involvement may place additional burdens on their care. Medical students have a right to a clinical education, but the obligation to fulfill this responsibility rests with the university, not its patients.[26]

In this case, the student must explain to the attending physician why she is refusing a simple request. Speaking up is not without risk, because these actions may affect her evaluation and status on the team. However, patients entrust physicians to exercise moral courage on their behalf.[27] Just as technical skills must be sought and practiced by future physicians, so too must habits of character and ethical conduct.

Peter King
Medical Student, Medical University of South Carolina

A Faculty Perspective

In his preoperative discussion, Dr. White would have ensured that the patient understood basic aspects of his disease and of the operation. During this conversation, the patient did not express to Dr. White the same thought he later mentioned to the resident and student: that he only wanted Dr. White to operate on him. If he had, the surgeon would have explained that he could not do the operation by himself: assistants – residents, medical students, physician's assistants, or nurses – would be helping him. They would sometimes hold tissue aside to allow him to see the blood vessels, and would sometimes be cutting or sewing, according to the usual routine that he employed in all of his operations. He would be physically present at the operating table during all the critical parts of the operation and would be fully responsible for every aspect of the procedure.[28] These were the very routines, he would have explained, that had led to his excellent surgical results. Nearly all patients gladly accept an explanation of this kind. If the patient insisted, however, that he and only he cut and sew, Dr. White would be bound to do just that (or to refer the patient to another surgeon).

Because medical students are not physicians, the patient should be made aware of their participation in operations: "In instances where the patient will be temporarily incapacitated (e.g., anesthetized) and where student involvement is anticipated, involvement should be discussed before the procedure is undertaken whenever possible."[25] Dr. White probably introduced the resident and the student to the patient when they entered the room, but, failing that, his mention of student assistants would have satisfied this ethical guideline. The patient could ask for further discussion and could, if he wished, exclude students from participating in the operation.

The resident's response to the patient's question is inappropriate. The patient is naïve about operating room procedures, so the resident's succinct reply misled him into false beliefs: Dr. White would be the only one cutting and sewing, assistants do not perform these acts, and the student, merely "watching," would not be scrubbed at the operating table. In reality, the lines between roles are not nearly so plainly drawn in the operating room.

Because Dr. White did not talk with the patient about operating room personnel, the student was ethically obligated not to help close the incision, just as described in the above essay. Indeed, the student should not even be scrubbed in at the operating table; rather, she should watch the operation from the best available vantage point. When asked to help close, the student should demur, repeating the resident's comments to the patient. Dr. White should then excuse the student from participating further in the operation. Later, in private, he should have an edifying conversation with the resident, explaining how to talk with patients about surgical assistants.

Robert Sade, M.D.
Professor of Surgery
Director, Institute of Human Values in Health Care
Medical University of South Carolina

SOCIAL JUSTICE 1

A second year student is doing a longitudinal patient care elective with a faculty member in obstetrics/gynecology. After several sessions he realizes that his participation is limited to the "non-private" patients, who had Medicaid or no insurance. He was not invited to see "private" patients, who had commercial insurance. He also noted that Latina and African-American patients were more likely to be non-private patients. One of his friends, when asked, was having the same experience with a surgery attending.

A Medical Student Perspective

This scenario gives cause for concern in that the patients are being stratified into two categories: those whom the medical student is and is not "allowed" to examine. From an educational standpoint, the groups break down into those from whom the medical students can "learn" and those from whom they cannot. Without proper explanation from the attending physician, this second year student is left to wonder why he is only allowed to see the non-private patients. Is it because those of lesser means do not have the right to object to being seen by a junior medical student? This student's experience is similar to that reported in the literature. In a study of student experience in an ambulatory clinic, students were significantly more likely to see patients with Medicaid insurance and of a minority group.[29]

Working with those of lesser financial means is not new for most medical students. Some volunteer at free clinics, while others offer assistance at homeless shelters or community-based programs. For most students who enter medical school, pursuing a career in medicine is accompanied by a deep-seated desire to help those in need. Now for a second year medical student, "those in need" are those in need of medical care. Imagine a private and non-private patient with beds right next to each other in the hospital. Repeat this situation several times, and the message being reinforced to the student may be that being a private patient earns certain privileges, one of which is the privilege of not to being "practiced on" by a medical student.

"Practicing" on patients, some of whom may not fully understand the extent of our inexperience, may pose ethical challenges. Even while getting proper supervision, are we putting our patients at risk? Perhaps not. Studies have shown that student involvement in indigent care may benefit both patient and student.[30] Studies of patients in an outpatient setting,[29] maternity ward,[30] and inpatient surgical setting[31] have reported that they appreciate that students can give them more time than other members of the health care team. Over 90 percent of surgical patients "agreed" or "strongly agreed" when asked if they had benefited from student involvement.[31] Among maternity patients, there was a significant trend for patients from lower social class groups to have a more positive attitude toward student doctors.[30] Another benefit of working with indigent patients may be that the cultural barriers between patients and students break down. Students then may become more likely to work with the poor after their training ends.[32]

As students, we can't control which patients faculty direct us to see. We should, however, appreciate the altruism of those patients who generously allow us to see them. And while working with patients, we can be reassured that our efforts often improve their health care experience.

Anthony Farah
Medical Student, Jefferson Medical College

A Faculty Perspective

The prevailing paradigm of clinical medical education, beginning with the clinical clerkships and ending after residency or fellowship, involves caring for patients under supervision. Graded authority and responsibility marks this phase of professional maturation. The result of this gradual assumption of authority and responsibility is a clinician with proficiency in the six domains of clinical competence in their chosen specialty.[33]

Clinical experience for medical students occurs in the unique setting of the systems of care endogenous to the teaching hospitals of their medical school. These systems have evolved over generations, and are usually based in settings where resident training also occurs.[34] This "continuum" of medical education places the resident in a position of teacher and supervisor, as well as trainee.

Residency programs developed in many institutions with the dual purpose of training the next generation of medical staff, as well as providing care for the indigent. Teaching hospitals affiliated with medical schools often provide care for a disproportionate share of the uninsured and underinsured of their service area. The structures of care often involve private services and non-private services, or entire hospitals dedicated to uninsured or underinsured patients coupled with hospitals dedicated to insured patients.

The altruistic delivery of patient care is seen in both settings. Physicians care deeply about the care provided to the patients they serve. Some physicians make the care of the indigent their life's work. Others provide care to all who come to their door, regardless of their insurance or economic status. Finally, some physicians provide care only to those economically capable of affording their services.

Certain concepts are important to understand in relation to learning in the clinical setting. First, it is a privilege to participate in a patient's clinical care. There is no "right" that accrues to an individual when they enter medical school that entitles them to participate in the care of all patients. Some patients do not wish to have their care directly managed by trainees. Those with choices are largely those with health insurance. The institutions caring for the uninsured and underinsured utilize residents and fellows to provide much of the hands-on aspects of patient care, with more distant supervision provided by faculty. The students in this case are observing the impact of this care dichotomy.

Second, trainees aspire to train in settings where they are granted greater autonomy earlier in training, which is usually seen in settings where the uninsured and underinsured receive care.

Third, the provision of care by individuals not competent to provide that care is unjust. The bravado of "see one, do one, teach one" referred to nostalgically by senior faculty, where learning and care is haphazard, and often at the patient's expense, is distinctly non-altruistic. Thus, the needs of the patient for expert care, and the needs of the student or resident to acquire knowledge and experience, must be balanced. This is the role of the faculty.

Fourth, most conceptual systems of social justice do not require equal care for all, but rather some level of care for all. These dichotomous settings are not, of their nature, unjust. The teaching hospitals in the United States are now a major component of the safety net for those Americans who are less fortunate, in addition to being the quaternary centers for high intensity, research-based care.[35] Indeed, the majority of the Medicaid admissions to hospitals occur in the less than 20 percent of hospitals that are teaching institutions, and the roughly 120 major academic medical centers associated with medical schools. In most cities, teaching hospitals have completely replaced indigent care institutions. In cities such as Chicago or Houston, where separate county facilities exist, they are associated with medical schools that provide students, residents, and faculty to care for the indigent.

The net result of this system is the altruistic provision of patient care to those who are less fortunate in teaching hospitals by teachers and students of medicine. We have long believed that this environment would permit them to learn that each person is unique, of value, and worthy of our best effort. Indeed, for many students, that is the lesson they learn. However, what unintended message might it send when students and residents are encouraged to "learn by doing" in the context of caring for patients in one setting, yet are not permitted to perform the same tasks in a private practice setting? What message does it send when the faculty are more directly involved in caring for their private patients than for their "unassigned" patients?

I fear that at least some of the students and residents get a very non-altruistic lesson. That lesson goes something like this: "We learn on *these* patients, so we can go out and care for *those* patients when we are finished training." And we all know who the *these* and *those* are.

These are not the lessons we intend. We prevent this unintended consequence of the altruistic provision of patient care through education of our trainees, and modeling of altruistic behaviors in all settings. The students in this case must first recognize that it is a privilege to participate in the care of any patient. Second, they must explore their reaction to this educational setting, share their reactions to the dichotomy they are observing, and reinforce those positive attributes that lead to both the development of clinical competency and altruism. Third, they must understand that the laudable

goal of gaining clinical competence must not occur at the expense of provision of excellent patient care to all.

Thomas J. Nasca, M.D.
Chief Executive Officer
Accreditation Council for Graduate Medical Education
Professor of Medicine
Formerly the Gertrude M. and Anthony F. DePalma Dean (2001–2007)
Jefferson Medical College

SOCIAL JUSTICE 2

A third year medical student struggles with her specialty choices. She was
inspired to go to medical school by her family physician, Dr. Dunn, who had
written one of her letters of recommendation for medical school. Her family in
rural Pennsylvania and Dr. Dunn expect that she will come home after
residency and join this practice. The student loved her family medicine
rotation, and to a lesser extent enjoyed her ophthalmology elective. With
a student debt of over $100,000, however, she is increasingly considering
ophthalmology.

A Medical Student Perspective

I have spent the past three years struggling to choose a specialty. With no
preconceived notions of my ideal fit, I found myself wanting to practice
whatever I was studying. My indecisiveness forced me to examine my
career goals and underlying motivations. I narrowed it down to internal
medicine and emergency medicine by the end of third year and arranged
a rotation in each for the beginning of my senior year. Emergency medicine
felt like a perfect fit from my first day. Although I wish I had discovered my
niche earlier in my training I am grateful for the lessons I learned from my
struggle.

While each student makes a decision with a unique set of priorities, the
factors can be separated into intrinsic and extrinsic. Intrinsic properties of
a specialty are inevitable: disease processes, organ systems, patient population, procedures, level of continuity, and breadth of scope. Extrinsic properties of a specialty are to an extent within a physician's control: salary, work
hours, call schedule, location, and academic opportunities. Within each specialty there are different practice environments that suit personal priorities.

Examining the intrinsic features of family medicine and ophthalmology
should help our student with her decision. She "loved" her family medicine

rotation so presumably she enjoys a broad scope encompassing preventative health care, managing chronic diseases, working with all ages, continuity with her patients and the role of a generalist. In stark contrast, she enjoyed ophthalmology, which involves a very deep knowledge of a single organ system, opportunities for complex procedures, a lack of continuity and the role of a consultant.

Comparing the extrinsic features of these specialties may explain her temptation to choose ophthalmology. The average salary in 2006 for a family physician is $150,000 vs. $280,000 for an ophthalmologist.[36] Furthermore the family physician works an average of 52.5 hours per week compared to the 47 the ophthalmologist works.[37] What would you do with an extra $130,000 and 250 hours of free time every year? It could determine whether your spouse has to work, where your children go to school, or whether you can retire early.

In the few short years of medical school, students learn that time is their most valuable commodity. While our friends are starting families, buying houses, and traveling the world we go over $100,000 in debt so we can spend the better part of our twenties in lectures, libraries, and hospitals. By the time students have to choose a specialty they have more debt and less free time than any other point in their lives. With student debt outpacing inflation[38] and physician salary stalling behind,[39] is it any wonder that our student is considering ophthalmology?

Yet choosing a career solely on salary is risky. The pecking order of physician salaries will change several times throughout one's career. Furthermore, everyone reading this book can think of at least one job they would not do for any amount of money. No matter what specialty a medical student chooses, he or she is going to be in the top 10 percent of American incomes. After they pay off their student loans and mortgage and send their children to college, physicians still have to wake up every morning and go to work. When money is no longer a problem what will keep you going every day? The bonds you've created with your patients? The fascination with a certain disease? The immediate gratification of procedures? In the end it is the intrinsic features of a specialty that become most important. After going through this difficult decision myself, my advice for this student is to schedule electives for the beginning of her fourth year and see which one feels right.

Kevin M. Eanes
Medical Student, Jefferson Medical College

A Faculty Perspective

Choosing a medical specialty and practice location represent two of the most important professional decisions that medical students and physicians make. This vignette raises a number of important issues focusing on an individual's career choices: issues related to social justice, balancing self-interest with the needs of others, the role of income and debt, and the role of faculty and mentors in advising future physicians.

Although a fundamental principle of medical professionalism is social justice – which includes working toward improving the fair distribution of health care resources[40] – most of the longstanding and serious issues related to the shortage of primary care physicians and those working in underserved rural and urban areas do not represent a major factor in individual physician career decisions. As with most helping professionals, medical students and physicians struggle with the balance between service to others and their own self-interest, though in reality, physicians have the luxury of usually doing both – no matter what specialty or practice location they choose. Rather, the national maldistribution of physicians is best addressed at a national and regional level by government, medical institutions, and the broader health care system.

Substantial research is available regarding individual physician career choice, and a myriad of factors have been identified as having an important influence.[41] These include: background and demographic factors related to the individual; the influence of friends, family, and faculty; prior experiences; issues related to finances, and, finally, the era in which we live.[42] In this scenario, we are presented with three items of information. First, the medical student feels somewhat obligated to her family doctor and her family, who expect her to return home and become a family doctor. Second, we are told that she "loved" her family medicine rotation, and "to a lesser extent enjoyed" her ophthalmology elective. And finally, she has over $100,000 in debt and this appears to be an important factor in her "increasingly considering ophthalmology" as a career choice.

This scenario is not uncommon. And with increasing levels of debt, students often feel substantial pressure to consider their debt burden as they choose a future specialty. Those advising students have a responsibility to present evidence-based information in order for students to make their own best decisions. In some instances, however, students have shared that faculty try to recruit them into various specialties, or to impose their own specialty selection values or income expectations upon them. While it is important for students to listen to the opinions and wishes of family, friends, and other physicians – as they often provide important insights from their own experience – it is critical that students balance the importance of these factors themselves, according to their own individual experiences and values, and make their own decisions. It is also important for students to seriously consider all aspects of their potential career, including the actual professional work and the satisfaction and frustrations involved, as well as the associated lifestyle (including income, hours worked, etc.). Students also need to have an accurate understanding of themselves, including their own income and lifestyle expectations (which differ widely among individuals), in order to know how to personally weigh the relative importance of all these issues.

Regarding debt, most students seem to feel this burden disproportionate to its actual financial implications, given the available data. In this instance, for example, repaying a $100,000 debt over twenty-five years will reduce annual income by about $10,000 per year.[43] While substantial, this pales in comparison to the differences in yearly income between the two specialties: family medicine $150,000 vs. ophthalmology $280,000.[36]

In summary, it is critical that all students make the important decisions of specialty choice and practice location for themselves, considering the available evidence, collective experience, and advice of others. This student needs to know herself, and identify what represents the best overall career match with her own career and life goals. Only each individual student can make the best decision for his or her career and life.

Howard K. Rabinowitz, M.D.
Ellen M. and Dale W. Garber Professor of Family Medicine
Director, Physician Shortage Area Program
Jefferson Medical College

COMMITMENT TO PROFESSIONAL COMPETENCE 1

A first year student, attending a medical school that uses the Honors-Pass-Fail grading system, has nearly completed his microbiology course and has an average of eighty. He realizes that it is not possible to obtain Honors in this course and all he needs is a score of fifty on the final exam to pass. He therefore decides to not attend many of the classes during the last week and to not study the section on parasitology.

A Medical Student Perspective

As an individual who strives to do her best regardless of subject matter, I find it difficult to accept the behavior of the student in this scenario. Although I recognize that one cannot realistically master all of the information presented, I also believe that one should try to succeed to one's fullest extent. However, for the sake of evaluating our current methods of grading students and teaching professionalism, I would like to consider other viewpoints. There are two reasons I have identified why the behavior of this student may not be as uncommon or unprofessional as it may initially seem.

Although the student does not perform his best, he does do what the faculty asks of him and masters 70 percent of the material. Similar to this scenario, numerous medical schools today use the Honors-Pass-Fail grading system where the faculty requires students to know 70 percent of the material presented in order to advance in school.[44,45] If faculty want students to know everything presented, then the requirement should be to know 100 percent of the material. Obviously, this is not realistic, and therefore is not currently in place. However, schools can continue to keep the 70 percent as a threshold for advancing in schooling, and simultaneously encourage students to learn all that they are able to master. As noted by the study from Stern et al.,[46] it is crucial for medical educators to clearly state what is professional behavior so that students are fully aware of what is expected. If faculty believe professional behavior includes students learning all that they can, then that should be clearly stated in the syllabus, along with the reminder that 70 percent is the minimum standard required for passing.

The second point is that the student faces a common, yet rarely discussed or developed, decision – which material *not* to master. It is not only impossible for medical students to master 100 percent of the material presented, but also in the future it will be challenging if not impossible to learn all of the details about new advances in one's own specialty. Therefore, it is left up to each future physician to decide what she or he will not learn. This is, in a sense, one of the skills inherent in becoming self-directed learners.

Ultimately, I do not endorse the student's behavior for he seems to have made a decision based on his own short-term needs, rather than on commitment to professional competence.[40] However, I do think that his behavior challenges us to find better ways of expressing to students what we deem as professional. If it is professional to learn all of the information that one can possibly learn, then we should clearly state that. And if there are ways to appropriately choose what material to not learn, then we should provide students with tools on how to make that decision.

Elizabeth Norheim
Medical Student, Jefferson Medical College

A Faculty Perspective

Faculty expend great care and deliberation in the development of medical school curricula. Clearly, all medical knowledge cannot be taught in four years to a medical student. Critical judgment is required to select those topics which are essential for the transformation of medical students into physicians. The objective is to train physicians with sufficient knowledge to treat their patients in all areas of medicine. Faculty struggle to teach and examine only areas of significant importance for the practice of medicine and the objective is that all students should achieve competence in all of those critical areas. Realistic minimum criteria have been identified for determining a student's knowledge of each medical school course and achieving a passing grade signifies that a student has met these minimum criteria.

There are several aspects regarding the behavior of the student described in this scenario that display an absence of the professional conduct expected of a practicing physician. The student used his judgment to decide that certain aspects of the curriculum were not important to him and could therefore be skipped. One of the key elements in proper patient care is to know when to trust your own judgment as opposed to the judgment of another. In this case the student trusted his own judgment and disregarded the opinion of the faculty. The student will pass the course, meeting minimum standards, yet demonstrated poor and potentially dangerous judgment by deciding to intentionally skip a significant portion of the curriculum. The ability to judge and then trust the opinion of others is crucial for making medical decisions. If the second year medical student does not trust the faculty to teach him what he needs to know to practice medicine, it is hard to imagine who he will trust as he progresses in his career as a physician.

Patients expect and deserve a 100 percent effort at every encounter with their physician. The medical student described in the scenario has started down the dangerous path of striving to meet minimum standards. Instead of trying to learn 100 percent of the material, he has decided to be satisfied with 70 percent. This attitude is not acceptable in patient care and is therefore unacceptable in attaining the knowledge required for appropriate patient care.

It is understood that medical students cannot know everything that is taught to them in their classes. Patients have the right to expect that their physicians will know where their limitations are and will know how to reach out to those more experienced in those areas. Furthermore, patients have a right to expect that their physician will expend a 100 percent effort to deliver optimal medical care to each of their patients. These behaviors do not suddenly appear when a student gets a medical degree. They are difficult to learn and require patterning, time and experience to perfect. The behaviors of good judgment, trust in deserving mentors and colleagues as well as a striving for excellence in patient care are learned as medical students and practiced by physicians. The student described in the scenario will have passed the course, yet will have failed in the critical demonstration of professional behaviors required of practicing physicians.[46]

David Abraham Ph.D.
Professor, Department of Microbiology and Immunology
Jefferson Medical College

COMMITMENT TO PROFESSIONAL COMPETENCE 2

A fourth year student, working with a primary care internal medicine practice over the past four weeks, has observed that the physicians, as well as the nurse practitioner, usually prescribe antibiotics for patients who have signs and symptoms of viral upper respiratory infections.

For a video of the vignette, see http://professionalism.jefferson.edu/.

A Medical Student Perspective

I entered medical school, like most of my classmates, with an idealistic vision of what I was hoping to accomplish with my degree. However, it has been increasingly difficult to hold on to this idealism throughout school. This case is one of those situations which seem to cause that idealism to slowly leak out. Antibiotics will probably not cause the patient any immediate harm but are not necessarily indicated. Are we, as students, in a position to question the physician's actions? How should we approach the discrepancy between what we learn in lectures and what we observe in the clinic?

It is clear that students' views of medicine change as they move through school and especially through their residencies. They tend to become more jaded and end with a paternalistic approach instead of a patient-centered approach to medicine.[47] As a student, I tried to approach this case from both the doctor's and patient's perspective. What is medically best for the patient and at the same time satisfactorily meets their expectations?

Current research indicates that even if patients expected antibiotics (regardless of whether they received them or not) the patients will leave the office satisfied if the physician educates them on the appropriate use and misuse of antibiotics. A comparison of patient education programs with physician continuing education programs on the guidelines for antibiotic usage found that programs involving patient education had the greatest decrease in unnecessary prescription writing.[48] Thus, if the physician takes an extra minute to educate and explain to the patient why antibiotics are not indicated, patients tend to accept this decision and leave the visit feeling satisfied.[48–50]

It also helps to prevent antibiotic resistance, which is a growing and imminent danger in today's medical world.

As a medical student still learning how to negotiate the clinical world, I can begin to understand how it might be difficult to practice evidence-based medicine while still meeting patient expectations and satisfaction. When we observe a case such as this, what are we to do? Who are we to model ourselves on as we grow as clinicians? How often are we told "it's something you will learn as you get more experience?" Does this fall under the "clinical experience" category that we will only be privy to as we move forward in our careers? As I took a step back and thought about how I have been learning throughout school, I realized that seeing what should not happen has often left more of an impression on me than seeing what should happen during a patient encounter. This physician, instead of prescribing antibiotics for the upper respiratory infection, should have taken the time to educate the patient about the risks and benefits of taking antibiotics in this situation. Such an approach demonstrates to the student both an excellent patient encounter as well as how to practice evidence-based medicine in the face of opposing patient expectations, something most of us are yearning to understand.

Anna Filip
Medical Student, Jefferson Medical College

A Faculty Perspective

Acute upper respiratory infections are the most frequent reasons for seeking medical attention in the United States. Although most of these infections are viral in origin and self limited in nature, they account for up to 75 percent of total antibiotic prescriptions written yearly.[51–53] Many randomized, placebo-controlled trials of upper respiratory illness have found no benefit for patients taking antibiotics compared with placebo. Yet, of 51 million visits for "colds," upper respiratory tract infections, and bronchitis in the United States in a year, 50–66 percent culminated in an antibiotic prescription.[54] The consequence of this excessive use of unnecessary antibiotics has been an epidemic spread of antibiotic resistance not only in the United States, but worldwide.[51] Why physicians continue to prescribe antibiotics when they are not clearly indicated is a complex issue.

Though guidelines for diagnosis and treatment of upper respiratory infections have been developed, physicians often prescribe antibiotics that are not clearly indicated.[55] It is difficult for a physician to be in a position where an illness might be made worse by inaction or where a chance to relieve symptoms might be missed. Though we can stratify patients based on symptoms and estimate the probability of bacterial infection, symptoms are often non-specific and we are still left with uncertainty. Some clinicians prescribe antibiotics believing that a fraction of their patients will obtain benefit. By prescribing antibiotics, we hope to prevent the remote case of a bad outcome.[51] How do we know how to proceed? Very often we don't. Medicine is an uncertain art and clinical judgment develops with time and experience.

In many cases, the physician's decision has more to do with the physician–patient relationship than the physician's diagnostic skills. The concept of antibiotic resistance is abstract and the patient's perceived need is immediate. Giving an antibiotic is a personal act, one which shows the patient that the doctor is involved and that he or she cares. It also means that the physician has made a diagnosis and knows what to do to make the patient better. It has been said that "the drug prescription prolongs the physician–patient encounter by enabling the patient to ingest a 'dose of the doctor'several times a day."[54] Patients can be quite vocal with demands for an antibiotic, especially if they have received one in the past. Sometimes it is easier to avoid a confrontation by giving in to a patient's demand for an antibiotic.

Also it is time consuming for the physician to explain why an antibiotic is not indicated and to reassure the patient that this is the right decision. Writing a prescription for an antibiotic is much faster. It completes the encounter and terminates the visit.

Yet, as a physician in practice, I feel that my integrity is at stake when I prescribe an antibiotic, or any intervention that is not indicated. The risk of doing harm and of further increasing worldwide antimicrobial resistance must take precedence. As stated in the student commentary, studies have shown that patient satisfaction is correlated with physician time spent and with the patient's understanding of their diagnosis to a greater extent than the receipt of a prescription for an antibiotic.[53] In my practice, I find that patients truly are more satisfied and actually more appreciative when I listen to and understand their concerns. Their trust is reinforced when I hold true to my principles and explain to them my clinical reasoning. Rather than an unnecessary antibiotic, I can offer them a decongestant for symptomatic relief, and reassurance of my availability in the unlikely event that they do not improve.

Carol Reife, M.D.
Clinical Associate Professor of Medicine
Jefferson Medical College

HONESTY WITH PATIENTS 1

A third year student, Rebecca Green, is near the end of her pediatrics clerkship and is asked by her resident if she wants to perform a lumbar puncture (LP) on an infant with a fever. Rebecca has observed lumbar punctures twice during the past month and understands how to perform the procedure. Yet she is concerned that her inexperience may cause harm to the child and that the parents may not want an inexperienced student performing an invasive procedure on their child. The resident, after encouraging Rebecca to be assertive and that she should perform the LP, introduces her to the parents as "student doctor Green." During the informed discussion, the resident tells the parents that "Dr. Green will do the procedure and I will be there if there is any problem."

For a video of the vignette, see http://professionalism.jefferson.edu/.

A Medical Student Perspective

As a fourth year medical student, Dr. Wilfond's essay below struck a chord. He makes a compelling case for full and complete disclosure by a student doing a first-time procedure. Then why, I wonder, when I found myself in a similar situation, was acting ethically neither clear nor easy?

During my recent Emergency Medicine rotation I saw a middle-aged man with AIDS and severe neck pain. When I presented to my preceptor, he responded, "So you'll do the LP." We briefly discussed that this would be my first time doing the procedure, although I had watched plenty. He assured me that he would lead me through it. I reflexively took his offer as a sign that I was worthy to do the procedure. The desire for approval from respected preceptors goes beyond formal grading.

When I explained to the patient that I would be doing the procedure with my doctor supervisor close by, he laughed: "Oh yeah, last time the rookie couldn't get it, but neither could any of the old doctors." Clearly I was in a situation with an informed patient and a thoughtful preceptor, yet I still chose not to tell this patient it was my first time. He seemed to understand that I was inexperienced, but if I told him directly that this was my first time, would he still consent to the procedure? During our conversation, I was conscious of my own tug between wanting to be honest and my near-desperate desire to try the LP. By making my inexperience explicit, I worried I would not only make the patient more nervous, but also risk having this learning opportunity taken away.

Should a patient be given the opportunity to opt in or out of having a medical student doing a procedure for the first time? We typically learn using patients until someone objects. Hospital employees or physicians' family members often avoid care by a student. Conversely, families who do not speak English are rarely informed or empowered enough to opt out of student care. When students like Rebecca are put in the awkward position of being called "student doctor," our participation verges on deception.

During my clinical rotations, I became aware of a perceived race to learn procedures. Learning how to do a paracentesis seemed like less of a learned skill and more of a badge of honor. On rotations lacking hands-on practice with procedures, I feared I was falling behind my classmates. In reality, we all need to learn procedures on some patients in order to perform them competently on future patients. The potential risks and benefits justifies a medical student's participation in some cases while not in others.

In the end, I attempted but did not get the LP. The attending guided me until it was time for his hands to take over. I felt indebted to the patient for allowing me this chance to learn. In return, I spent time giving careful answers to his questions and smuggled graham crackers from the nurses' stations. I hope that despite a few extra pokes in his back, his overall experience was enhanced by my participation. As medical students, we continually struggle to find our role; what do we do *for* patients, and not just *to* patients. While we lack experience, we should not underestimate what we can offer: time, compassion and a fresh perspective. Ultimately, honest communication may go farther to help patients than whether or not we "get the LP."

Sarah Bergman Lewis
Medical Student, University of Washington School of Medicine

A Faculty Perspective[11,56–62]

Medical trainees need to learn to do clinical procedures to become competent physicians, and the learning process will expose some patients to additional harm and discomfort because of the trainees' inexperience. Rebecca's situation raises questions related to trainee qualifications and the appropriate disclosure to patients. In the pediatric setting, these issues are complicated because of the unique characteristics of procedures in children and the reliance on parents to protect the child's interests.

The first question for Rebecca is whether she is at the point in her own professional development that she is technically prepared to do the procedure. Has she mastered requisite procedures, such as drawing blood and the use of sterile techniques? Does she understand the cognitive aspects of the procedure, i.e., the anatomy, the risks, etc.? Some trainees may have excessive exuberance for procedures while others demonstrate persistent avoidance. Supervisors of trainees must play a role in determining if a student is prepared, rather than just relying on the trainee's personal assessment. Rebecca may be ready, but the supervisor would have to ask about her experience to make this assessment.

A second question for Rebecca is whether this procedure is necessary for her specific professional development. The impact of a failed or bloody LP on an infant with a fever can include prolonged antibiotic treatment or selecting the wrong antibiotic. Given these serious consequences, compensating benefits are necessary. LPs should only be performed by those trainees who are likely to be doing LPs on infants as part of their career. As a third year medical student, Rebecca does not need to do this LP. However, if she were planning on a career in pediatrics, the risk could be justified.

So when Rebecca becomes a pediatric intern, should she inform the mother that this is her first LP and should she ask for permission? More central to pediatric training than learning to do an LP is learning to respect families, to communicate effectively, and to build trust with parents. Such disclosure and permission can help Rebecca achieve those goals, regardless of whether the mother agrees to allow Rebecca to do the LP.

Some trainees may worry whether a patient would ever agree to be the intern's first spinal tap. But disclosure is particularly important for those parents of patients who would not agree, so they can have their wishes respected. The challenge for Rebecca and her resident is for them to communicate confidence, care, and respect, so that the parent might agree. It will be important to explain not only the risks of the procedure itself, but also the nature and likelihood of those risks for a first time procedure (in this case, an inconclusive diagnosis), that Rebecca will be supervised, and replaced, if she is having difficulty. Parents must also be given the alternative of having the supervisor do the LP. This discussion can increase the therapeutic alliance between the medical team and the mother and will permit Rebecca to ask questions while she is performing the procedure without having to pretend she knows what she is doing. Learning how to communicate with parents about uncertainty, inexperience, and the need for consultation and advice, is much more challenging and more important to learn than doing a spinal tap on an infant.

Benjamin S. Wilfond, M.D.
Department of Pediatrics, University of Washington
School of Medicine
Director, Treuman Katz Center for Pediatric Bioethics,
Seattle Children's Hospital

HONESTY WITH PATIENTS 2

A student on a fourth year gynecology rotation observed a vaginal hysterectomy. The following morning on rounds, the attending reviewed the prior day's orders and asked the house-staff team why prophylactic antibiotics were not given. The resident and intern replied that it was an oversight and that they would be more careful with future patients. The intern, after listening to the discussion on rounds, included in his progress note the error of the missed antibiotic and the concern about an increased risk of postoperative infection. Later in the day the resident, when meeting with the student and intern, reprimanded the intern for including the antibiotic omission in his note and said: "So you want to be sued? You should know that this is just what plaintiff attorneys look for."

A Medical Student Perspective

Malpractice. It is a word that scares all physicians, and as a student with limited knowledge about the medical-legal system, I am terrified at the prospect of being involved in a lawsuit. In this case, both the intern and the resident are the student's superiors, making the decision of whom to listen to even more difficult. The intern has just begun his training in the hospital, whereas the resident already has some experience under her belt. Who should the student believe as she makes her way towards her professional career, and models her own behaviors after those she observes in her clerkships?

As a student, I find this situation confusing and frightening, but feel that honest documentation is the best strategy. It is important to realize that careful recording of the events that occurred while the patient was in your care is needed for the credibility and validity of the record should the patient's chart ever be requested for legal examination. In this case, prophylactic antibiotic treatment is the standard of care for a vaginal hysterectomy as recommended by the American College of Gynecologists.[63] By noting the omission of the antibiotic, one can show honesty and awareness of good medical practice, both of which will lend credibility to the physician. In an article on avoiding lawsuits, Rice argues that a physician's record is his or her best argument in court, but if it is inconsistent, a plaintiff's attorney will immediately go after the doctor's credibility.[64] In all likelihood, there will be documentation elsewhere in the chart listing other medications given to the patient during treatment; thus, a missing medication will catch the eye of anyone closely combing the record. At least if the omission is noted, a person reading the records will see that the physician attempted to follow recommended guidelines, but accidentally forgot to dispense the antibiotic.

Furthermore, and possibly most critically, it is important to note the missing dose of antibiotic because the chart is the centerpiece of communication for the entire team. The patient's treatment regimen has changed because the antibiotics were not dispensed, and the rest of the team must be made aware of this. In this situation, where an omission has occurred, guidelines have been set forth by the American Health Information Management Association to produce consistent standards of medical record keeping.[65] These guidelines recommend that documentation of the missed antibiotic should be identified as a "late entry." The time and date of the additional entry must be noted, and a reference to the date of the incident should be documented. The source of the information on the omission should be included in the note. Under no circumstances should the chart be altered in any way to hide any missed medical care, as this is definitely a misstep plaintiff attorneys look for in their searches.[66]

Unfortunately, in an age of the highly charged medical-legal environment, it is often difficult for anyone practicing medicine not to feel as though their every move is under a microscope. As a student learning to practice within the ever-changing legal atmosphere of medicine, one should seek the counsel of the clerkship director if ever confused, and if still unable to get an answer, then the question should be brought to the hospital's ethical board.

Lee Rabinowitz
Medical Student, Jefferson Medical College

A Perspective from an Attorney

Documentation in the hospital chart is critical. Documentation should be accurate, comprehensive, legible, and contemporaneous. The chart should be able to tell other caregivers in a concise way the status of the patient, treatment, and medical decisions. The chart is not, however, a place for caregivers to argue with one another, or fix blame.

The medical student's perspective above sets forth all of the salient issues. The progress note written by the intern was accurate and truthful. The information about the failure to give the antibiotic could have been gleaned from a careful review of the chart, including the medication orders, medication administration document, and nurse's notes. The intern's note highlights the failure to provide the antibiotics when they should have been given and may be helpful for future caregivers. This accurate and complete documentation could affect the patient's subsequent treatment and possibly prevent actual infection and injury – which would be the most effective way to avoid a potential lawsuit.[67]

The resident's reaction was probably an overreaction. Certainly, a plaintiff's attorney reviewing the case may zero in on the antibiotic omission as set forth in the note, but a note such as this is certainly not as harmful as a less than truthful notation in the chart, or, much worse, an altered record. An alternate option – and likely preferable reaction to the error – would be for the physician not only to document it accurately in the chart but to inform the patient and discuss it with her. While the natural reaction to a medical error may be to withhold information and hope that no one discovers it, there is a school of thought in both medical and legal circles that honest communication with a patient, even in the face of an error that causes injury, may decrease the likelihood of a lawsuit. If there is a lawsuit, jurors certainly are likely to view honesty on the part of the doctor more favorably than they are any suggestion of a cover up or outright dishonesty.

The comment by the resident, as well as the medical student's perspective, sets forth the highly charged atmosphere dealing with the repercussions of medical errors and medical malpractice. From a learning, patient safety, and risk management perspective, the entire system would be better served by a shift in focus from a culture of blame to a culture of learning.[68]

Perhaps the resident's comments and inquiry would have been better served in determining why the antibiotics were not administered, and attempting to have everyone learn from what was apparently a system failure to correct it from occurring again.[69]

Peter J. Hoffman, Esq.
Eckert, Seamans, Cherin & Mellott, LLC, Philadelphia, PA

PATIENT CONFIDENTIALITY 1

Following a lecture in which a patient is interviewed in front of the class, two medical students meet with a friend at lunch. The friend is not a student. While dining, one of the student talks about the lecture and mentions specific details of the patient's medical condition.

For a video of the vignette, see http://professionalism.jefferson.edu/.

A Medical Student Perspective

As medical professionals, we balance benefit and risk every day in our efforts to help patients while doing them no harm. Every clinical action – every test, every intervention, every piece of advice – is a human one and bears the potential to harm as well as the possibility to help. Sharing information is a necessary risk in medicine. Patients share a wealth of sensitive data about their bodies and their lives so that we may fully understand their health problems and diagnose and treat them properly. In doing so, they trust that we will handle their confidences with the utmost respect for the hurt, embarrassment, and personal, professional, and financial catastrophe that their disclosure might cause.

Each time confidential information goes beyond the physician–patient covenant, the possibility of breach and resultant harm is amplified, but clearly some disclosure is necessary. Medicine is a team endeavor – patient data must be shared freely with nurses, staff, and other physicians in order to deliver the highest quality integrated care. All members of the team are similarly sworn and legally bound to maintain patient confidentiality. The flow of information within the team is necessary to benefit the patient.

In this scenario, however, the students are privy to patient information for the benefit of their education, and they reveal details in front of a non-medical friend. It is clear that sharing in this situation is not for the purpose of helping the patient. It is unclear, though, whether the students in the vignette have revealed anything identifying about the patient. Patient confidentiality is only breached if the listening party can connect the material to an individual. Unfortunately, discerning how much can be revealed without compromising patient confidentiality is tricky. Is it worth the risk if there is no possibility or intention to benefit the patient?

Although discussing patients outside the professional context is inherently risky, I believe it is unrealistic to expect medical professionals never to speak about their work outside of the office or hospital. We must all cope with the emotional consequences of our professions, and healthcare workers have the special burden of dealing with issues of life and death every day. In addition, I believe it is integral to our own well-being that we are able to share our experiences with our loved ones to maintain our personal relationships and support systems. Ultimately, essential to ensuring that we are fit to take care of patients is taking care of ourselves.

The challenge, then, is how to talk about our professional lives without jeopardizing patient privacy. It is a difficult undertaking; often it is hard to predict what number of details will be identifying, as outsiders might already be familiar with some cases from the news or through connections in the community. The struggle to find a solution, however, is worthwhile. In my own experience, physicians and medical students handle this quandary in ways that span the spectrum, with some choosing to share whole case reports with loved ones, omitting only the patient's name, and others exercising varying tactics of discretion. Institutions, therefore, would serve their health care workers and patients both by working with practitioners to achieve more uniform approach. A realistic set of guidelines would acknowledge that clinicians are humans with personal lives of their own while helping them guard their patients' privacy as strictly as possible.

Amanda Lerman
Medical Student, Jefferson Medical College

A Faculty Perspective

Confidentiality is typically the first crucial concept to learn in the process of the professionalization of medical students. It is an early chapter in all the textbooks for a reason: Before you learn anything about a patient, you must understand the importance of having the right to that information.[70] The information to which it applies can be defined thus: If you would not have known that information were you not a medical student, then you cannot share that information with anyone who does not share your oath to confidentiality.

To first year medical students, the expectations placed upon them often seem unfair. This is totally natural: One cannot change one's sense of personal identity or self-image overnight. Yet that is what the faculty often appears to expect. The gap in expectations can be so great that some explanation may be needed for both groups to understand each other.

Here is my suggestion for how to mediate between medical student self-image and faculty expectations of professionalism with regards to confidentiality. First, the faculty must understand that professionalization is a gradual psychological process, and one that begins in the first year but is not complete until the third year (or later). If there is reason to worry about whether students can maintain patient confidentiality, then the faculty might be burdening students with confidential information too early in their training. It might be better to offer only paper cases and standardized patients for the first semester or the entire first year while the students begin to make the adjustment to their new professional responsibilities.

Second, to take the student's perspective, I would suggest that we can help them understand their responsibilities with the following metaphor. Applying to medical school is not just applying to get into a highly competitive undergraduate institution. It is also akin to proposing to marry someone. When a school interviews you, it is like a first date. Much of what they are looking at is what sort of a person you are, and whether they would like to be seen with you in various settings. When they admit you, it is like accepting your proposal: They don't just like your grades, they like you.

Once you are admitted you still have a chance to change your mind, rather like getting cold feet from the cost and complexity of wedding planning. But if you don't cancel your wedding plans, then you are making a lifetime commitment to another person. You will care what they think of you, and will be willing to make some personal changes to meet their expectations. Becoming a doctor is not just getting a degree, or learning a lot of new information. It also means a change in your identity. First others will start to see you differently, and later you will start to think differently and see yourself differently as well.

So what should you say to your friend at that lunch? You can tell them that medical school is harder than you thought, but it isn't just the science courses, it's learning how to react to the stories patients tell – what to say, and what not to say. Tell your friends about confidentiality, and how that's an important part of becoming a doctor. It is possible to keep your old friends, but gradually you will probably find, as have many others, that you have less in common with your old friends and more in common with your fellow medical students. And it isn't about science; it's about your developing new professional identity.

Jeffrey Spike, Ph.D.
Professor and Director, Campus-Wide Ethics Program
McGovern Center for Health, Humanities and the Human Spirit
University of Texas Health Science Center, Houston

PATIENT CONFIDENTIALITY 2

A medical student, nearing the end of her third year, is curious about the outcome of a patient who she became close with and helped care for during her pediatric clerkship nine months previously. The patient is a fourteen- year- old girl who was diagnosed with acute renal failure from glomerulonephritis. The student accesses the hospital electronic medical records, which contains inpatient and outpatient records, to understand how the patient has been over the past nine months.

A Medical Student Perspective

Having spent most of the preceding two years in the classroom, third year medical students have been seasoned with a myriad of facts, lectures, and exams. Eager to test the real-world applications of extensive historical medical knowledge and contemporary scientific research, they enter the wards to learn firsthand about patient care. Witnessing how medical intervention can influence the course of disease and affect patient outcomes is a powerfully rewarding and sometimes humbling experience. As fresh and enthusiastic members of the health care team, it is natural for students to want to follow patients' long-term progress, especially when electronic medical records make access readily available.

Even though the student in this case was directly involved in the care of the patient, for how long is it morally permissible to access medical records in order to follow her progress? What influence do – and should – patients, and in this case, parents have in deciding this? And if access were more restricted or more difficult, would the student still pursue follow-up?

It is important to think about the intent of the student in this case. Most likely the student would feel she wants to check on the patient out of genuine concern for the well-being of her former patient. Part of the reward in providing care is seeing how you have improved the quality of life for another. As long as the student is not hurting the patient or indulging ulterior motives, she is acting appropriately.

However, in my experience on the wards, verbal interaction with patients is frequently impersonal. It is often limited to eliciting critical information for a diagnosis rather than fostering any appreciable discussion about what the patient wants, needs, thinks, or feels. I believe that the focus of modern medicine in this country has shifted too far away from the patient, and centered too much on the disease. I recall the feeling of being categorized as an illness when I was a patient myself; I felt very protective of my personal information and did not want anyone accessing it without my consent. If I were the medical student in this case I would have to ask myself exactly why I wanted to follow up on that patient, and, if I were the patient, if I wouldn't want my wishes to be assigned more importance.

As medical students we must reclaim the heart of medicine by serving patients and focusing our efforts primarily on them. We must treat each encounter as a sacred experience, and allow those decisions best made by patients to remain in their hands. A brief phone call to the family to obtain permission would be the most appropriate thing to do. If concern about the patient is truly at the heart of the matter, talking directly to the family would be most ethical. And if there were more information available only in the medical record, permission to access it could be given during that phone call. Even though we have an obligation to improve our medical education, our highest obligation is to the wishes of the patients who allowed us the opportunity to become involved with their care in the first place.

Mark Sylvester
Medical Student, University of Miami Miller School of Medicine

A Faculty Perspective

Medical privacy and confidentiality are neither courtesies offered by the powerful to the embarrassed, nor administrative pains in the neck endured for the sake of compliance with regional or national laws imposed by legislative busybodies. They are, rather, ancient duties identified by physicians as essential to high-quality medical practice. Put differently, the values of privacy and confidentiality are *internal* to the medical profession. Protecting them has good consequences and helps physicians treat patients with respect.[71]

Medical education and the privileges it affords are likewise ancient. Patients, who might prefer that only seasoned physicians care for them, often come to appreciate their crucial role in the fledging years of future doctors. And patients generally understand that medical students are competent to do comparatively little, but that in order to learn how to do most anything they must be included as members of a team, and so allowed access to intimate personal information.

That right to access information is, however, not eternal; it ends after – well, when? Perhaps the best answer to this question is to be given by the patient herself (or parent or guardian; or both). That is, the foundation of privacy protections in ethics and the law rests on the idea that patients ought to control who has access to their information.

It is good that medical students bond with patients and come genuinely to care about them; and it is good that such caring does not expire. But this is not to say that caring for patients entitles students (or trained physicians, for that matter) to look around in the electronic medical record after a formal relationship has ended. Medical records, whether paper-based or electronic, are tools for patient care, not resources to be used to gratify personal interests or curiosities, no matter how benign or even noble.

Moreover, "curiosity" and "caring" do not necessarily overlap. One could argue that if our third year medical student were truly interested in the welfare of a former patient she should seek permission to visit her; the electronic record is a poor medium for staying in touch. In the other direction: Suppose the student did not care at all about the former patient (she did wait nine months for her curiosity to get the better of her in a case involving a malady with as much as a 7 percent mortality rate), but thought there might be something of importance or medical interest to learn from the review of a former patient's chart. In that case, the student might still want to seek permission, though in the environment of a teaching hospital such permission could be given by an attending or resident.

The role of medical students is special and privileged: Society needs physicians, and it is prepared to give students access to patient secrets while they learn their profession at the bedsides of sick people. But in the absence of an ongoing clinical relationship or of a bona fide learning moment, access to more patient information should be controlled by those at the center of the health care universe: patients.

Kenneth W. Goodman, Ph.D.
Professor of Medicine, Miller School of Medicine
Director, Bioethics Program
University of Miami

MAINTAINING APPROPRIATE RELATIONS WITH PATIENTS 1

A second year medical student visits her mother, who was admitted to the hospital thirty-six hours earlier with chest pain. The student is concerned that her mother is not getting timely and appropriate care. She tells her mother about these concerns and asks the hospital house physician why a CT scan of the chest has not yet been performed.

A Medical Student Perspective

As a second year medical student, the daughter does not have the competence or knowledge of a fully trained physician, nor is she likely to be familiar with the workings of the hospital. But as long as the best interests of her mother are served, she has every right to ask questions about the medical management. Some individuals thrust into this scenario might be hesitant to use their medical knowledge for fear of doing more harm than good or of acting unprofessionally. Such hesitation, however, unfairly holds individuals who happen to be medical professionals to a different standard than that of any other family member who has a sick loved one.

Whether one is a physician or medical student, most individuals would feel overwhelmed in this scenario, and might seek to gain some amount of control over the situation by trying to understand what had happened. And whether our student's concerns over delay stem from spurious or genuine knowledge, asking questions, unless done without tact, represents a way of understanding and aiding both patient families and, conceivably, the medical team.

Why then might advocating or asking questions in the interest of a sick parent or spouse be labeled as inappropriate intervention? For instance, when does advocacy become interference? Perhaps the concept of "do no harm" applies here to worried family members just as to medical professionals.[72] Family members, especially medical professionals, must realize that despite whatever they may advocate, advise or ask for, they are ultimately neither the person being treated nor the physician doing the treating. Some actions by the student, even with the best of intentions, may constitute inappropriate intervention and predispose to harm. These actions include looking at the medical chart or looking up study results, without permission of her mother. More alarming would be if the daughter somehow went against her mother's wishes to exert her own clinical beliefs. To exceed the normal role of a family member or to essentially treat or practice medicine rather than solely advocate creates worrisome ethical quandaries. In short, do all one can to advocate but leave the stethoscopes at home when visiting a loved one in the hospital.

Rather than chastise the daughter for "meddling" in this scenario, the house physician should take time to explain the clinical thinking and plan so as to better include both mother and daughter in the medical management of the chest pain. It is likely this daughter simply wants the best care for her mother, not to medically manage. Though we may be medical professionals, we are sons and daughters first.

Dylan Kann
Medical Student, University of California, Davis School of Medicine

A Faculty Perspective

There have been some prevalence studies and analyses in the literature about physicians treating their own families (many, probably most, do at one time or another), with arguments back and forth about how appropriate this is.[73–76] Currently, while it is generally advised against, there can be no absolutism in an ethical prohibition to this behavior, since its probity is much dependent on individual circumstances (is another competent, non-relative doctor readily available or not? Is the complaint of the family member straightforward or complex? Is the physician in the family expert enough in the suspected illness to do the best job possible for his or her loved one? Is he or she so emotionally involved as to have impaired judgment in the choices of diagnosis and therapy?) The outcomes of such in-family therapy are, so far as I could find, undocumented in the literature in any systematic way, and so the theoretical ethical rectitude of physicians treating their own families is difficult to judge in evidence-based terms of risk and benefit to the patients involved.

Our scenario, however, is a different one. This is not a case of a doctor treating her own family. It is, rather, a daughter, who happens to be a medical student, making inquiry of the treating team of the care provided to her mother. She is, in this scenario, not very different from "lay" individuals who, having equipped themselves with some information from the neighbors, other doctors and students, and/or the Internet, question the treating physician about options for diagnosis she has heard are used in others who have the same complaint as her mother.

Her role as medical student should not, indeed cannot, disenfranchise her from pursuing what she naturally sees as her filial duty to her mother. In fact, when a family member (including a medical student or physician) is too hesitant to "interfere" with the treating doctors' care of a loved one (even though one has some concern about it) and things subsequently go badly for the patient, terrible self-recrimination may follow. An essay by a cardiology fellow published in the *Annals of Internal Medicine*[77] poignantly tells the story of her reluctance to challenge her teachers in their approach to her beloved father's therapy, and how she now believes that her "non-interference" eventuated in his premature and unnecessary death from heart disease. She says, "I have yet to overcome the failure, sorrow, loss and despair that descended on me when my father died."

There is another aspect to this scenario, however, that must be addressed. As I read our case, the student "tells her mother about these concerns" before discussing them with the hospital house physician. In doing this, the student may have inadvertently increased her mother's anxiety and unnecessarily decreased her mother's confidence in her physicians' skill and knowledge. Since sustained patient trust in her doctors, if merited by them, can significantly ameliorate suffering and be a major contributor to therapeutic success, the student may have undermined the very thing she wanted to assure: her mother's best care. She should have discussed her misgivings about the absence of CT scan with the treating physicians (who might have either alleviated her concerns by their explanations of their chosen approach or agreed with her and ordered the CT scan) before sharing her doubts with her mother. Since it is the duty of both family members and doctors to promote rather than erode the patient's comfort, there would be no conflict to our student, nor to any caring family member, in pursuing this clarification. The medical student was not, therefore, unethical, but simply inexperienced and mistaken in this specific act in her attempt to contribute to her mother's care. And if she did this to demonstrate to her mother how knowledgeable and in-charge she was, to show off her medical sophistication a little, then her error was that she acted more from pride, or a desire for approval for herself, than from a daughter's thoughtful concern about her parent.

Faith Fitzgerald, M.D.
Professor, Internal Medicine
Asst. Dean of Humanities and Bioethics
University of California, Davis School of Medicine

MAINTAINING APPROPRIATE RELATIONS WITH PATIENTS 2

A fourth year medical student is asked by his sister-in-law if she should have a prophylactic mastectomy. Her mother and grandmother both had breast cancer at an early age and she has just learned that she carries a mutation in the BRCA1 gene. The sister-in-law's physician discussed the risks and benefits of a mastectomy, but did not give a firm recommendation for or against it, only stating that she would need to consider both options, talk to family members, and make an informed decision.

A Medical Student Perspective

From the day I was accepted into medical school, my family considered me a doctor. It did not matter that I had many years ahead of me before becoming a physician; in their eyes I was already able to accurately diagnose and treat any number of maladies. I was, and am, continually honored to be asked for medical advice: It tells me that my family trusts me. There are, however, certain personal and professional concerns that accompany giving medical advice to family members, especially when we are still in training.

It is important to recognize what role family members expect us to play when they ask our advice. Are they looking for professional opinions about medical care, or are they approaching us solely as a family member? If we are being asked for medical advice, the burden of maintaining a proper patient–physician relationship falls on us.[78] For example, as a medical professional the student ought not discuss the sister-in-law's medical problems with anyone else in the family – doing so would break doctor–patient confidentiality.

When a person is accepted into medical school, families feel a certain pride, which can motivate the student to succeed. When family members ask for medical advice, however, this sense of pride can become a hindrance. As students not wanting to disappoint our families, we may feel tempted to exaggerate our clinical knowledge. This can result in us offering incorrect advice, which can end up hurting our families. It is our responsibility to recognize our limitations so we can avoid risking complications in the care of our loved ones.[79]

The student may have never encountered a situation like the one his sister-in-law is facing and may not be qualified to offer medical judgment. Even some experienced physicians do not adequately prepare women for decisions about prophylactic mastectomies. A 2007 study found that 81 percent of women reported not having sufficient counseling before undergoing the procedure.[80] If fully trained doctors do not adequately counsel patients about these decisions, it is unrealistic to assume that students will be able to sufficiently answer all the relevant medical questions.

Also, it can be awkward when family members seek our medical advice, particularly when we need to ask them sensitive or embarrassing questions. Without this information, however, we will not have a complete history, and will be at risk for providing inaccurate advice.[81] A mastectomy can result in long-term psychological effects such as changes in emotional stability, sexual relationships, and feelings of femininity. Will the student be prepared to talk to his sister-in-law about topics such as the possibility of future breastfeeding or breast implants? Is he able to address the possible psychological ramifications of this surgery, such as anxiety and loss of femininity? If not, then it will be very difficult to offer useful and accurate medical advice.

One study reported that 99 percent of physicians received requests from family members for medical advice.[74] As we move through our medical education and into our careers, we not only have to accept the challenges of treating our patients but also of responding to requests from our family members. It is important to set boundaries with our families early in our training to avoid conflicts in the future. If we are unable to offer medical advice, we are still able to offer time, empathy, and a listening ear.

Christine Lee Ruehl, M.D.
Medical Student, Penn State College of Medicine

A Faculty Perspective

What should a medical student do when a family member seeks health-related advice? Should the student decline on the grounds that he or she is not yet a physician, or that it is inappropriate to have a therapeutic relationship with a relative? Or should students use their knowledge and expertise (limited as it is) to consult and advise, since they likely know (and care) more about the family member than an impartial physician? Such requests are commonplace[74] and challenging,[82] typically beginning early in a student's career and continuing until (or past) retirement. Yet they can be awkward for the student, who has one foot in the world of doctors and the other in the world of patients, all the while knowing the limits of his or her knowledge.

As is often said, good ethics starts with good facts, so to address this question, some clarifications are in order. First, it is important to understand of *whom* this question is being asked. Is the request for advice being directed to the student in his role as medical expert, or supportive family member? Professionalism is about many things, not least of which is behaving in a manner consistent with one's role. What is expected and ethical in one role may differ from that in another,[83] and it is crucial to clarify roles and obligations up front.

Second, it is important to clarify *what* is being asked. Is the sister-in-law looking for empathy and reflective listening, or medical advice? A fourth year medical student may have more of the former to offer, although it's possible that the latter is what is really wanted. Given the potential discomfort of having expertise sought that is not yet present, it behooves the student to find out what the sister-in-law hopes to achieve through their conversation, and to establish clear and appropriate expectations.

Third, it is important to note that this particular request would be challenging even if the student *did* have advanced knowledge about breast cancer, since decisions regarding genetic testing and prophylactic mastectomy are particularly value driven,[84] and students (as well as the physicians) generally have no particular expertise about a patient's risk tolerance, values, or preferences.

Furthermore, while we might fantasize that a person facing the choice of whether to undergo prophylactic surgery is a rational decision maker who systematically weighs all the pros and cons and then decides through a dispassionate and deliberate process, the literature on decision making shows this is seldom the case.[85] Rather, such choices are governed by many factors, including fear, past experience, personal appeals, and anecdotes.[86] In this context, the views of an individual who is both a close family member and a novice medical expert could potentially receive disproportionate weight, and inappropriately influence the decision.

In addition to the empirical question of whether the student has sufficient knowledge to offer substantive medical advice in this situation is the normative question of whether he ought to advise, regardless of his knowledge level. Professional organizations have opined about the role physicians should play in providing treatment to family members, and in general, have argued that they ought to avoid doing so. For example, the AMA *Code of Medical Ethics*[81] states that physicians generally should not treat their close family members because "the physician's personal feelings may unduly influence his or her professional medical judgment." Likewise, the American College of Physicians' *Ethics Manual*[87] states "physicians should avoid treating themselves, close friends, or members of their own families," because "the physician's emotional proximity can result in a loss of objectivity." Such guidelines would apply to students as well.

So, what's the student to do in this case? In my view, the student should help in a way that is consistent with his professional obligations and role, clearly delineating boundaries and clarifying expectations. What might such help look like? First, listen carefully and be empathic, by reflecting the sister-in-law's feelings and being non-directive. This can help the sister-in-law articulate her concerns and uncertainties, and may aid her deliberation. Second, help the sister-in-law gather more information, by providing readings, credible Web sites, information about support groups, and perhaps putting her in contact with others who have made similar decisions. Third, encourage her to speak with her physician and a genetic counselor, and offer to help her generate a list of questions. If these individuals are not responsive, offer to help her find others who are, either for a second opinion or to transfer care. In summary, there are many ways a student can help family members with their medical concerns without directly telling them what to do. Learning such skills early in one's career is vital if one is to avoid perpetual expectations for medical advice in subsequent years.

Michael J. Green, M.D., M.S., FACP
Professor of Medicine and Humanities
Director, Penn State Bioethics Program
Penn State College of Medicine

IMPROVING THE QUALITY OF CARE 1

A medical student is on her first clinical rotation. On morning rounds with her team she notices that several of the residents – including the senior supervising resident – neglect to clean their hands between patients. When she observed this on the first day of her rotation, the student assumed that the residents failed to clean their hands because the team was rushing to complete rounds before a teaching conference. The next day, however, she again saw the same individuals examine three patients in a row without cleaning their hands. The student wonders whether and how she should address this with the residents who are supervising her during this rotation.

A Medical Student Perspective

The first exposure to clinical rotations can be an extremely disorienting time for a medical student. How else can one explain the confusion that this student felt when observing others deliver flawed health care? Being exposed to a completely unfamiliar system in which we are constantly judged and evaluated places us in a precarious position. This clinical vignette highlights the constant conflict that we face between pleasing those around us and pleasing our ethical compass. It can often feel as though we are being forced to choose between promoting our own success and promoting the success of our patients.

Today, no clinician can deny that hand cleaning is a critical part of patient care. Infections due to resistant bacteria have become common and the rate of nosocomial infections is rising. Thus, inattention to hand hygiene is simply bad medicine. Intellectually, we are all aware of this. Everyday, however, up to 50 percent of doctors fail to clean their hands prior to examining a patient.[88]

As medical students, our job is to observe the various physician models and pick and choose those attributes we would like to incorporate into the physician we hope to become. These lessons are learned from both the good and the bad role models. Multiple studies have shown that the poor hand hygiene of our role models can leave a lasting impression. In an observational study performed in 2006, Snow and colleagues found that mentor hand hygiene was the strongest predictor of student hand hygiene.[88] Nonetheless, students and trainees do have the ability and the responsibility to increase awareness among their more experienced colleagues. Observing, but not addressing, suboptimal clinical care allows this behavior to continue and permits our own ethical vigilance to deteriorate. Each time such an issue goes unchallenged, we slide deeper into the system we hope to improve.

I believe that people enter the field of medicine with the intent to take good care of their patients. I also believe that physicians know that hand washing improves patient care. However, in the chaos of day-to-day medicine it is easy to develop a disconnect between these two concepts. As medical students with a fresh perspective, we are in the unique position to remind our more experienced colleagues what they knew at our stage – that they are too busy not to wash their hands. Without the nosocomial spread of resistant bacteria, we would all be less busy.

Yet, within the medical hierarchy, there are appropriate ways to address the residents' behavior. Making an obvious show of stopping to wash your hands reminds all the team members of the importance of hand hygiene. Carrying around sanitizing hand gel and offering it out to others at regular intervals makes it hard for other team members to refuse. This can be accomplished without shaming or accusations and makes it easy for increased compliance to happen more naturally. Most importantly, we need to take the negative influence and learn from it, so that those who come after us are not negatively influenced by us, the mentors and role models of the future.

Kiona Allen
Medical Student, University of Pennsylvania School of Medicine

A Faculty Perspective

Although hand hygiene is the bedrock of infection control practice, many clinicians fail to recognize its importance. Breaches in hand cleaning have led to hospital-based outbreaks of serious viral infections, spread of resistant bacteria to vulnerable patients, and transmission of infections from patients to health care workers. Nonetheless, observational studies suggest that in some intensive care units compliance with basic hand hygiene practices may be as low as 30 percent and that physicians are less likely to perform appropriate hand hygiene than other members of the medical team.[89]

So why does the scenario described occur everyday at virtually every hospital? Barriers to hand hygiene have been studied extensively and include convenience, workload, and knowledge.[90,91] Surveys of health care workers revealed that the mere placement of sinks and alcohol hand rub dispensers can make a significant difference in the frequency of hand cleaning. Some clinicians reported that they had too many patients or that a patient was "too critical" to permit hand cleaning prior to delivering care. Finally, clinicians often underestimated the significance of hand hygiene, stating that hand cleaning was unlikely to improve the health of their patients.

The culture of academic medicine, which often entails strict attention to hierarchy, may also play an important role in undermining the delivery of the high quality medical care. Many of the basic practices associated with good medical care are simple to perform but require vigilance to ensure they are consistently done. Thus, members of a team of health care workers are in an ideal position to remind each other when an important facet of care – such as hand hygiene – has been inadvertently overlooked. Sadly, many of us work in hospitals and health care settings where we worry that a gentle reminder to a colleague, such as "I think you might have forgotten to clean your hands", would not be well received. Studies have demonstrated, however, that verbal reminders are remarkably effective at improving compliance with hand hygiene and that their impact is more lasting than educational interventions.[92]

Delivering high quality medical care is difficult, surprisingly difficult. Ironically, many of the practices that determine the quality of care – such as hand hygiene and other infection prevention activities – require little or no specialized knowledge or skill. Thus, the potential for delivering high quality care is available to all members of the health care team, regardless of their education or position within the medical hierarchy. Although uncomfortable, I would encourage the student in this scenario to find a graceful but direct way to remind her senior resident, and all other members of the team, to clean their hands. This simple intervention might save her patient's life.

Susan Coffin, M.D., M.P.H.
Medical Director, Infection Prevention and Control,
Children's Hospital of Philadelphia
University of Pennsylvania School of Medicine

IMPROVING THE QUALITY OF CARE 2

A fourth year student is doing an office-based primary care clerkship. In this very busy practice, the student typically sees every third patient and presents the information to the physician and they then see the patient together. Today they are forty-five minutes late. The student and physician see an elderly man who has atrial fibrillation and has had difficulty staying at a therapeutic anticoagulant level while on warfarin. The physician evaluates the patient and adjusts the warfarin. After the physician leaves, the student elicits the additional history that the patient consumes about six beers daily.

For a video of the vignette, see http://professionalism.jefferson.edu/.

A Medical Student Perspective

Many medical students on their core clinical rotations see their work on a clinical team as redundant. Every note they write is rewritten or co-signed not only by the intern, but by the resident and often by an attending. Every order they place must also be reviewed/co-signed up the chain of command. As a third year medical student, it is easy for one to be disenchanted with one's place on the team and feel trivialized.

In today's health care climate, physicians are under pressure to see a large volume of patients more efficiently. Overall time spent seeing the patient is further reduced due to increased administrative duties. Primary care physicians may spend an average of ten to twenty minutes per patient.[93] As medical students, we are in a unique position. Given our lighter patient load, we have the luxury of spending more time with our patients than our mentors. In this particular case, the extra time the student spent with the patient shed light on a probable cause for the patient's inability to maintain a therapeutic dose of warfarin – his alcohol consumption.

On my first day of an inpatient rotation during my third year – my first day on the "ward" – I was in a pediatric unit, examining my first patient and noticed a heart murmur on physical exam. The patient had been on the floor for two days, but in looking over the previous notes, I noticed that neither the resident nor the attending documented this murmur. Since it was my first day, I was still unsure of myself. Summoning the little self-confidence I had, I presented my findings to the resident. Thankfully, the resident not only appreciated my input but also went over to the patient with me, performed a cardiac exam, and also noticed the murmur. This experience showed me how important it is to the team environment to have encouraging leaders who provide a safe setting for the other members of a team to voice their opinion.

Though we do not know the result of the vignette, the student will next present his findings to the physician. As Dr. Holmboe highlights below, an important part of health care education in the clinical setting is having team leaders, the physicians, in facilitating roles, where the other members of the team can approach them with their opinions.

Similarly, the medical student needs to demonstrate an adequate level of development as a team member – and demonstrate competence and a willingness to take responsibility.[94] The student can assist the physician's role as a leader and facilitator. After identifying the patient's alcohol consumption as an important modifier of his anticoagulation status, the student should relay the importance of this information to the physician. In an ideal environment, the physician would facilitate this communication and, if necessary, act on the new information.

However, practical situations are hardly ideal, and there are team settings where lines of power and authority are clearly drawn. It is my hope that our educational system will continue to improve, and in much the way we have fostered interdisciplinary care on the floors – integrating different specialties as well as different professions (nursing, medicine, pharmacy, social services, etc.) – we will continue to tread towards integration amongst the lanes of hierarchy, as seen in the relationship between the student and attending physician.

Neerav Goyal, M.P.H.
Medical Student, Jefferson Medical College

A Faculty Perspective

Medicine is, and always has been, a team activity. We are only now beginning to understand how important teamwork is in providing patient-centered, effective and safe care. In both inpatient and outpatient academic settings, students are an important member of the interdisciplinary team. As Mr. Goyal points out above, students are often in a position to spend more time with patients. This "extra" time with patients can have several positive consequences. First, students can develop a meaningful, human relationship with patients as they learn more about who the patients are as people; this is especially true during a chaotic hospital admission. Second, students will often explore medical histories and physical exams in greater depth, and as a result may uncover findings missed by others on the health care team.

One might assume that students may uncover historical and physical exam findings missed by others simply because they may have more time to conduct a thorough history and exam. However, some evidence suggests that students may be every bit as competent as their attendings in some skills. For example, Vukanovic-Criley and colleagues found the cardiac examination skills of both full-time and volunteer faculty were no better than those of third or fourth year students.[95] Mr. Goyal's experience with the heart murmur is certainly testament to this research finding. Students were also found to be positive contributors to quality improvement in community-based faculty outpatient offices, helping those practices identify opportunities for improvement through medical record audits.[96] Thus, students bring important and useful knowledge and skills to the care of patients.

However, the hierarchical nature of physician and local medical culture can have a pernicious effect on students wanting to point out potential problems, errors, or unique information about patients. Students clearly see themselves as the bottom of the academic food chain; much in their environment supports this perception. First, students are highly dependent on faculty for grades and may be reticent to point out an oversight or missed finding by an attending. Second, faculty often spend limited time with students, and that time is often shared with other learners on the team. Third, as Mr. Goyal points out, physicians in the outpatient setting are often harried in today's practice environment, and students may perceive any disruption to workflow as unwelcome.

However, beyond issues associated with hierarchy, one of the biggest barriers to the professional development of medical students is the hidden curriculum. The hidden curriculum is defined as "the set of influences that function at the level of organizational structure and culture, including for example, implicit rules to survive the institution such as customs, rituals, taken for granted aspects" – a set that can be positive and/or negative.[97] In our current vignette, an attending and office staff dismissive of the student's concern about the patient's drinking would be sending a strong message to the student to "stay out of the way," at substantial risk to the patient. On the other hand, an attending that acts on the information uncovered by the student, even if she neglects to give the student positive feedback, is sending a powerful message that the student is a valued member of the office team.

In a recent review, Baker and his colleagues developed a core set of team-work competencies.[98] Three of these competencies are pertinent to our vignette: team leadership, mutual performance monitoring and mutual trust. In Baker's model of team competencies several key leadership behaviors include facilitating problem solving and synchronizing the individual team member contributions. Clearly both behaviors apply to the student's role in caring for this at-risk patient.

For mutual performance monitoring and trust, identifying mistakes and lapses in other team member actions, sharing information (in this case the alcohol use) and the willingness to admit mistakes and accept feedback are crucial behaviors to ensure patient safety and effective care. Imagine the powerful message sent if the attending admitted his or her own mistake to a student but more importantly acted on the event to learn and improve their own future performance.

Professionalism can only be known in and through action. This vignette highlights the important potential behaviors by both the student and the attending that are essential to ensure this patient receives patient-centered, effective, and safe care.

Eric Holmboe, M.D.
Senior Vice President for Quality Research and Academic Affairs
American Board of Internal Medicine

IMPROVING ACCESS TO CARE 1

A first year medical student's school and the Liaison Committee on Medical Education requires that all students have health insurance. Students can opt out of the insurance plan offered by the school with proof of other insurance. In order to save money, the student elects to stay with his family's plan, which covers children up to the age of twenty-three. The family plan does not have prescription or mental health coverage, and stipulates that the non-emergency care he receives must be from a provider close to his parents' home, which is a hundred miles away from the medical school. The student affairs dean contacts the student to discuss her concern about the limitations of this plan and to recommend he obtain a more comprehensive plan offered by the school.

A Medical Student Perspective

The conflict between the student and his school resembles the struggle between autonomy and paternalism in the patient–physician relationship. It is unrealistic, however, to expect that an institution would know its students as intimately as a physician would know his patients. And it is unreasonable for the school to justify the imposition of this policy in a pa-ternalistic manner.

In electing to stay with his family's health plan, a justification the student provides is that this plan is cheaper. The implied fault of this decision is that the student is jeopardizing his access to health care to cut costs – yet research has shown that student debt creates stress that can contribute to burnout.[99] Financial stress, when manifesting as clinical symptoms, can adversely affect academic performance.[100] A 2006 study found that there was a direct corre-lation between students' perceptions of their own debt and their perfor-mance in school.[101] The student in this vignette may perceive his debt as a source of stress that could be exacerbated by a more expensive plan. A cheaper plan might elicit less stress and, subsequently, not risk poor aca-demic performance.

Another discrepancy between plans is the coverage of mental health. Though mental illness is a serious concern, access to mental health care may seem less of a necessity from the student's perspective. Several studies have shown that medical students are reluctant to acknowledge mental ill-ness and pursue the appropriate treatment because they are apprehensive of the repercussions for their continued medical training and career.[102] Though there has been an increasing awareness of mental health concerns, some of the stigmas remain, even among medical students. As a consequence, 47 percent of medical students still sought mental health care outside the uni-versity and 19 percent explored other avenues of care.[103]

Finally, there is concern that this student's choice of insurance does not provide access to care locally. Several studies have found that, even in instan-ces where insurance coverage was not a concern among students, there still exist obstacles to seeking primary care. One study found 55 percent of med-ical students were "too busy," 43 percent self-diagnosed and anticipated the problem resolving on its own, 31 percent were concerned with cost, and 12 percent worried about confidentiality.[103]

In isolating the potential motivations behind this student's choice of in-surance, the struggle again between the principles of autonomy and pater-nalism is evident. The school is not in a position to understand the student's consideration of all these variables and, therefore, cannot hope to advise him with his own interests and concerns in mind. Only the student is aware of these subtler influences, risks, and benefits. The medical school ought to fully respect the student's autonomy and therefore recognize him as an individual uniquely capable of making the most appropriate decision for himself.

Christopher H. Henry
Medical Student, Jefferson Medical College

A Faculty Perspective

Health care costs rise each year, and medical students, most of whom are in considerable debt from education loans, increase their indebtedness further from rising health care premiums. It is no wonder that students look for ways to trim expenses. Therefore, saving money by limiting health insurance coverage becomes an easy target.

Medical students are, by and large, a young healthy group of individuals. Many have not sought medical care in years, so typically they do not think they'll ever "need" a more comprehensive and more expensive health plan. "I don't ever get sick" is a phrase used by some students as they try to opt for an inexpensive catastrophe-only plan in order to save hundreds of dollars annually.

The Association of American Medical Colleges (AAMC) recommends that every medical school provide its student body with health insurance. Although it is often joked that second year students believe they have many of the diseases they learn about in pathology, the truth is medical students do actually frequent physicians and use medications more than the general population in the same age group. An analysis among nearly a thousand medical students at Jefferson has shown an increased health care utilization compared to aged-matched controls.

The AAMC also recommends that medical school health care plans include mental health services, prescription drug coverage, and access to care in the vicinity of the medical school. Yet these components of health insurance add significantly to the cost of the plan, and make most "affordable" plans found elsewhere unacceptable. Some students may argue that they don't need mental health coverage, but, indeed, I have found that they often do. With the stress of medical school, the pressure of exams, the volume of information to be learned – all in students in an age group where we are likely to see new onset depression, anxiety, and even bipolar disorder, the need for mental health coverage seems obvious. Students need access to mental health for test-taking anxiety, insomnia, depression, anxiety, and other mental health concerns without having to worry about whether or not it is covered. A 2008 report underscored the importance of such coverage. In this cohort study of over 4,000 medical students, the investigators found that 10 percent of students experience suicidal ideation during medical school.[103]

As a student affairs dean who manages a medical school insurance plan, I have struggled over the years with the requirement that a health care plan allow students to be seen by physicians in a non-emergency setting in the vicinity of the medical school. Students may argue that they will continue to use their physician "back home" who will take care of anything while on break, and if they are sick they can be seen at student health or the emergency room. While this may hypothetically sound reasonable, in reality, this does not work out. Over the years, I have seen enough injuries and illnesses to conclude that such a geographic restriction sacrifices care and adds to the already stressful life of a medical student.

As stated in the Physician Charter, physicians need to be committed to improving the access of care for their patients, must strive to reduce barriers to equitable health care, and eliminate barriers to care based on financial considerations.[40,103] While medical students learn how to promote the best care for their patients and adhere to the many tenets of medical professionalism, they ought to be concerned about their own welfare and not limit their own access to care. I therefore believe that students should make a relatively small financial sacrifice, and obtain the comprehensive insurance coverage that is recommended by their school.

Kristin DeSimone, M.D.
Assistant Dean, Student Affairs and Career Counseling
Jefferson Medical College

IMPROVING ACCESS TO CARE 2

A fourth year medical student working in a homeless shelter clinic observes the difficulty that some of the patients have in accessing physicians at his medical school. Each of the patients has chronic and disabling medical problems, has Medicaid insurance, and has been referred by their primary doctor at the clinic to a subspecialist at the medical center. The patients have included a man with refractory seizures (referred to a neurologist), a woman with sickle cell anemia and severe avascular necrosis who needs a hip replacement (referred to an orthopedic surgeon), and a woman with poorly controlled type I diabetes and recurrent diabetic ketoacidosis (referred to an endocrinologist). In each case, the patient had been informed that they could not be evaluated by the subspecialist because the practice did not accept Medicaid insurance.

For a video of the vignette, see http://professionalism.jefferson.edu/.

A Medical Student Perspective

As a third year medical student one will certainly witness the inequalities of the U.S. health care system. In this vignette, patients are denied visits to subspecialists because they have Medicaid insurance. As a student, it is always disheartening to witness the health care system fail a patient. It is intellectually satisfying to make a diagnosis and effective treatment plan, but demoralizing for yourself and the patient when the treatment is unattainable because of insurance. Speaking with individual specialists does not solve the problem, because the policy regarding which insurances to accept is usually made by the practice administration and not an individual physician. It is not the place of a third year medical student to navigate the labyrinth of reimbursement and coverage.

Unfortunately, rejection by specialists is becoming even more common for Medicaid patients, which covered 15 percent of non-elderly Americans in 2003.[104] Among specialists, about 20 percent of medical specialists and surgical specialists are no longer accepting Medicaid patients.[105] Physicians commonly note low reimbursement rates, excessive administrative demands, delayed reimbursements, full practices and the high clinical burden as common reasons for not accepting Medicaid patients.[105]

As in this vignette, most medical students will participate in a student-run clinic where many patients either have Medicaid or are uninsured.[106] At these clinics, students have the opportunity to act as an advocate, which may entail speaking with a caseworker, contacting specialists directly, or providing patients with information about outside resources. Learning to become a physician-advocate is becoming increasingly important in securing the best health care for your patients. In fact, advocating not only for individual patients but also for larger projects (local public health projects, policy changes, and global health) related to health is part of a physician's professional responsibility.[107]

As the next generation of physicians, we must collectively remember that the only way to effect permanent change is to become more involved in advocacy beyond individual patients. If the current health care system remains, we will have an increasing number of uninsured and underinsured patients, a high average of student debt, and declining real incomes.[108] The challenge that lies before us is to balance our principles of equal access, social justice and integrity with the practicality of earning an income that provides us with a comfortable lifestyle. We need to learn from and look to those physicians already in practice on how to handle these issues. By observing the behavior of our physician-colleagues, we can begin to develop our own guiding principles regarding balancing care for people and financial reimbursement. During my own practice, I hope to treat and be an advocate for many insured as well as uninsured and underinsured patients. Ultimately, one will have the choice to provide or deny care to certain populations. The question one must start answering now is: what kind of physician will you become?

Kimmie Pringle
Medical Student, Jefferson Medical College

A Faculty Perspective

Medical student-run clinics in homeless shelters are common throughout the United States.[109] They provide hundreds of students with opportunities for valuable and substantive service-learning experiences that enhance their clinical training, augment team-building and leadership skills, and foster their role as patient/societal advocates. The stories and problems of the homeless population are complex and reflect the growing divide between "those who have, and those who have not."[110] Homeless men and women have a significant burden of chronic disease, with increased morbidity and mortality,[111] much of which is preventable and/or treatable. For a myriad of reasons, the "system" of care for the homeless is often the student-run shelter clinic, the emergency room and/or a hospital bed. Access to specialty services is limited, particularly for the uninsured or those with Medicaid.

The Medicaid program was created in 1965, in part to increase access of low income people to mainstream medical services. However, over the years, office-based physicians have reduced their treatment of Medicaid patients, and many have withdrawn from the program altogether.[112] In addition, specialty physicians are much less likely than primary care physicians to accept new Medicaid managed care patients.[113] The inadequacy of Medicaid payment rates, in comparison with those of Medicare and private insurance, is often cited as a major factor contributing to low levels of Medicaid participation by physicians.[114] In fact, adverse selection may present serious financial risks for academic medical centers participating in Medicaid managed care.[115]

The question is, can physicians refuse to accept patients who have Medicaid? Certainly they can. But should they refuse to accept Medicaid patients, particularly when these patients have been seen and evaluated by medical students from their institutions? Again, they can. But what message is this sending to the medical students, who rely on their faculty to model medical professionalism?

Medical educators are increasingly focusing on medical professionalism as a key element in the curriculum. As Inui writes:

> And how are we faring as medical educators in preparing future physicians for professional roles in our complicated world? I would conclude that the "formative arc" of education today is strong on the acquisition of technical knowledge and weak-to-negative on the acquisition of values and moral formation. While preparing successfully to pass tests of knowledge, our students measurably move from being open-minded and curious to test-driven and minimalistic, from open-hearted and idealistic to self-centered and well-defended, and from altruistic to cynical. In the course of their educational experience with us, they also

move from taking notes and focusing on the explicit curriculum (what we say) to learning most from what we do. Here, then, is the greatest challenge of educating for professionalism. If we wish to change our students' preparation for their careers, we ourselves will need to change.[116]

Medical professionals and educators should look to *Medical Professionalism in the New Millennium: A Physician Charter*[40] as a guide to their work and actions. The preamble to the Charter is that *professionalism is the basis of medicine's contract with society*. Fundamental principles of professionalism are the primacy of patient welfare, patient autonomy, and social justice. "The medical profession must promote justice in the health care system, including the fair distribution of health care resources. Physicians should work actively to eliminate discrimination in healthcare, whether based on race, gender, socioeconomic status, ethnicity, religion, or any other social category."[40]

Specialists should follow the tenets of the Charter and live by these precepts. They should resist efforts to impose a corporate mentality on a profession of service to others.[40] Students should not have to work in a system that models behavior which disregards the precepts of medical professionalism, and contributes to the erosion of their idealism and altruism. Instead, students should be afforded opportunities to be effective "community oriented primary care advocates."[117]

James Plumb, M.D., M.P.H.
Professor, Department of Family and Community Medicine
Jefferson Medical College

COMMITMENT TO A JUST DISTRIBUTION OF FINITE RESOURCES 1

A third year student working with a gastroenterologist observes the physician ordering CT scans for most patients he sees for abdominal pain. The physician explains that ever since he "was burned in the past" because of missed pancreatic cancer, which can be difficult to diagnose, he usually orders CT scans for patients with abdominal pain.

A Medical Student Perspective

The majority of formal education in professionalism occurs in the first two years of medical school. Some of what students learn during the pre-clinical years, however, is inconsistent with what is observed in clinical settings. The practice of defensive medicine illustrates this point. Defensive practices, performed by medical students' clinical role models, have at least two broad ramifications. First, defensive practices have the potential to damage the patient–physician relationship. Second, medical students learn unprofessional values by observing physicians who practice defensive medicine.

The practice of defensive medicine often constitutes a breach of professional values. When a physician orders a test that is not medically indicated, but rather fulfills the desire for protection from the threat of litigation, the physician breaks the bond of professional trust that characterizes the patient–physician relationship. This bond is predicated on the belief that physicians will always act in the best interests of patients.[118] Some defensive practices subject patients to additional costs without additional risks. As illustrated by this case study, other practices expose patients to additional costs as well as potential risks associated with the invasive follow-up of an incidental finding.

While these practices may damage the trust between patients and physicians, they also have negative implications for medical students who observe this behavior. According to a study by Brownell et al., senior residents reported that their clinical role models were the best teachers of professionalism.[119] Because of the nature of medical training, these same role models may also influence medical students' values. When medical students observe unprofessional behavior, they learn distorted professional values. This has the potential to damage the culture of professionalism, which will ultimately be sustained by tomorrow's physicians.

The behavior of attending physicians may have positive or negative influences upon trainees. Medical students are assigned to clinical rotations, which means that they are not able to choose their preceptors. For this reason, medical students must identify what type of behavior is worthy of emulation. This is complicated by the fact that there is a spectrum of practice that constitutes defensive medicine. Some defensive practices have the potential to improve the quality of care. Thorough documentation, expanded informed consent, and positive interactions between patients and physicians are examples of these behaviors.[118] The motivations behind these practices are consistent with defensive medicine, but the end result is improved patient care. The challenge for medical students who are new to the clinical setting is to recognize when this boundary is crossed. Students need to identify the behaviors that are consistent with patients' best interests, which is a difficult task.

Justin S. Brandt
Medical Student, Jefferson Medical College

A Faculty Perspective

At first glance, the practice described by the practitioner in our hypothetical case seems stunningly inappropriate. How can a medical professional, who has taken an oath to provide altruistic care to his patients, make medical decisions so callously positioned to save his own skin? Wouldn't it be more appropriate to limit the use of expensive imaging utilizing ionizing radiation to those cases that clinically merit such intensity? Isn't this an example of "defensive medicine," clinical behavior designed to avoid liability? Doesn't this sort of indiscriminate use of medical technology add to the spiraling cost of medical care, leading to further inequity of services?

On closer inspection, however, the behavior of this physician needs to be interpreted in the context of modern practice of medicine. The use of medical technology, especially imaging, has greatly increased the cost of health care, but has also contributed to better outcomes.[120] Specifically, there is evidence that a lower threshold for the use of CT scanning in the evaluation of acute right lower quadrant pain leads to fewer laparotomies for suspected appendicitis.[121]

The case in point is not one of acute abdominal pain, however. Clearly the practitioner is ordering CT scans in patients who do not need them. Defensive medicine can be seen in two major forms. Assurance behavior ("positive" defensive medicine) is characterized by the provision of additional medical services that are of no medical value, often to document a legal standard of care. Avoidance behavior ("negative" defensive medicine) is characterized by physicians' attempts to distance themselves from risk by eschewing certain procedures, refusing to care for certain populations of patients, or even leaving clinical practice altogether.[122] The behavior of our hypothetical physician is far from an aberrant; defensive medicine is widespread. Defensive medicine is described in a variety of health care and legal systems around the world, including the United Kingdom, Australia, and Japan.[123,124] In the United States, self-estimates of defensive practice behaviors is well over 50 percent in generalists and as high as 90 percent in high-risk specialists. These behaviors are more common in those who lack confidence in their liability insurance or perceive a high insurance premium burden.[122]

Unless we accept that the majority of our colleagues, and ourselves, fall short in the department of professionalism, we must ascribe at least some of these defensive behaviors to the milieu in which we practice. It is clear that various reforms of the medical system can lead to decreases in defensive medical practices. For example, enactment of caps on damages reduced hospital expenditures up to 9 percent in the late 1980s, while adoption of direct liability reform led to growth in overall physician supply in the late

1990s.[123] Other measures that may have decreased the perceived need of physicians to practice defensively include restrictions on contingent fees, adoption of no-fault insurance instruments, and the use of alternative dispute-resolution systems. Systems utilizing these models already exist elsewhere in the world.

As physicians, we must never abrogate our professional responsibilities, nor should we deflect blame for our ethical transgressions to others. But part of our professional energies may be well spent on bringing positive change to the system in which we practice, allowing us more latitude for clinical judgment in our daily practices.

Steven K. Herrine, M.D.
Professor of Medicine
Assistant Dean for Academic Affairs
Jefferson Medical College

COMMITMENT TO A JUST DISTRIBUTION OF FINITE RESOURCES 2

A fourth year medical student on an ICU (intensive care unit) rotation is taking care of an elderly patient with severe dementia, admitted from a nursing home with sepsis and multi-organ failure. The family insists on pursuing all available interventions, including hemodialysis and mechanical ventilation.

A Medical Student Perspective

Contrast these scenarios: In a rural Mexican village, an elderly patient who has suffered multiple strokes spends her last months at home with family, passing her days in a hammock in the jungle instead of a wheelchair or hospital bed. Caregivers are present at all times; she is fed, washed, turned, and carried as needed. Her body eventually tires and she dies at home, without lines or machine attachments.

In an urban U.S. hospital, an elderly patient with severe dementia develops sepsis, survives, and requires prolonged hemodialysis and mechanical ventilation. His family wishes to care for him at home, but he is unable to be extubated. With his family nearby, he dies in the ICU two months later after dialysis, a tracheotomy, multiple infections, blood transfusions, and countless studies.

End-of-life care decisions are extraordinarily difficult and fraught with emotion. Families often wish to have every treatment available provided for their loved one, with the perception that more interventions and doing "everything possible" will mean better outcomes and offer the greatest chance for survival. Yet numerous studies, including the Dartmouth Atlas of Health Care's 2008 report, indicate that higher spending and more care are not associated with greater patient satisfaction, quality of care or improved health outcomes.[125]

How end-of- life care decisions in the ICU are made – who gets what care, when and why – is not readily transparent to medical students. Patients with little chance of recovery seem to receive intervention after intervention. Early on, every medical student learns certain degrading terms: "total flog," or "train wreck," and associates these names with unceasing care in the face of medical futility. Overworked residents, already stretched thin, really bear the brunt of such decisions, fully realizing that resources spent on patients with little hope of recovery are taken away from other patients who might indeed benefit. These resources are not only financial, but also labor intensive since they can involve time spent at a patient's bedside or reviewing a complex patient's chart. It becomes difficult to make sense of the efforts expended in certain clinical situations, as in the vignette, and patients become dehumanized and resented, seen as "cases" rather than as individuals.

As a medical student, I frequently wondered when I was going to receive instruction in the big picture. What were we doing and hoping to accomplish? Did our work seem as futile to my teachers as it sometimes did to me? If so, to prevent the next "wreck," who was going to "stop the train"? Interestingly, Barnato et al. found that elderly patients themselves preferred palliative treatments to life-extending ones.[126] If patients weren't demanding such interventions, whom were we treating – our patients' families? Ourselves?

We are a long way off from allowing our loved ones the peace to die while lying in a hammock. I left the ICU thinking that so much unnecessary treatment could have been avoided by advance planning. Early, frequent, and clear communication amongst family members and between patients and their primary care doctors is the most effective means to a just and transparent distribution of end-of-life resources.[127] And for the people I care about in my own life, I hope they would choose to spend their last days and weeks with family, at home, as unencumbered as possible by tubes, lines, and hourly vitals checks.

Patty Frew
Medical Student, Oregon Health and Science University

A Faculty Perspective

This vignette illustrates two dilemmas facing modern medicine – how to best care for a patient with severe dementia when the family insists on pursuing all available interventions, and how to model professional behavior in this teaching setting. My approach, as an intensivist, is to develop a framework for the medical student to use in the ICU, to provide ethical guidelines for admitting and discharging ICU patients and for the use of scarce ICU resources.[128]

In this framework, I lay out the missions of the ICU: to (1) preserve meaningful human life, (2) provide palliative care, and (3) provide compassionate care at the end of life. I point out to the student that patients who suffer from severe irreversible lack of cognitive function rarely benefit from ICU care, so the reasons for the family's insistence need to be carefully explored.[129]

I also review the ethical principles of beneficence, nonmaleficence, autonomy, and justice. These are all components of decision making for this patient. Students easily understand how beneficence and autonomy support the request for initial use of ICU care. Nonmaleficence often needs further explanation, a reminder that ICU care is invasive and uncomfortable, as are invasive procedures such as mechanical ventilation and hemodialysis. Finally, I address justice, which I define as "just allocation of scarce resources." This should also be addressed at the institutional level, for example, the institution may have an explicit institutional policy for priority in admissions and discharges based on medically objective criteria.[130]

I review with the student the steps I take to recommend goals of care to a family. I first identify my own recommendation. For the patient in this vignette, I would recommend limiting ICU care. This is at variance with family goals, so I then determine whether or not other health care providers, for example, nurses, respiratory therapists, consultants, agree with my recommendation. Once I have consensus, my team holds a family conference.[131] At this conference, my initial goal is to identify the concerns of the family. Often there are good reasons for insistence on "doing everything," and if we can understand these, we can reassure and support families. In defense of this approach, families rate clinicians' communication skills as equally or more important than clinical skills.[132] Let me give several approaches I often take:

1. Clear and understandable explanations of dialysis and ventilation are important. We can reassure the family that they have done all that should be done in this situation. When families recognize this, there is considerable relief, and often a decision to withdraw support

follows. It is vital to invest time on these family dynamics, both for the student to see, and to minimize post-bereavement complications for the family.[133]

2. The family may not understand the discomfort the patient experiences in the ICU. I encourage them to visit if they have not done this. Often the family will recognize that the comfort of good palliative care will offer the patient greater benefit than an invasive procedure or ongoing treatment.

3. The family needs guidance to express what the patient would want in this situation, not what they would want. Often this redirection helps the family say "no, she/he wouldn't want this," and move toward palliative care.

In summary, teaching students the mission of the ICU, reviewing ethical principles, and modeling family conferences, can help students to work with a family, such as the one described in the vignette, with greater compassion. It will also allow students to feel more comfortable working as part of the ICU team.

Molly Osborne, M.D., Ph.D.
Professor of Medicine and Associate Dean Student Affairs
Oregon Health and Science University

COMMITMENT TO SCIENTIFIC KNOWLEDGE 1

Nearing the end of his third year, a student recalls many outpatients during his medicine, family medicine, and obstetrics-gynecology clerkships who requested diagnostic tests learned about through the media, advertisements, or friends but not recommended by their physician. These tests included CT scanning for lung cancer screening, CA-125 testing for ovarian cancer screening, virtual colonoscopy for colon cancer screening, and cardiac calcium scoring for coronary artery disease.

A Medical Student Perspective

Medical students are often asked questions about the latest screening recommendations. It seems inevitable that patients will request medical tests, which have no known benefit as screening tools. Understanding the evidence and guidelines regarding health care screening is essential to fulfilling a critical role as part of the medical team. The United States Preventive Services Task Force (USPSTF) is an excellent resource for the latest evidence-based medicine

(EBM) recommendations on screening.[134] However, using EBM to support or refute tests to screen for pathology is limited by the amount of available research. Studies illustrate about 30 percent of patient care is based on randomized clinical control trials.[135] Therefore, utilizing evidence, when it does exist, is of the utmost importance in the consideration of such requests.

EBM-based screening is poorly implemented for a variety of reasons.[136] Patients are increasingly knowledgeable and vocal about their wants and needs regarding health care. Often patients confuse a screening test with a diagnostic test. An astute medical student will guide the history taking with specific questions to address the patients' underlying concerns. An appropriate screening test looks for disease not expected to be present, has a high sensitivity and specificity, and an available treatment able to change the overall outcome.[137] Diagnostic tests are used when symptoms or disease are identified during the history and examination.

While it may seem easier for a physician to comply with such requests to satisfy the patients' desires, there is the potential for numerous harmful consequences. These include false positive results (causing anxiety), false negative results (causing false reassurance from future screening), and expense, as the patient may have to bear some or all of the costs.

Acquiescing to patients' requests for screening tests can damage trust in the patient–physician relationship. For example, if a clinician orders a test for screening purposes without supporting evidence, the results could lead to doubt and confusion. Professional autonomy dictates the ability to apply knowledge as a means to benefit the patient.[136] The refusal to perform laboratory or radiographic tests that have no evidence as an appropriate screen falls under the practice of professional autonomy.

When encountering this situation, a medical student needs to prepare the patient for the attending physician's ultimate decision. Thoughtful interaction with patients allows for further explanation and education. A medical student needs to anticipate the patient's response to why tests will be refused and discuss the request with his or her attending physician. Patient acceptance of a screening test refusal may be variable. If the patient remains unconvinced regarding the lack of evidence, one could consider counseling the patient about potential harmful consequences.

Finally, some physicians could err on the side of pleasing their patients. Medical students can address this by asking the attending physician questions which would elicit the reasoning guiding the decision. The opportunity may arise for medical students to illustrate the current evidence-based recommendations to both the medical team and patients. Through being inquisitive, being concerned, and using an evidenced-based approach, medical students may then be able to engage both the patient and physician in an important dialogue about the best use of screening tests.

James J. Buchino
Medical Student, University of Louisville

A Faculty Perspective

Patients ask physicians for medical screening tests for many reasons. Requests may be based on a personal health history or experiences of family or friends. Interest in screening may also come from media coverage or perceptions of marketing, Internet Web sites, and special interest groups. Such tests are not necessarily beneficial to the patient. The number of screening examinations proven as beneficial by randomized controlled trials is far fewer than patients and physicians would imagine.[137] Nevertheless, physicians often acquiesce in ordering tests that have not been proven to be of benefit due to concerns of patient dissatisfaction.

Acquiescence fails on two counts. First, when a test is proposed, it should be of benefit to that patient; that is, the test has been shown to be of more gain than harm in discovering disease (with parameters of prevalence, detection, and ability to treat upon discovery) to warrant screening. Second, many requested screening tests have no empirical foundation in evidence for their support, with many known to be *ineffective* or *more harmful than beneficial*. Such tests are not acceptable per the USPSTF standard of evidence.[134] There are other factors, though, that may have bearing on one's willingness to order a test.

Family history or individualized occupational hazard histories may warrant a consideration of *elevated-risk screening*. Having in-depth discussion of family history or aggravating co-factors may even result in the discovery of symptoms that warrant diagnostic testing – a different matter, as testing for disease in the presence of symptoms alters the calculus whereby the pathophysiologic rationale for testing enters into the hunt for the sought disease.

Physicians can best role-model how to respond to patients requesting possibly non-beneficial screening tests when working with medical students by using a virtue- and principle-based approach to patient care. Physicians' efforts should be directed toward promoting medical goals that benefit patients, while also acknowledging their own professional integrity and prudence. The medical student can then observe and learn those skills necessary in declining requests for non-beneficial screening tests. Patients may balk when physicians refuse to order tests. Role-modeling to medical students a sensitive refusal may still uncover any additional mitigating history, risk factors, or symptoms that they have not disclosed. In their absence, patients have no ethical claim to a test that is without proven benefit (e.g., "I want it and I deserve it"), and medical students need to learn how to convey this message.

An essential tenet for physicians refusing to order unproven screening tests is professional integrity.[138] Professional integrity is the virtue that guides the physician to use established values, standards, norms of medicine with which the individual practitioner acknowledges and accepts. The physician needs to convey those aspects of medicine that are standard of care and those that are not. The patient – and medical student – need to comprehend why a request is outside the doctor's perception of professional integrity if it is judged to be without merit. Education of both patients and medical students is key – physicians need to convey why something may be helpful or not, rather than "will the doctor order it or not?" The physician is steward of the patient's medical care in promoting his or her benefit through the prudent use of testing while minimizing harm, and medical students need to have this demeanor role-modeled to them.

David John Doukas, M.D.
William Ray Moore Endowed Chair of Family Medicine and
Medical Humanism
Professor and Director of the Division of Medical Humanism
and Ethics
Department of Family and Geriatric Medicine
University of Louisville

COMMITMENT TO SCIENTIFIC KNOWLEDGE 2

A fourth year student on an otolaryngology clerkship works with a physician who frequently recommends complementary/alternative medicine (CAM) to patients. The student observes the physician suggesting B vitamins, gingko, and black cohosh for a woman with tinnitus. During other patient visits, the physician recommends acupuncture and therapeutic bodywork for a man with temporomandibular pain and butterbur for a woman with chronic allergic rhinitis. The student, while recalling the evidenced-based lectures he had the last three years, wonders how the otolaryngologist can recommend these CAM treatments without clear data supporting their benefit.

A Medical Student Perspective

The student should be applauded for being critical of the otolaryngologist's CAM treatment recommendations. With an increasing emphasis on the importance of practicing evidence-based medicine (EBM), it is crucial for medical students to develop and start practicing an analytical mindset with encountered medical practices. In this situation, the student has an opportunity to practice this approach – it is certainly appropriate for the student to politely question the doctor's recommendations. However, the student must make sure that any conversation about this be approached in a professional manner. To avoid an awkward patient–doctor interaction, it would be best to ask such a question outside of the clinical exam room. It might also be helpful to conduct some research on your own, allowing for a better-informed discussion with the doctor. As long as discretion is appropriately practiced, most physicians would be open and happy to explain their decisions and recommendations.

It is always in our patients' best interests that we, as their health care providers, constantly strive to provide treatments that have been scientifically shown to be beneficial. However, this dedication to EBM must be applied to all medical decisions we make for our patients, whether "allopathic" in nature or not. CAM therapies should not receive a reprieve from the rigorous standards of EBM. However, the inherent nebulous and somewhat foreign quality of CAM modalities has prompted most of us, as Western-trained practitioners, to artificially develop a hypercritical attitude when evaluating such options.

When interacting with some of my fellow classmates or even other non-medical friends (or even within myself), I can sometimes notice a mindset that subconsciously promotes a relatively unquestioning acceptance of Western medicine, especially when compared to CAM. As evidenced by the data shown from *Clinical Evidence* as laid out in Dr. Rindfleisch's commentary below, there is still a large portion of Western interventions that have not been scientifically proven to be effective. These data illustrate the importance of our needing to utilize the same critical eye for all medical recommendations we make for our patients.

This scenario focuses on the health care provider being an advocate for CAM therapies, but a more common situation would be for the patient to initially inquire about such options. With over one-third of Americans reporting CAM use at least once over the past twelve months in 2002, CAM modalities have become oft-accessed treatment options.[139] It is inevitable that we will encounter patients who have utilized or have questions about CAM treatments.

Overall, a delicate balance needs to be attained that allows one to be open-minded about the use of CAM therapies, but also to remain critical and offer evidence-based opinions on these modalities whenever possible. Working towards this equilibrium would be a big step towards improving our ability to provide well-informed patient-centered care.

James Wu
Medical Student, University of Wisconsin School of Medicine

A Faculty Perspective

People frequently use complementary/alternative medicine (CAM) modalities. A 2002 survey revealed that over 50 percent of U.S. adults have ever used CAM, not including prayer and megavitamins.[139] A 2005 study reported that 37 percent of respondents had recently taken botanicals.[140] However, many people choose not to tell their health care providers about CAM use. For example, a 2001 study indicated nearly half of the respondents felt their physicians were "prejudiced" against supplement use and one-third (and the percentage is higher in other studies) had not disclosed to their doctor that they took supplements.[141] I would posit that we as providers will offer better care if we are aware of what CAM therapies our patients are using and if we can offer them knowledgeable guidance that accounts not only for research findings, but also for safety of CAM interventions, patient autonomy, and cultural and other influences shaping the choices patients make.

Increasing numbers of physicians are incorporating CAM into their practices. This is one part of the approach used in integrative medicine which, among other things, "focuses on the least invasive, least toxic, and least costly methods to help facilitate health by integrating both allopathic and complementary therapies."[142] Most proponents of integrative medicine argue it should not be considered as a specialty unto itself, but rather as "good medicine" that can be practiced by all medical practitioners, regardless of specialty.

This case exemplifies a situation that can commonly arise in an integrative practice. Like the surgeon in the scenario, I often recommend CAM treatments. Many of these approaches may not have randomized, controlled trials supporting their use, though it should be noted that many do. When possible, evidence-based data should of course be weighed into decision making, but if such data are not available, how might decisions be made?

The availability of 'clear data' supporting therapeutic interventions is an issue that extends beyond the use of CAM. I was quite surprised the first time I opened BMJ's *Clinical Evidence*, a comprehensive, evidence-based review of the medical literature.[143] Ratings are assigned to all interventions reviewed, and then a summary is provided of "the state of our current knowledge." This summary indicates that:

- 13 percent of interventions used by healthcare providers are beneficial
- 23 percent are likely to be beneficial
- 8 percent show a tradeoff between benefits and harms
- 6 percent are likely to be ineffective or harmful
- 6 percent are unlikely to be beneficial
- 46 percent are classed as "unknown effectiveness."

As providers, we owe it to those who seek our care to advise them openly and honestly about what is known and not known about any therapies they might use. That requires that we keep ourselves updated on the current state of the research. Ultimately, we must acknowledge that the final decision about use of a treatment is the patient's.

In this scenario, I would encourage the student to review the data about such therapies and talk to the surgeon about them in more depth. The student would do well to note what criteria he or she will follow when deciding whether or not to recommend various therapies. How much should such decisions be based on one's knowledge of the literature? How much should one draw from personal experience? Where does familiarity with the treatment fit in? The experiences and wishes of the patient? Our intuition and gut instincts about what the patient needs? Answering such questions falls into the realm of the "art of medicine," and different providers will answer those questions differently. Regardless of the answers, exploration of these questions will help us grow as practitioners and enhance our capacity to meet our patients' needs.

J. Adam Rindfleisch, M.D., M.Phil.
Assistant Professor, Department of Family Medicine
Consultant, Integrative Medicine
University of Wisconsin School of Medicine

MANAGING CONFLICTS OF INTEREST 1

A student attends a pharmacology lecture given by a psychiatrist who discusses the medical treatment of depression and anxiety. He is very enthusiastic about a new drug. In the syllabus, it is noted that the psychiatrist is also a consultant for the company that manufactures this drug.

A Medical Student Perspective

With the increasing trend for academic physicians to serve as consultants for industry, the lines which define conflict of interest have become less and less distinct. Industry has an important place in health care. Pharmaceutical and medical device companies develop new products and support clinical trials as well as post-marketing surveillance. However, the influence of industry at the medical student level can only be detrimental.

As students we trust that what our mentors and professors teach us is accurate to the best of their knowledge. It is this inherent trust which necessitates proper modeling from the institutions and faculty whom we turn to for our curricula. In this case, when the psychiatrist includes a disclaimer in the syllabus stating that he has a conflict of interest, how should we apply this to our interpretation of his lecture? Should we consider him biased or should we consider him better informed than someone who does not serve as a consultant? Despite the ambiguity of this question, the solution is clear – students should not be placed in the position of having to speculate as to the validity of this lecture.

During the clinical years, it is common for students to witness and participate in drug lunches and to be offered designer pens and other flashy devices which bear the name of some new and expensive drug. At first glance, it seems that there may be no harm in a free lunch for house staff and samples of expensive drugs for patients who may not otherwise be able to afford cutting edge medicine.

But the truth is – there is no such thing as a free lunch. Gifts engender a sense of loyalty which can quickly transform into a prescription for the latest, most expensive drug when the generic standard of care may have been more appropriate. A patient who receives a free "new" drug sample can later be left in a difficult situation when the samples run out and she cannot afford the "new" drug once no longer free.

I believe there is a balance that must be struck between industry and academics. Institutions must insure that those privileged with the task of teaching future generations of physicians eliminate sources of bias and confusion regarding relationships with industry. This can be accomplished by developing clear guidelines for what is acceptable to be included as part of the curriculum and what is not. Additionally, as recommended by the Association of American Medical Colleges,[144] medical schools must recognize and mandate that gifts, meals, and free samples are not appropriate and should be eliminated. Guidelines set by academic institutions can help faculty understand what is appropriate with regards to medical school education while outlining what is acceptable in terms of physician participation as consultants or clinical trial investigators. Finally, there needs to be open discussion regarding the concept of disclosure. Conflict of interest disclosure needs to become a process rather than the last slide of a presentation or a line in a syllabus. Mistrust flourishes in the unknown and so we need to be clear and open so that students, when presented with material which contains disclosures, can learn how to process the information.

As a profession, we must continue to recognize those specific situations in which the influence of industry is harmful to medical education. As the relationship between pharmaceuticals companies and academic institution changes, we will need to re-evaluate and maintain open forums for discussion. This will allow us to keep our institutions unbiased so that a person in a teaching position does not need to offer a disclaimer. Because when he does, what is really being disclaimed is the trust which is vital to this great profession.

Shanu Kohli Kurd
Medical Student, Jefferson Medical College

A Faculty Perspective[145]

Medical school faculty have the daunting task of fostering the knowledge, attitudes, and skills that students under their tutelage will need to become physicians. The medical school faculty's job is to teach, the students', to learn. There exists an unspoken bond of trust between the students and faculty that to the best of the faculty members' ability they will teach those "truths" of knowledge and experience, that will help the students to best care for their patients.

A conflict of interest is "a set of conditions in which professional judgment concerning a primary interest tends to be unduly influenced by a secondary interest." In the case vignette, the astute student will call into question the "truths" purportedly spoken in the lecture on depression and anxiety treatments because the student has reason to be concerned that the faculty member's professional judgment has been affected by a secondary interest, namely, the faculty member's consulting relationship with the company that manufactures a drug discussed during the lecture.

Medical schools have developed mechanisms to manage faculty members' relationships with the pharmaceutical industry for the purpose of conducting clinical trials, including conflict of interest policies, institutional review boards, and patient informed consent. These mechanisms serve to protect the patients' welfare in the setting of a faculty member's potential conflict of interest. Additionally, many medical schools have adopted policies which significantly limit the potential influence of commercial entities on campus, such as prohibiting gifts and meals.

Given the inevitable interdependence between health care providers and the industries which test and sell health care products, at a minimum, it is necessary that medical schools address related issues, such as bias in research and conflict of interest, through the curriculum. Medical schools should also insist on transparency and disclosure to students of faculty's potential conflicts of interest. These approaches, while important, do not really address the primary issue raised in the vignette.

When students begin to doubt the motivations of the faculty and a breach in trust in the student–faculty relationship occurs, the medical school will have failed in an important component of the student's education. Medical school faculty have a duty to model the attributes of proper professional behavior. As altruism, or the demonstration that patient interest comes before self interest, is arguably one of the most important attributes of the professional behaviors expected of a physician, faculty should be advised to avoid not only real conflicts of interest, but the appearance of them as well.

Karen Novielli, M.D.
Professor of Family and Community Medicine
Senior Associate Dean, Faculty Affairs
Jefferson Medical College

MANAGING CONFLICTS OF INTEREST 2

During a small group discussion on the subject of conflict of interest, third year students were divided on the ethics of receiving lunches and gifts from pharmaceutical companies. Many students felt that there was nothing ethically wrong with this practice since they were unable to prescribe drugs. Also, many students appreciated the money saved on lunches.

A Medical Student Perspective

The onslaught of pharmaceutical lunches began in my sophomore year of college when I only thought how great it was these people gave me free food. I felt detached from the influence on patient care. This detachment was easily maintained through the beginning of medical school, but as I progressed,

I began to sense how this idea was flawed and that as a medical student, I do have a significant effect on patient care – I have an effect on their outlook, family perspectives, communication, occasionally treatment, and overall quality of care.[146–150] I realized that what is shaping me now will be what affects the future care of my patients. The bottom line is that, like any education, it is most effective for pharmaceutical companies to gain influence early in a physician's career. It is likely well worth a few sandwiches to pharmaceutical companies to create a favorable outlook for future medical students and beyond.[31]

So when does our education cover this issue? At my school, it is in our first year Physician and Society course, with the topic stuck somewhere between the discussion on abortion and how capitation works. Aside from an occasional lunch lecture (student group funded), the discussion is largely lost until we see how ubiquitous it is in the hospitals.[151]

This process seems inherently backwards to me: discussion (class) followed by observation (clinic). I emphasize observation because very often, as students, we feel powerless to question an attending physician on ethics – after all, they are grading us. I remember a recent conversation between three surgeons about a "great" vendor-sponsored dinner they had attended. I wanted to ask about their feelings in attending such an event regardless of the value to patients. I did not, however, pose this question as I was not comfortable questioning their morals. At the very same time, I remember thinking it must be terrific to be treated to a $100 meal. And herein lies the problem. During our training, often tacitly, students are made to feel entitled to these perks, gently having their egos massaged and being reassured that it is all for the good of the patient. And when it is not done to us directly, we see and hear it in conversations between our mentors: the physicians who train us on rotations.

I feel lucky to have had time to think about conflict of interest (COI) using good evidence, objectivity, and transparency before I am put in the position where this may seriously impact my patients' care. I hope that my future actions will be dictated by objectivity and good evidence. Indeed, maybe this is all any of us need to sort out the topic for ourselves: time to reflect and form our own opinions about what is best for our future patients.

Phil Barbosa
Medical Student, University of Minnesota School of Medicine

A Faculty Perspective

Conflict of interest has been a long-standing issue within medicine. In its most generic (and historically situated) form, COI is framed as a clash between commercialism and the image of the physician as a professional person. The Prayer of Maimonides, for example, exhorts physicians not to "allow thirst for profit, ambition, for renown and admiration, to interfere with my profession."

Our case study is of interest for several reasons. First, most medical students do not receive their principal instruction in COI issues within the formal curriculum. Instead, much of what students learn about COI (e.g., what is defined as a COI within medicine; what should one's response be when an issue arises) takes place within medicine's informal and hidden curriculums.

Second, while commercialization and the influence of "big pharma" are substantive issues, they are by no means the only COI issues. Other important topics are the integrity of research findings, hospital administration policies, efforts to control the cost of care, self-referral and physician ownership of hospitals, clinics, and labs, and publication (journal) policies.

Third, while discussions about free lunches and gifts are a necessary part of any professionalism curriculum, the most intimate and personal COI issue for medical students remains essentially unaddressed – and thus remains an invisible part of one's learning about COI. This is the conflict between the patient as a recipient of health care and the patient as a learning tool. How students/physicians learn, both formally and informally, to negotiate this tension (e.g., "When does patient safety and quality of care take precedence over my learning?") sets both the tone and the stage for how students/physicians respond to and define other COI issues. Because all this takes place largely on a tacit and unconscious level means that the lessons learned have an invisible and often insidious effect on student socialization.

The ubiquity of tacit learning around COI issues brings us to a fundamental conundrum. Although organized medicine is taking significant steps to curtail COI within medical schools and academic health centers (see below), and although research on COI clearly documents the biasing impact of industry funding and sponsorship on physician prescribing behavior and medical research findings, many physicians flatly reject the idea that their personal decision making can be dictated by outside influences. The typical rationale/response is: "Yes, COI is real – yes, my peers can be influenced – but not me."

This refusal to personalize the corrosive power of COI remains a major barrier to COI reform.[151,152]

The potential impact of several publications bear watching. Most recent (2008) are two reports, the first, a comprehensive set of recommendations [144] from the Association of American Medical Colleges (AAMC) on COI within educational settings, and the second a report from the Macy Foundation on continuing education in the health professions.[153] Both reports were preceded by another AAMC report[154] summarizing research on the interpersonal dynamics and psychological effects of social reciprocity. Other influential publications include the American Medical Student Association's (AMSA) second-generation report card on "U.S. medical schools' policies on pharmaceutical company access and influence" (eight schools received A while forty-seven received F)[155] and the widely cited policy proposal published in JAMA urging academic health centers to curtail COI.[156] Finally, laws have been passed at the state level (e.g., Minnesota, Vermont) requiring industry to report gifts/payment to physicians, while Congress is debating a similar statutory approach to transparency at the national level. All of this scrutiny is creating waves of discussion and discord within physician ranks.[157]

As for the case itself, believing that lunches and gifts are permissible because one is not yet able to prescribe is a rationalization unworthy of medical students – and their instructors. The fact that a group of highly educated individuals would unabashedly offer such tortured and "distancing" logic is testimony to the power and pernicious impact of medicine's informal and hidden curriculums and how distorted COI issues can become within these subterranean learning environments.

Frederic W. Hafferty, Ph.D.
Professor of Behavior Sciences
University of Minnesota School of Medicine – Duluth

COMMITMENT TO PROFESSIONAL RESPONSIBILITIES 1

After the anatomy final, a first year medical student returns to her college alma mater to attend a fraternity party. That night she is arrested for drunk driving and disorderly conduct. A mutual friend from college informs one of her medical school classmates about the incident, which is later confirmed by the classmate's review of the local paper's Daily Record. The medical school's policy states that all violations of the student conduct policy including misdemeanor arrests must be reported to the school.

A Medical Student Perspective

How would you feel about your child's pediatrician if he or she had been arrested for drunk driving and disorderly conduct? As future physicians, our reputation and character will be significant factors in building relationships with our patients.

For a medical student, this case raises several issues. The first relates to the importance of medical students acting professionally as they represent their schools and the profession. Roberts and Dyer[158] defined professionalism as "those attitudes and behaviors that serve to maintain patient interest above physician self-interest. Accordingly, professionalism ... aspires to altruism, accountability, excellence, duty, service, honor, integrity, and respect for others."

As medical students, we experience significant stress. Many students drink alcohol to cope with the stressors within and outside of medical school and some students experience deleterious consequences associated with its use. As medical students entering the profession of medicine, we must move beyond self-interest to accountability to the school, colleagues, the profession of medicine, and ultimately our patients. Therefore, we are accountable to a higher standard both inside and outside of the classroom. By doing this, we earn the respect of those we work with, including our patients.

The second professionalism issue entails the duty to address unprofessional behavior of medical school classmates by confronting the student or reporting the incident to the school. The American Medical Association *Code of Medical Ethics*[81] emphasizes the importance of safeguarding the health of patients by identifying and helping impaired physicians to return to optimal functioning. As professionals, medical students should also be accountable for confronting colleagues and superiors in any case of gross professional misconduct. Anonymous reporting opportunities within the medical school would certainly facilitate medical student reporting. This would also assure that impaired students get the help they need and eliminate any repercussions to the student reporting the problem.

The third professionalism issue relates to the institutional response toward the student exhibiting unprofessional behavior. In essence, this involves the perspective of the medical academic community and its obligation to address unprofessional conduct. Stern and Papadakis[46] emphasize the importance of immediate action by licensing boards against unprofessional behavior because "public safety and the public's trust of our profession are at stake." Medical schools overseeing the professional development of students should take the same position. Early intervention for student problems with professionalism is essential and may be helpful in decreasing future physician disciplinary action by medical boards.[159] Medical students behaving unprofessionally, such as the student in this case, must be identified and then given an opportunity to undergo counseling to address behavioral changes with the understanding that the next incident will result in dismissal.

In summary, as future physicians, we are held to an even higher standard by taking an oath to conduct ourselves with dignity and professionalism. It is incumbent on medical students to act responsibly and on medical schools to assist in our development of professionalism through an appropriate reporting structure and early intervention for students experiencing problems with professionalism.

Danielle Ku'ulei Potter
Medical Student, Creighton University School of Medicine

A Faculty Perspective

A 2006 study[160] found that 89 percent of medical students had used alcohol over the previous year. Whereas this rate is higher than in the general population or in those who are college educated,[161] at-risk and binge drinking among medical students is lower than age-matched peers.[7] The fact that alcohol and drug abuse are among the leading reasons for disciplinary action against physicians[162] makes it imperative for us to closely monitor our students' use and its consequences.

The student affairs dean would likely consider several issues regarding this case scenario. To begin, the classmate has been placed in a difficult predicament. She can protect the student from untoward consequences by saying nothing or adhere to her professional responsibilities to the school and ultimately the profession by reporting this incident to the administration. As students matriculate into medical school and enter the profession of medicine, many take an oath during a white coat ceremony that stresses professionalism. Key components of professionalism include self-regulation and accountability for actions, both of which enhance a commitment to professional responsibilities, engender patient trust, and assure patient well-being. With this in mind, students should not only be encouraged to discuss professionalism issues directly with their classmates, but also to report incidents that violate school policy. In this case, self-reporting of the arrest would likely result in a referral for a substance abuse/dependency assessment and possibly treatment with monitoring thereafter, which could benefit the student and prevent future problems. Far more negative consequences would likely be associated with the school's independent discovery of the arrest.

In order to foster accountability for actions and professionalism, it is incumbent upon student affairs administrators to create a reporting structure and environment perceived as safe by students. Schools should have an effective mechanism in place that provides a supportive and confidential manner for handling student conduct problems. These policies should not only be clearly advertised, but they should also provide maximum opportunities for rehabilitation and treatment as they minimize potentially career-threatening consequences, for example, notation on the Medical Student Performance Evaluation (a.k.a. Dean's Letter). In doing so, students will be more willing to self-report or to report concerns about classmates.

Finally, professionalism, like any other behavior, may be learned through coursework and the hidden curriculum. Professionalism must be thought of as a skill set that may be specifically taught within the medical school curricula. Training should take into account the many real-world ethical dilemmas, challenges, and stressors that our students are likely to encounter when deciding to take action. Educators and administrators must also model professionalism in interactions with students, colleagues, and patients.[163] In addition, schools must support substance abuse prevention programs along with activities and wellness-oriented functions that are alcohol free or stress the appropriate use of alcohol. In the end, students with proper training, a supportive environment, and exposure to role models who exhibit professionalism will not only be more committed to acting professionally, but will also be more likely to work effectively through difficult professionalism dilemmas.

Michael G. Kavan, M.D.
Associate Dean for Student Affairs
Professor of Family Medicine
Creighton University School of Medicine

COMMITMENT TO PROFESSIONAL RESPONSIBILITIES 2

A third year student, on his surgical clerkship, sees a newly hospitalized patient with his resident. The patient had a history of inflammatory bowel disease and is now admitted with increased pain and diarrhea. The student observes the resident as he completes a cursory history and exam and then presents findings to the attending, many of which have been fabricated.

For a video of the vignette, see http://professionalism.jefferson.edu/.

A Medical Student Perspective

Grades, respect of peers and residents, a future in surgery; all seem at risk by simply considering the consequences of reporting the incident. Fortunately, I am yet to face this dilemma in real life, but each year up to 75 percent of graduating students state they have personally witnessed medical errors.[164] Disappointingly, but not surprisingly, fewer than half of these errors are reported.

From the reading of the Hippocratic Oath on the first day of class, students understand professionalism: competently caring for patients, maintaining accountability, humility, and an altruistic attitude all while respecting collegial relationships and the academic atmosphere.[165]

The student role in the hospital, though, is often ill defined.[166] Not quite a doctor but more than a passive observer, contributions are difficult to measure. SOAP (subject, objective, assessment, and plan) notes are often discarded, presentations ignored, and attempts to "help" frequently seem burdensome. Is it your role to be an active patient advocate? Do the same rules of professionalism govern students, residents, and attendings?

Society, as Arnold points out, tends to frown at whistle-blowers.[167] In general, remaining quiet is preferred to questioning a peer. Formal, anonymous methods of incident reporting exist, but are often written off as too severe a penalty, leaving simple avoidance as the most commonly chosen alternative.

From a selfish point of view, avoidance is easily justified. Third year students lack confidence in their knowledge and place supreme importance on grades and evaluations. With minimal stress, it is easy to assume the patient will be cared for properly. But what if they aren't?

As students, we strive to embody the ideals of medicine. We are eager to show empathy, professional ethicality, and maintain an absolute desire to help others.[167] Every missed opportunity for professional behavior, though, serves as justification to repeat the infringement in the future. Doing the right thing is always difficult but is part of what defines professionalism, and if approached appropriately, can maintain our ideals while limiting adverse consequences.

Personally, I am best suited to a subtle approach. I would avoid confronting the resident in the presence of others, as embarrassment and lost trust can irreparably damage relationships and opinions. As students, we follow a fraction of the patients covered by house staff, providing ample opportunity to complete the history and physical and discern the patient's true issues. Briefly presenting all new and pertinent findings to the resident will draw attention to previous misrepresentations. Further, I would take advantage of my status as a student to ask the resident to repeat and teach troubling parts of the patient's exam and history.

These cautious approaches provide the opportunity to correct mistakes without blatantly challenging the resident. I believe most mistakes are products of fatigue and stress rather than true shortcomings in ethical fiber. A tired resident will always appreciate help in averting disaster, and in the end the patient will receive appropriate care.

In the rare case of an unresponsive resident, buckle your seat belt and stick to your professional values. The character of all involved will be exposed and everyone will be better for it.

Chris Yingling
Medical Student, Jefferson Medical College

A Faculty Perspective

On one level, the responsibility of the student is simple. As a member of the health care team, he or she is morally obliged to make certain that accurate information is passed among team members to ensure optimal care of the patient. If we wish to incorporate the aviation concept of crew resource management into medical practice, then any member of the health care team, no matter how junior, should feel free to speak up and note an incorrect piece of data that is being shared.

However, the scenario portrayed here is not the simple matter of a single test result being mistakenly recounted by a busy resident. Nor is it an example of "roundsmanship" where the resident smoothly throws out a ballpark number – "the potassium was 4.3" when the result was actually 4.1 – in order to give the appearance of total control of their service. The latter is a somewhat less egregious, although still not completely innocent, behavior.

Rather, this resident is engaged in a behavior which is, at the very least, unethical, and is, very likely, potentially dangerous for the patient. A missed element of the history of present illness, of past history, or of a pertinent physical finding, could lead to a very real error in diagnosis or a delay in care. It is also likely that this episode does not represent just a one-time misstep. A resident who glibly fabricates false information has probably done so many times before.

I believe that it is a lot to ask of a student to try and to remediate this problem on his or her own and I am not confident that the efforts described by the student in the commentary above would be successful. Although an adept student may be able to artfully work the true details (or lack thereof) during the rounding session with the resident and attending, the underlying behavior of the problem resident has not been addressed. Furthermore, it is unlikely that a junior student would be able to discuss this problem meaningfully with the resident after the event occurred. The well-established medical hierarchy almost certainly ensures that counseling efforts will not be accepted or viewed constructively when directed up the chain of command.

Therefore, the student is placed in the very uncomfortable position of acting as a whistle-blower. He or she must bring the problem to the attention of a superior, at the risk of jeopardizing that resident's job or professional standing in the program. Not understanding how a residency program or, indeed, how the entire medical profession, deals with ethical problems such as these, adds to the student's unease in this situation. Further, the student may believe that by being a "snitch" they are jeopardizing their own standing within the department, with a resulting negative impact on his or her own career.

My recommendation for the student in this case is to immediately bring this episode to the attention of the clerkship or program director. Trying to directly report the misbehavior to the particular attending could, depending on that attending, lead to a less than ideal handling of the situation. Rather, the clerkship director or program director should hear the student's concerns. Then, in collaboration with the patient's attending, a re-interview and examination of the patient can elicit what was or wasn't performed by the resident. Directed questions such as "And when the resident asked you about . . . " or "When the resident performed the rectal examination . . . " will quickly expose the fabrications of the resident. The problem can then be addressed directly by the attending or the program director, without exposing the student to undue retribution or recriminations by the resident, or by others in the program. The behavior of the problem resident can then be closely reviewed and, hopefully, appropriate remediation may be achieved.

We must educate our clerkship directors and prepare them to handle these ethical dilemmas. We must also let our students know that they have a safe pathway through which they can share their concerns and encourage them to make the morally correct choices. By working together, we can develop the just culture that will allow medicine to provide safe and ethically sound care for all patients.

John C. Kairys, M.D., FACS
Assistant Dean for Graduate Medical Education and Affiliations
Vice Chairman for Education, Department of Surgery
Jefferson Medical College

REFERENCES

1. Rosenthal JM, Okie S. White coat, mood indigo – depression in medical school. *N Engl J Med.* 2005;**353**(11):1085–1088.

2. Swinker ML. Should doctors call in sick? *Am Fam Physician.* 2004;**69**(1):219–20, 223.

3. Kim JJ, Diamond DM. The stressed hippocampus, synaptic plasticity and lost memories. *Nat Rev Neurosci.* 2002;**3**(6):453–462.

4. Miller NM, McGowen RK. The painful truth: Physicians are not invincible. *South Med J.* 2000;**93**(10):966–973.

5. Vander A, Sherman J, Luciano D. Defense mechanisms of the body. In: *Human Physiology: The Mechanisms of Body Function.* New York: McGraw-Hill; 2001:729–731.

6. Special Report: Discouraged Doctors. http://www.acpe.org/education/surveys/Morale/morale.htm. Accessed May 6, 2007.

7. Dyrbye LN, Thomas MR, Huntington JL, et al. Personal life events and medical student burnout: A multicenter study. *Acad Med.* 2006;**81**(4):374–384.

8. Roberts LW, Warner TD, Carter D, Frank E, Ganzini L, Lyketsos C. Caring for medical students as patients: Access to services and care-seeking practices of 1,027 students at nine medical schools. Collaborative research group on medical student healthcare. *Acad Med.* 2000;**75**(3):272–277.

9. Hilgenberg S. Transformation: From medical student to patient. *Ann Intern Med.* 2006;**144**(10):779–780.

10. Dyrbye LN, Thomas MR, Shanafelt TD. Medical student distress: Causes, consequences, and proposed solutions. *Mayo Clin Proc.* 2005;**80**(12):1613–1622.

11. Christakis DA, Feudtner C. Ethics in a short white coat: The ethical dilemmas that medical students confront. *Acad Med.* 1993;**68**(4):249–254.

12. Caldicott CV, Faber-Langendoen K. Deception, discrimination, and fear of reprisal: Lessons in ethics from third-year medical students. *Acad Med.* 2005;**80**(9):866–873.

13. Halbach MM, Spann CO, Egan G. Effect of sleep deprivation on medical resident and student cognitive function: A prospective study. *Am J Obstet Gynecol.* 2003;**188**(5):1198–1201.

14. Barger LK, Cade BE, Ayas NT, et al. Extended work shifts and the risk of motor vehicle crashes among interns. *N Engl J Med.* 2005;**352**(2):125–134.

15. Dyrbye LN, Thomas MR, Shanafelt TD. Systematic review of depression, anxiety, and other indicators of psychological distress among U.S. and Canadian medical students. *Acad Med.* 2006;**81**(4):354–373.

16. Mountain SA, Quon BS, Dodek P, Sharpe R, Ayas NT. The impact of housestaff fatigue on occupational and patient safety. *Lung.* 2007;**185**(4):203–209.

17. Myers JS, Bellini LM, Morris JB, et al. Internal medicine and general surgery residents' attitudes about the ACGME duty hours regulations: A multicenter study. *Acad Med.* 2006;**81**(12):1052–1058.

18. Arora VM, Seiden SC, Higa JT, Siddique J, Meltzer DO, Humphrey HJ. Effect of student duty hours policy on teaching and satisfaction of 3rd year medical students. *Am J Med.* 2006;**119**(12):1089–1095.

19. Nixon LJ, Benson BJ, Rogers TB, Sick BT, Miller WJ. Effects of accreditation council for graduate medical education work hour restrictions on medical student experience. *J Gen Intern Med.* 2007;**22**(7):937–941.

20. Zahn CM, Dunlow SG, Alvero R, Parker JD, Nace C, Armstrong AY. Too little time to teach? Medical student education and the resident work-hour restriction. *Mil Med.* 2007;**172**(10):1053–1057.

21. White CB, Haftel HM, Purkiss JA, Schigelone AS, Hammoud MM. Multidimensional effects of the 80-hour work week at the University of Michigan Medical School. *Acad Med.* 2006;**81**(1):57–62.

22. Van Eaton EG, Horvath KD, Pellegrini CA. Professionalism and the shift mentality: How to reconcile patient ownership with limited work hours. *Arch Surg.* 2005;**140**(3):230–235.

23. Bernat JL, Peterson LM. Patient-centered informed consent in surgical practice. *Arch Surg.* 2006;**141**(1):86–92.

24. Ubel PA, Silver-Isenstadt A. Are patients willing to participate in medical education? *J Clin Ethics.* 2000;**11**(3):230–235.

25. Council on Ethical and Judicial Affairs. Opinion E-8.087, medical student involvement in patient care. In: *Code of Medical Ethics of the American Medical Association: Current Opinions with Annotations.* 2006–2007 ed. Chicago: AMA Press; 2006.

26. Pelligrino ED. Medical education. In: Reich WT, ed. *Encyclopdia of Bioethics.* New York: Macmillan Library Reference; 1995.

27. Dwyer J. Primum non tacere. An ethics of speaking up. *Hastings Cent Rep.* 1994;**24**(1):13–18.

28. American College of Surgeons Statements on Principles. http://www.facs.org/fellows_info/statements/stonprin.html#anchor172771. Accessed September 14, 2007.

29. Frank SH, Stange KC, Langa D, Workings M. Direct observation of community-based ambulatory encounters involving medical students. *JAMA.* 1997;**278**(9): 712–716.

30. Richardson PH, Curzen P, Fonagy P. Patients' attitudes to student doctors. *Med Educ.* 1986;**20**(4):314–317.

31. York NL, DaRosa DA, Markwell SJ, Niehaus AH, Folse R. Patients' attitudes toward the involvement of medical students in their care. *Am J Surg.* 1995; **169**(4):421–423.

32. Dodson JA, Keller AS. Medical student care of indigent populations. *JAMA.* 2004;**291**(1):121.

33. The ACGME General Competencies, as contained in the ACGME Common Program Requirements. http://www.acgme.org/outcome/comp/GeneralCompetencies Standards21307.pdf. Accessed December 4, 2008.

34. LCME Standard ER-8. Liaison Committee on Medical Education Web site. http://www.lcme.org/functionslist.htm#structure. Accessed December 4, 2008.

35. Hill LD, Madara JL. Role of the urban academic medical center in US health care. *JAMA.* 2005;**294**(17):2219–2220.

36. Tolkoff M. Exclusive earnings survey: How are you doing? *Med Econ.* 2006; **83**(20):74–6, 78–80, 82–3.

37. Dorsey ER, Jarjoura D, Rutecki GW. Influence of controllable lifestyle on recent trends in specialty choice by US medical students. *JAMA.* 2003;**290**(9): 1173–1178.

38. 2003 Report of the American Medical Association Medical student Section Task Force on Medical Student Debt. http://www.ama-assn.org/ama/pub/category/ 5349.html. Accessed October 15, 2007.

39. Lowes R. The earnings freeze: Now it's everybody's problem. *Med Econ.* 2005;**82**(18):58–62, 64, 66–8.

40. ABIM Foundation. American Board of Internal Medicine, ACP-ASIM Foundation. American College of Physicians-American Society of Internal Medicine, European Federation of Internal Medicine. Medical professionalism in the new millennium: A physician charter. *Ann Intern Med.* 2002;**136**(3):243–246.

41. Ernst RL, Yett DE. *Physician Location and Specialty Choice.* Ann Arbor, Michigan: Health Administration Press; 1985.

42. Funkenstein DH. *Medical Students, Medical Schools and Society during Five Eras: Factors Affecting the Career Choices of Physicians, 1958–1976.* Cambridge, Massachusetts: Ballinger; 1978.

43. American Association of Medical Colleges. AAMC MEDLOANS Program: Educational Debt Manager. http://www.aamc.org/programs/medloans/ debtmanager.pdf. Accessed October 15, 2007.

44. Hughes RL, Golmon ME, Patterson R. The grading system as a factor in the selection of residents. *J Med Educ.* 1983;**58**(6):479–481.

45. Magarian GJ, Mazur DJ. A national survey of grading systems used in medicine clerkships. *Acad Med.* 1990;**65**(10):636–639.

46. Stern DT, Papadakis M. The developing physician – becoming a professional. *N Engl J Med.* 2006;**355**(17):1794–1799.

47. Haidet P, Dains JE, Paterniti DA, et al. Medical student attitudes toward the doctor-patient relationship. *Med Educ.* 2002;**36**(6):568–574.

48. Macfarlane J, Holmes W, Macfarlane R, Britten N. Influence of patients' expectations on antibiotic management of acute lower respiratory tract illness in general practice: Questionnaire study. *BMJ.* 1997;**315**(7117):1211–1214.

49. Harris RH, MacKenzie TD, Leeman-Castillo B, et al. Optimizing antibiotic prescribing for acute respiratory tract infections in an urban urgent care clinic. *J Gen Intern Med.* 2003;**18**(5):326–334.

50. Webb S, Lloyd M. Prescribing and referral in general practice: A study of patients' expectations and doctors' actions. *Br J Gen Pract.* 1994;**44**(381):165–169.

51. Gonzales R, Bartlett JG, Besser RE, et al. Principles of appropriate antibiotic use for treatment of acute respiratory tract infections in adults: Background, specific aims, and methods. *Ann Intern Med.* 2001;**134**(6):479–486.

52. Scott JG, Cohen D, DiCicco-Bloom B, Orzano AJ, Jaen CR, Crabtree BF. Antibiotic use in acute respiratory infections and the ways patients pressure physicians for a prescription. *J Fam Pract.* 2001;**50**(10):853–858.

53. Mostov PD. Treating the immunocompetent patient who presents with an upper respiratory infection: Pharyngitis, sinusitis, and bronchitis. *Prim Care.* 2007;**34**(1):39–58.

54. Avorn J, Solomon DH. Cultural and economic factors that (mis)shape antibiotic use: The nonpharmacologic basis of therapeutics. *Ann Intern Med.* 2000; **133**(2):128–135.

55. Snow V, Mottur-Pilson C, Gonzales R. Principles of antibiotic use for treatment of nonspecific upper respiratory tract infections in adults. *Ann Intern Med.* 2001;**134**(6):487–9.

56. Botkin JR. Informed consent for lumbar puncture. *Am J Dis Child.* 1989; **143**(8):899–904.

57. Feudtner C, Christakis DA. Making the rounds. the ethical development of medical students in the context of clinical rotations. *Hastings Cent Rep.*1994; **24**(1):6–12.

58. Feudtner C, Christakis DA, Christakis NA. Do clinical clerks suffer ethical erosion? students' perceptions of their ethical environment and personal development. *Acad Med.* 1994;**69**(8):670–679.

59. Gamulka BD. The need for true informed consent in pediatric teaching hospitals. *Acad Med.* 1998;**73**(6):628–629.

60. Gordon HH. Advice to medical students preparing for clinical clerkships. *Pharos Alpha Omega Alpha Honor Med Soc.* 1979;**42**(2):9–16.

61. Wendler DS, Shah S. How can medical training and informed consent be reconciled with volume-outcome data? *J Clin Ethics.* 2006;**17**(2):149–157.

62. Williams CT, Fost N. Ethical considerations surrounding first time procedures: A study and analysis of patient attitudes toward spinal taps by students. *Kennedy Inst Ethics J.* 1992;**2**(3):217–231.

63. ACOG Committee on Practice Bulletins. ACOG practice bulletin no. 74. Antibiotic prophylaxis for gynecologic procedures. *Obstet Gynecol.* 2006;**108**(1):225–234.

64. Rice B. 10 ways to guarantee a lawsuit. *Med Econ.* 2005;**82**(13):66–69.

65. Foundation of Research and Education of AHIMA. Update: Maintaining a legally sound health record – paper and electronic. *J AHIMA.* 2005;**76**(10):64A–64L.

66. Kern SI. Malpractice consult. Alter the records? Bad idea. *Med Econ.* 2007; **84**(10):26.

67. Wu AW. Handling hospital errors: Is disclosure the best defense? *Ann Intern Med.* 1999;**131**(12):970–972.

68. Leape LL. Statement before United States Senate subcommittee on labor, health and human services, and education. 2000.

69. Leape LL, Woods DD, Hatlie MJ, Kizer KW, Schroeder SA, Lundberg GD. Promoting patient safety by preventing medical error. *JAMA.* 1998;**280**(16): 1444–1447.

70. Bernard L. *Resolving Ethical Dilemmas: A Guide for Clinicians.* 3rd ed. Baltimore: Lippincott, Williams, and Wilkins; 2005.

71. Cushman R. Privacy / Data Protection Project. http://privacy.med.miami.edu/. Accessed July 9, 2008.

72. Jonsen AR. Do no harm. *Ann Intern Med.* 1978;**88**(6):827–832.

73. La Puma J, Stocking CB, La Voie D, Darling CA. When physicians treat members of their own families: Practices in a community hospital. *N Engl J Med.* 1991;**325**(18):1290–1294.

74. La Puma J, Priest ER. Is there a doctor in the house? An analysis of the practice of physicians' treating their own families. *JAMA*. 1992;**267**(13):1810–1812.

75. Dusdieker LB, Murph JR, Murph WE, Dungy CI. Physicians treating their own children. *Am J Dis Child*. 1993;**147**(2):146–149.

76. Mailhot M. Caring for our own families. *Can Fam Physician*. 2002;**48**:546–7, 550–2.

77. Van Spall HG. When my father died. *Ann Intern Med*. 2007;**146**(12):893–894.

78. Carroll R, Tulsky J, Shuchman M, Snyder L. Should doctors treat their relatives? *ACP Observer*. 1999.

79. Oberheu K, Jones JW, Sade RM. A surgeon operates on his son: Wisdom or hubris? *Ann Thorac Surg*. 2007;**84**(3):723–728.

80. Rolnick SJ, Altschuler A, Nekhlyudov L, et al. What women wish they knew before prophylactic mastectomy. *Cancer Nurs*. 2007;**30**(4):285–9.

81. American Medical Association. *Code of Medical Ethics of the American Medical Association: Current Opinions and Annotations. 2006–2007* ed. American Medical Association; 2006.

82. Chen FM, Feudtner C, Rhodes LA, Green LA. Role conflicts of physicians and their family members: Rules but no rulebook. *West J Med*. 2001;**175**(4):236–9; discussion 240.

83. Hardimon MO. Role obligations. *The Journal of Philosophy*. 1994;**91**(7): 333–363.

84. van Dijk S, Otten W, Zoeteweij MW, et al. Genetic counselling and the intention to undergo prophylactic mastectomy: Effects of a breast cancer risk assessment. *Br J Cancer*. 2003;**88**(11):1675–1681.

85. Redelmeier DA, Rozin P, Kahneman D. Understanding patients' decisions. Cognitive and emotional perspectives. *JAMA*. 1993;**270**(1):72–76.

86. Ubel PA. Is information always a good thing? Helping patients make "good" decisions. *Med Care*. 2002;**40**(9 Suppl):V39–44.

87. Snyder L, Leffler C, Ethics and Human Rights Committee, American College of Physicians. Ethics manual: Fifth edition. *Ann Intern Med*. 2005;**142**(7):560–582.

88. Snow M, White GL, Alder SC, Stanford JB. Mentor's hand hygiene practices influence student's hand hygiene rates. *Am J Infect Control*. 2006;**34**:18–24.

89. Watanakunakorn C, Wang C, Hazy J. An observational study of hand washing and infection control practices by healthcare workers. *Infect Control Hosp Epidemiol*. 1998;**19**(11):858–860.

90. Pittet D. Improving compliance with hand hygiene in hospitals. *Infect Control Hosp Epidemiol*. 2000;**21**(6):381–386.

91. Pittet D, Simon A, Hugonnet S, Pessoa-Silva CL, Sauvan V, Perneger TV. Hand hygiene among physicians: Performance, beliefs, and perceptions. *Ann Intern Med*. 2004;**141**(1):1–8.

92. Seto WH, Ching PT, Fung JP, Fielding R. The role of communication in the alteration of patient-care practices in hospital – a prospective study. *J Hosp Infect*. 1989;**14**(1):29–37.

93. Gottschalk A, Flocke SA. Time spent in face-to-face patient care and work outside the examination room. *Ann Fam Med*. 2005;**3**(6):488–493.

94. Hersey P. *The Situational Leader*. Escondido, CA: Center for Leadership Studies; 1984.

95. Vukanovic-Criley JM, Criley S, Warde CM, et al. Competency in cardiac examination skills in medical students, trainees, physicians, and faculty: A multicenter study. *Arch Intern Med*. 2006;**166**(6):610–616.

96. Gould BE, Grey MR, Huntington CG, et al. Improving patient care outcomes by teaching quality improvement to medical students in community-based practices. *Acad Med*. 2002;**77**(10):1011–1018.

97. Hicks LK, Lin Y, Robertson DW, Robinson DL, Woodrow SI. Understanding the clinical dilemmas that shape medical students' ethical development: Questionnaire survey and focus group study. *BMJ*. 2001;**322**(7288):709–710.

98. Baker DP, Salas E, King H, Battles J, Barach P. The role of teamwork in the professional education of physicians: Current status and assessment recommendations. *Jt Comm J Qual Patient Saf*. 2005;**31**(4):185–202.

99. Heins A, Keehn C. Financial crisis for medical students and residents. *Ann Emerg Med*. 2003;**41**(5):733–735.

100. Pasnau RO, Stoessel P. Mental health service for medical students. *Med Educ*. 1994;**28**(1):33–9; discussion 55–7.

101. Ross S, Cleland J, Macleod MJ. Stress, debt and undergraduate medical student performance. *Med Educ*. 2006;**40**(6):584–589.

102. Roberts LW, Hardee JT, Franchini G, Stidley CA, Siegler M. Medical students as patients: A pilot study of their health care needs, practices, and concerns. *Acad Med*. 1996;**71**(11):1225–1232.

103. Dyrbye LN, Thomas MR, Massie FS, et al. Burnout and suicidal ideation among U.S. medical students. *Ann Intern Med*. 2008;**149**(5):334–341.

104. Chua K. Overview of the U.S. *Health Care System*. http://www.amsa.org/uhc/HealthCareSystemOverview.pdf. Updated February 10, 2006. Accessed July 21, 2008.

105. Cunningham PJ, May JH. Medicaid Patients Increasingly Concentrated among Physicians. Tracking Report No. 16. http://www.hschange.com/CONTENT/866/. Accessed June 24, 2008.

106. Simpson SA, Long JA. Medical student-run health clinics: Important contributors to patient care and medical education. *J Gen Intern Med*. 2007;**22**(3):352–356.

107. Gruen RL, Pearson SD, Brennan TA. Physician-citizens – public roles and professional obligations. *JAMA*. 2004;**291**(1):94–98.

108. Ha TT, Ginsburg PB. Losing ground: Physician income. Tracking Report/Center for Studying Health System Change, June 2006.

109. Plumb JD, McManus P, Carson L. A collaborative community approach to homeless care. *Prim Care*. 1996;**23**(1):17–30.

110. Plumb JD. Homelessness: Care, prevention, and public policy. *Ann Intern Med*. 1997;**126**(12):973–975.

111. Hibbs JR, Benner L, Klugman L, et al. Mortality in a cohort of homeless adults in Philadelphia. *N Engl J Med*. 1994;**331**(5):304–309.

112. Davidson SM. Physician participation in medicaid: Background and issues. *J Health Polit Policy Law*. 1982;**6**(4):703–717.

113. Backus L, Osmond D, Grumbach K, Vranizan K, Phuong L, Bindman AB. Specialists' and primary care physicians' participation in Medicaid managed care. *J Gen Intern Med.* 2001;**16**(12):815–821.

114. Rowland D, Salganicoff A. Commentary: Lessons from Medicaid – improving access to office-based physician care for the low-income population. *Am J Public Health.* 1994;**84**(4):550–552.

115. Bailey JE, Van Brunt DL, Mirvis DM, et al. Academic managed care organizations and adverse selection under Medicaid managed care in Tennessee. *JAMA.* 1999;**282**(11):1067–1072.

116. Viewpoint: Educating for Professionalism in Medicine. AAMC Web site. http://www.aamc.org/newsroom/reporter/sept03/viewpoint.htm. Accessed August 11, 2007.

117. Sandy LG, Schroeder SA. Primary care in a new era: Disillusion and dissolution? *Ann Intern Med.* 2003;**138**(3):262–267.

118. De Ville K. Act first and look up the law afterward?: Medical malpractice and the ethics of defensive medicine. *Theor Med Bioeth.* 1998;**19**(6):569–589.

119. Brownell AK, Cote L. Senior residents' views on the meaning of professionalism and how they learn about it. *Acad Med.* 2001;**76**(7):734–737.

120. Dunnick NR, Applegate KE, Arenson RL. The inappropriate use of imaging studies: A report of the 2004 intersociety conference. *J Am Coll Radiol.* 2005;**2**(5):401–406.

121. Lee CC, Golub R, Singer AJ, Cantu R, Jr, Levinson H. Routine versus selective abdominal computed tomography scan in the evaluation of right lower quadrant pain: A randomized controlled trial. *Acad Emerg Med.* 2007;**14**(2): 117–122.

122. Studdert DM, Mello MM, Sage WM, et al. Defensive medicine among high-risk specialist physicians in a volatile malpractice environment. *JAMA.* 2005; **293**(21):2609–2617.

123. Kessler DP, Summerton N, Graham JR. Effects of the medical liability system in Australia, the UK, and the USA. *Lancet.* 2006;**368**(9531):240–246.

124. Hiyama T, Yoshihara M, Tanaka S, et al. Defensive medicine practices among gastroenterologists in Japan. *World J Gastroenterol.* 2006;**12**(47):7671–7675.

125. Wennberg JE, Fisher ES, Goodman DC, Skinner JS. Tracking the care of patients with severe chronic illness. *The Dartmouth Atlas of Health Care 2008 Web site.* http://www.dartmouthatlas.org/atlases/2008_Atlas_Exec_Summ.pdf. Accessed May 31, 2008.

126. Barnato AE, Herndon MB, Anthony DL, et al. Are regional variations in end-of-life care intensity explained by patient preferences?: A study of the US Medicare population. *Med Care.* 2007;**45**(5):386–393.

127. Lilly CM, De Meo DL, Sonna LA, et al. An intensive communication intervention for the critically ill. *Am J Med.* 2000;**109**(6):469–475.

128. Fair allocation of intensive care unit resources. American Thoracic Society. *Am J Respir Crit Care Med.* 1997;**156**(4 Pt 1):1282–1301.

129. DNR in the OR and Afterwards. AHRQ Web M&M Web site. www.webmm.ahrq.gov/case.aspx?caseID=135. Accessed November 16, 2008.

130. ATS Bioethics Task Force. Witholding and withdrawing life-sustaining therapy. *Ann Int Med.* 1992;**115**:478–485.

131. Curtis JR. Communicating about end-of-life care with patients and families in the intensive care unit. *Crit Care Clin.* 2004;**20**(3):363–80, viii.

132. Molter NC. Needs of relatives of critically ill patients: A descriptive study. *Heart Lung.* 1979;**8**:332–339.

133. Lautrette A, Darmon M, Megarbane B, et al. A communication strategy and brochure for relatives of patients dying in the ICU. *N Engl J Med.* 2007; **356**(5):469–478.

134. Health Care: U.S. Preventive Services Task Force (USPSTF) Subdirectory Page. http://www.ahrq.gov/clinic/uspstfix.htm. Accessed 7/21/2008, 2008.

135. Slowther A, Ford S, Schofield T. Ethics of evidence based medicine in the primary care setting. *J Med Ethics.* 2004;**30**(2):151–155.

136. Reinertsen JL. Zen and the art of physician autonomy maintenance. *Ann Intern Med.* 2003;**138**(12):992–995.

137. Ewart RM. Primum non nocere and the quality of evidence: Rethinking the ethics of screening. *J Am Board Fam Pract.* 2000;**13**(3):188–196.

138. Doukas DJ, Fetters M, Ruffin MT, 4th, McCullough LB. Ethical considerations in the provision of controversial screening tests. *Arch Fam Med.* 1997; **6**(5):486–490.

139. Barnes PM, Powell-Griner E, McFann K, Nahin RL. *Complementary and alternative medicine use among adults: United States*, 2002. advance data, no. 343.

140. Rogers G. Herb consumers' attitudes, preferences profiled in new market study. *HerbalGram.* 2005;**65**:60–61.

141. Blendon RJ, DesRoches CM, Benson JM, Brodie M, Altman DE. Americans' views on the use and regulation of dietary supplements. *Arch Intern Med.* 2001;**161**(6):805–810.

142. Rakel D, Weil A. Philosophy of integrative medicine. In: Rakel D, ed. *Integrative Medicine.* 2nd ed. Elsevier: Philadelphia, PA; 2007.

143. *BMJ Clinical Evidence Handbook.* London: BMJ Publishing Group; 2007.

144. *Report of the AAMC Task Force on Industry Funding of Medical Education to the the AAMC Executive Council.* Washington, D.C.: Association of American Medical Colleges; 2008.

145. Watson PY, Khandelwal AK, Musial JL, Buckley JD. Resident and faculty perceptions of conflict of interest in medical education. *J Gen Intern Med.* 2005; **20**(4):357–359.

146. Swenson SL, Rothstein JA. Navigating the wards: Teaching medical students to use their moral compasses. *Acad Med.* 1996;**71**(6):591–594.

147. Wolfe SM. The destruction of medicine by market forces: Teaching acquiescence or resistance and change? *Acad Med.* 2002;**77**(1):5–7.

148. Lemmens T, Singer PA. Bioethics for clinicians: 17. Conflict of interest in research, education and patient care. *CMAJ.* 1998;**159**(8):960–965.

149. Coleman DL, Kazdin AE, Miller LA, Morrow JS, Udelsman R. Guidelines for interactions between clinical faculty and the pharmaceutical industry: One medical school's approach. *Acad Med.* 2006;**81**(2):154–160.

150. Schneider JA, Arora V, Kasza K, Van Harrison R, Humphrey H. Residents' perceptions over time of pharmaceutical industry interactions and gifts and the effect of an educational intervention. *Acad Med.* 2006;**81**(7):595–602.

151. Campbell EG, Gruen RL, Mountford J, Miller LG, Cleary PD, Blumenthal D. A national survey of physician–industry relationships. *N Engl J Med.* 2007;**356**(17):1742–1750.

152. Chimonas S, Brennan TA, Rothman DJ. Physicians and drug representatives: Exploring the dynamics of the relationship. *J Gen Intern Med.* 2007;**22**(2):184–190.

153. Harger M, Russell S, Fletcher SW. *Continuing Education in the Health Professions: Improving Healthcare through Lifelong Learning.* New York: Josiah Macy Jr. Foundation.

154. Association of American Medical Colleges. The scientific basis of influence and reciprocity: A symposium. 2007.

155. American Medical Student Association. *AMSA's 2007 PharmFree Scorecard.* Washington, D.C.: American Medical Student Association; 2007.

156. Brennan TA, Rothman DJ, Blank L, et al. Health industry practices that create conflicts of interest: A policy proposal for academic medical centers. *JAMA.* 2006;**295**(4):429–433.

157. Harris G, Roberts J. Doctors' ties to drug makers are put on close view. New York Times Web site. www.nytimes.com/2007/03/21/us/21drug.html. Updated 2007. Accessed July 29, 2008.

158. Roberts LW, Dyer AR. *A Concise Guide to Ethics in Mental Health Care.* Arlington, VA: American Psychiatric Publishing; 2004.

159. Papadakis MA, Teherani A, Banach MA, et al. Disciplinary action by medical boards and prior behavior in medical school. *N Engl J Med.* 2005;**353**(25):2673–2682.

160. Baldwin JN, Scott DM, Agrawal S, et al. Assessment of alcohol and other drug use behaviors in health professions students. *Subst Abus.* 2006;**27**(3):27–37.

161. Department of Health and Human Services, Substance Abuse and Mental Health Services Administration. *National Survey on Drug Use and Health: National Findings.* Department of Health and Human Services; 2006.

162. Holtman MC. Disciplinary careers of drug-impaired physicians. *Soc Sci Med.* 2007;**64**(3):543–553.

163. Goldstein EA, Maestas RR, Fryer-Edwards K, et al. Professionalism in medical education: An institutional challenge. *Acad Med.* 2006;**81**(10):871–876.

164. Madigosky WS, Headrick LA, Nelson K, Cox KR, Anderson T. Changing and sustaining medical students' knowledge, skills, and attitudes about patient safety and medical fallibility. *Acad Med.* 2006;**81**(1):94–101.

165. Chard D, Elsharkawy A, Newbery N. Medical professionalism: The trainees' views. *Clin Med.* 2006;**6**(1):68–71.

166. Park J, Woodrow SI, Reznick RK, Beales J, MacRae HM. Patient care is a collective responsibility: Perceptions of professional responsibility in surgery. *Surgery.* 2007;**142**(1):111–118.

167. Arnold L. Assessing professional behavior: Yesterday, today, and tomorrow. *Acad Med.* 2002;**77**(6):502–515.

PART THREE

Cases Involving Physicians

3 Principle of Primacy of Patient Welfare

Cases and Commentaries

PATIENT WELFARE – ADULT PRIMARY CARE

A family physician recommends that an eighty-two-year-old woman with a history of coronary disease take the non-steroidal anti-inflammatory (NSAID) drug celecoxib (Celebrex) for osteoarthritis. The physician chooses celecoxib over a non-Cox 2 inhibitor because of his concern about NSAID-induced gastropathy. Celecoxib requires prior authorization and the physician is aware that the insurance company only allows use of this drug when a patient has tried and is intolerant of other NSAIDs. The physician forwards a note to the insurance company indicating this to be the case, despite the fact that the patient has not tried other NSAIDs.

A Perspective from a General Internist

Clinical Background

Each year, the use of NSAIDs, including aspirin, accounts for a significant amount of gastrointestinal complications, mainly gastric ulcers and gastritis. These complications lead to an estimated 7,600 deaths and over 70,000 hospitalizations in the United States.[1] Factors listed in Table 3.1 have been shown to increase the risk of NSAID-induced gastropathy.

The average duration of NSAID use before the onset of GI symptoms is twelve weeks. The longer the duration of NSAID use, the higher the risk of gastropathy.

There is an approximate 1 percent absolute risk reduction for symptomatic ulcer disease when using celecoxib compared to other non-COX-2 inhibiting NSAIDs over a one-month duration. Other methods to decrease NSAID-induced gastropathy include the concomitant use of proton pump inhibitors, high-dose H2 receptor antagonists (not standard dose), and the prostaglandin E analog misoprostol.[1,3]

Table 3.1. Risk factors for NSAID-associated gastropathy[2]

Risk factors for gastropathy	Increased risk
Prior history of an adverse GI event such as an ulcer or hemorrhage	4 to 5 fold
Concurrent use of glucocorticoids	4 to 5 fold
Age > 60	5 to 6 fold
High (more than twice normal) dosage of a NSAID	10 fold
Concurrent use of anticoagulants	10 to 15 fold

Risks for gastropathy with this patient include her age and the possibility that she may be on an NSAID long-term. Therefore, the family physician is appropriately concerned about risks to his patient while she is on an NSAID.

Professionalism Consideration

It is understandable that this family physician, as most other physicians, can become frustrated with the need to justify to his patient's insurance company why this patient should be on celecoxib.

First, there are many time-consuming administrative challenges that the physician experiences on a daily basis. This may involve running an office, managing employees, issuing referrals, and dealing with billing and coding concerns. Administrative burdens may also include filling out prior authorization forms not only for this class of drug, but also for medications to treat some of the most common conditions in primary care such as hyperlipidemia, hypertension, allergies, peptic ulcer disease, and depression. Additionally, prior authorization may be required for items other than pharmaceuticals, such as CT or MRI scanning and patient use of medical equipment. With these burdens, it may be understandable that a physician would want to fill out the prior authorization form quickly and not verify the intolerance by clarifying this with the patient or reviewing the patient's medical records.

Second, the physician may not want his clinical judgment to be "second-guessed" by an agent for the insurance company. The physician can reasonably argue that only he should be able to make clinical judgments regarding which medication a patient is placed on and this judgment should not be influenced by guidelines mandated by insurance companies. The physician's decision is solely guided by what is clinically best for the patient, whereas insurance company guidelines are often significantly impacted by cost considerations.

Last, this physician may be aware that prior authorization may lead to biases or potentially reduced treatment in certain patients. Traditionally, patients with Medicaid or other "less desirable" insurance plans may have a more restrictive prescription plan and therefore may have far fewer choices about what medications can be used. Also, patients who are required to have their medication prior authorized may discontinue the medication in that class of drugs entirely, thereby avoiding any potential benefit.

As noted in the commentary by Dr. Gordin that follows, prescription drugs continue to be a significant contributor to the overall costs of health care, an expense that is rising substantially more than inflation. Over 45 million Americans lack health insurance and, even for those with health coverage, insurance premiums are rapidly rising for individuals and employers. A 2006 study has shown that the average cost of a family insurance plan that Americans receive through their jobs has risen 7.7 percent between 2005 and 2006, to $11,500.[4]

Although it may be burdensome for physicians to regularly and honestly complete prior authorization forms, this process has been clearly shown to reduce health care expenses.[5,6] Physicians may prefer this form of cost containment rather than others, including decreased physician reimbursement or eliminating the coverage of the medication regardless of prior authorization. Patients may also prefer this form of cost containment by insurance companies, rather than even greater increases in their premium.

Most importantly, there is no evidence that mandating prior authorization results in any clinical sacrifice to the patient. If there is a true clinical benefit to the drug preferred by the physician, it should be easily explained on the authorization form and readily approved by the insurance company.

Opinion

Although it may be perceived as a harmless act, the physician has committed fraud. As noted in the commentary below, an act of fraud may place the physician at risk for contractual termination by the health plan. And it may lead to larger problems for the physician, such as loss of staff privileges and sanction by the state board of medicine. The physician may consider working within the system and the state medical society to ease the administrative burden on doctors. One solution may be to lessen the number of medications requiring prior authorizations. Another possibility may come through electronic prescribing, which may allow quicker recognition of medications requiring prior authorization as well as more efficient processing of the request – particularly while the patient is in the office for his or her visit.

John Spandorfer, M.D.
Associate Professor of Medicine, Jefferson Medical College

A Perspective from an Insurance Executive

While overall costs for prescription drugs have moderated, national prescription-drug spending accounts for about 10 percent of total health care costs.[7] Additionally, over the 2003–2014 period, national health care spending is forecast to continue to grow faster than gross domestic product (GNP), from 15.5 percent in 2003 to 18.7 percent in 2014.[8] Over the past twenty years there has been a substantial increase in the share of national health expenditures attributed to pharmaceutical costs, and total pharmaceutical spending for public and private payers. This trend is driven by new drug development, increased utilization, an aging population, and price inflation, as well as promotional spending, especially direct-to-consumer advertising.

To insure continued affordability and access to quality health care, evidence-based medicine must drive appropriate drug utilization to enhance patient outcomes and to reduce drug benefit costs. This is becoming increasingly important as employers move toward "consumer driven health care" benefits, such as Health Savings Accounts, which place a greater portion of the heath care cost burden on the patient.

Insurers and pharmacy benefit management companies utilize multiple approaches in balancing ways to provide affordable benefits for their members with managing pharmacy costs. The impact of these types of programs is demonstrated by a reduction in pharmacy spend trend to 8.2 percent in 2004, reflecting a ten-year low that was attributed in part to increases in use of generics and tiered co-payment structures.[7] Pharmacy utilization usually focuses on select drugs or drug categories known to have potential for misuse, abuse, or adverse effects. Utilization techniques include plan designs which encourage generic alternatives; formulary design and co-pay structure; specialty drug management; drug quantity management; prior authorization; and step therapy.

This particular clinical scenario highlights prior authorization and step therapy. Step therapy is a program designed to encourage the use of therapeutically equivalent, lower-cost drugs (first-line therapy) before stepping up to medications that are more expensive (second-line therapy). Because COX-2 drugs are several times more expensive than non-selective generic NSAIDs, COX-2s are only cost effective if used by patients who truly need them. Additionally, inappropriate use of drug therapies may result in unnecessary patient exposure to risk. In the case of COX-2s, this issue is highlighted by the continuing concerns over the cardiovascular safety of cyclo-oxygenase 2 inhibitors, which led to the market withdrawal of rofecoxib (Vioxx) in 2004 and of valdecoxib (Bextra) in 2005.

A 2003 report demonstrated 19 percent of patients in the study had no medical condition that would indicate the need for a COX-2 inhibitor; 65

percent of those new to COX-2 therapy did not have an indication of being at risk for GI events, and 68 percent had no history of trying a lower cost non-selective NSAID before beginning COX-2 therapy. Overall, 45 percent of new COX-2 users (individuals with no GI risk or prior traditional NSAID use) were given a COX-2 inhibitor as first-line therapy when lower cost nonselective NSAIDs might have been the most cost-effective approach.[9]

Prior authorization can help identify those patients who may have a contraindication for the non-selective NSAIDs and thus may require COX-2 therapy. Clinical criteria to support pharmacy management initiatives such as prior authorization are developed by an independent, multi-specialty pharmacy and therapeutics (P&T) committee, which includes practicing physicians who review drugs in all therapeutic categories, and evaluate them based on efficacy and cost.

Assuming these criteria were being utilized by the health plan to determine medical necessity for first-line use of COX-2 therapy, the patient would have received authorization secondary to the fact that she was eighty-two years old, irrespective of the fact that she did not have documented gastrointestinal intolerance to NSAIDs.

It should be noted that by misrepresenting the patient's clinical history in order to obtain an authorization, the physician risks contractual termination by the health plan. Additionally, the misrepresentation could potentially be considered heath care fraud, which is defined as knowingly and willfully falsifying, concealing, or covering up a material fact or making a false statement or representation, or submitting a document known to contain false information to a health care benefit program.

Stephen Gordin, M.D.
Director, Clinical Affairs, Horizon Health Care of New Jersey

PATIENT WELFARE – OBSTETRICS AND GYNECOLOGY

A thirty-year-old woman in her first pregnancy is sent for a routine ultrasound to evaluate fetal anatomy. The pregnancy has been uncomplicated. She has not had medical problems in the past nor had any surgeries. The only medication she takes is prenatal vitamins. She was sick at the time the ultrasound was first scheduled (twenty weeks of gestation) and is twenty-three weeks of gestation when the examination is finally rescheduled.

On the ultrasound, fetal anatomy appears normal. However, the maternal cervix appears shortened when imaged transabdominally and so a transvaginal scan is performed. This shows a cervical length of 0.5 cm (normal > 2.5–3 cm) with funneling of the amniotic membranes down to the level of the internal os. (Normally there should be no funneling.)

A high-risk obstetrician tells her that a shortened cervix with funneling is a risk for preterm delivery. He indicates that there is no intervention demonstrated to prevent preterm delivery in such cases but that he recommends strict bed rest and hospitalization at least until twenty-eight weeks of gestation to avoid a delivery at the extremes of prematurity.

The patient agrees to his plan and is admitted to the hospital and placed on strict bed rest. On rounds one afternoon after two days of hospitalization, the patient is in tears. Asked, she indicates that she has just been called by her insurance company to say they will not authorize a hospitalization for bed rest alone and that if she stays even one night more she will be personally liable for the resulting charges.

A Perspective from an Obstetrician

Clinical Background

Ten to twelve percent of deliveries in the United States are premature (<thirty-seven weeks of gestation) and preterm birth is the second leading cause of neonatal mortality in this country.[10] The majority of preterm deliveries, however, are the result of preterm labor. Risks for preterm labor include a history of preterm delivery and multiple gestations, but most preterm labor occurs in pregnancies with few recognized risks.

Labor is defined as a pattern of regular uterine contractions associated with cervical opening (dilatation) and shortening (effacement). Generally, such changes are evaluated using a vaginal, digital exam. Vaginal examination, however, only allows evaluation of that portion of the cervix that protrudes into the vagina. Recognizing that ultrasound may allow visualization of the whole cervix, researchers have recently studied the utility of measuring cervical length as a predictor of preterm delivery. In fact there is an inverse correlation between cervical length and risk of preterm delivery and a shortened cervix (< 2.5 cm) as a predictor of preterm labor and delivery.[11]

Unfortunately, although a short cervix is a recognized risk for preterm delivery, no intervention demonstrably improves outcome or increases the length of gestation. Initially, obstetricians hoped that a cervical cerclage (a stitch placed transvaginally to tie and hold the cervix shut) would improve outcome when a short cervix was detected, but carefully conducted, randomized trials have failed to show such a benefit.[12]

Faced with such patients, obstetricians often recommend bed rest. However, while activity has been associated with increased frequency of uterine contractions (irritability), little firm evidence is available to support bed rest (as compared to usual activity) to prevent preterm delivery.[13] These limitations of evidence aside, many patients and providers feel that reducing activity offers them the opportunity to "do something." After all, could they forgive themselves if they didn't change what they were doing and went on to have a very premature delivery?

Professionalism Considerations

Hospitalization, at least in theory, offers several advantages over at-home management: stricter limitation of activity, closer observation for concerning symptoms, and the availability of prompt evaluation, intervention and, potentially, delivery and newborn care. Yet even without treatments or other interventions, hospitalization is expensive, for a hospital bed has an overhead – associated staff and equipment – that one's bed at home does not. Insurers, recognizing cost and the absence of evidence of benefit may, not surprisingly, object to these hospitalizations.

When insurers and patients and providers disagree, education is a good place to start. Those caring for the patient should speak with those making coverage decisions (e.g., a medical director). These conversations can present patient and provider concerns, distinguish the patient's circumstances (a very short cervix as opposed to one just at the lower limit of normal) and detail alternate plans that have been tried or considered and rejected. Those making decisions may not be expert in the field and may mistake absent evidence (no appropriate trial conducted, given the challenges in recruitment and design) for negative evidence (a well-designed trial has shown no benefit). In my experience, conversation and education are strong persuaders. In an effort to make one's case and win over the insurer, however, one should not misstate facts, exaggerate risk, or misrepresent concern for adverse outcome as certainty.

Next, providers should consider and reconsider alternatives. Be creative! Is there a skilled nursing facility appropriate for the patient? Are there home services that can make being at home a safer, more comfortable and productive place? Perhaps a home health aid would make strict bed rest possible and have a lower cost that would make home care with an aid appealing to the insurer. If the issue of concern is child care, maybe there are others who can help or, again, professionals to hire. If the concern is distance from hospital, maybe a willing relative or friend lives closer. If admission is designed for education (imagine a patient with newly diagnosed gestational diabetes), visiting nurses or others might make in-home education possible. Frequent contact by phone might substitute for the questions asked on daily rounds. In my own years of practice, I've found that more is "do-able" at home and that more resources are available than I had once imagined.

In facing these challenging situations, it may be tempting to tailor the care plan to meet what insurance will cover. If daily intravenous therapy would meet the acuity required for coverage, why not add it? The ethical value of honesty argues otherwise. A provider's relationship with patients, other staff, and insurers is based on trust, and as others see or conclude that a doctor is stretching the truth or lying, the provider's position as a trusted resource and caregiver will be eroded. Even without making arguments invoking a slippery slope, a core ethical foundation of medical care is recommending and providing patients only with the care likely to improve their health and outcome.

Of course, the patient should be aware of all these discussions. In such conversations, providers should communicate concerns raised by and decisions of the insurer, avoiding the temptation to vilify them for their decision. After all, the patient (and the provider) is likely to continue to need to work with the insurer and changing coverage at this point is unlikely to be an option. Care also needs be taken to assure the patient that she will neither be abandoned nor her health compromised.

Opinion

If these alternatives have been explored and found to be unsatisfactory, the patient should not be discharged. Financial concerns are important but not paramount. Our primary professional obligation is to our patients, not their insurance providers. Providers can and should advocate for their patients and their needs at the hospital level; often fees can be waived or expenses covered by a pool set aside for such situations.

Jeffrey L. Ecker, M.D.
Associate Professor of Obstetrics,
Gynecology and Reproductive Biology
Harvard Medical School

A Perspective from a Health Care Attorney

The first and most important question is: "What does the doctor think is the best treatment?" If inpatient care best serves this patient, then the focus must be on reversing the non-approval of the admission by the insurer.

In order to get approval, one needs first to identify why it is not available. There is a practical and legal difference between services which are not covered by the insurance policy, and those which are subject to prior authorization. Non-covered services are services not included under the insurance contract. Generally, it is extremely hard, if not impossible, to get around the problem of a service being non-covered.

A more common scenario is that although covered, the recommended treatment requires prior authorization. After you have prescribed these services and your office or hospital administrator, who calls the insurance company for approval, has been turned down, you are entitled to a peer-to-peer conversation with a physician at the health plan. Much of the decision to authorize care is dependent on whether the care is medically necessary. Health plans typically use an algorithm to assess whether a given service is medically necessary. The algorithm and medical necessity definition should generally be made available to the physician by the plan upon request. You may be able to demonstrate that your patient's situation meets the criteria under the algorithm. If not, then you may convince the plan physician that your patient has special circumstances (i.e., she is pregnant, has a shortened cervix, and is at high risk for preterm delivery) that call for the exercise of good medical judgment to avoid a bad, and expensive, birth outcome. However, if the algorithm leads to "no" and the plan's doctor cannot be convinced that your patient's situation merits an exception, the question of whether the service is covered turns on whether the service is medically necessary as defined by the health insurance contract.

This is where many physicians lose an important opportunity to gain approval of a service. In their anger and frustration, they fail to address how their patient's situation meets the insurer's definition of medical necessity. "Medical necessity" is a legal term that varies from one health insurance contract to another. Whether a given service is medically necessary depends on how the insurer defines medical necessity in its insurance contract. For example, if a contract were to define medically necessary services as "those services which, if denied, would cause the demise of the patient in five days," it is unlikely that this patient (or any other patient for that matter) would get treatment. If the plan's medical necessity definition is more liberal, your chances of getting the service approved are greater.

In this vignette, the admission that you requested has been "not approved." Hospitalization is generally a covered service, so the dispute is likely over whether the admission is medically necessary. Federal Medicaid law requires states to establish a process for providing notice and an administrative hearing whenever a service is reduced or denied. You or your assistant need to file the appeal. The hospital may have someone who is able to file an appeal for you. The argument will be whether the admission is "medically necessary" under the terms of the insurance contract. Regulations may provide for expedited review in urgent cases, and generally the attending physician's opinion on whether a situation is urgent is controlling.

If this fails, look to see if there are patient advocates in the community who can help, such as the staff of the Pennsylvania Health Law Project. Other states also have legal advocacy groups. Isn't managed care beautiful, the way it gets doctors and lawyers working together?

Michael Campbell, Esq.
Reuschlein Clinical Teaching Fellow
Villanova University School of Law, Villanova, PA

PATIENT WELFARE – PEDIATRICS

The pediatric team is asked to evaluate a one-year-old child with asthma who is admitted by the orthopedic team for a femur fracture. The orthopedic surgeon is a neighbor of the child's family. On evaluation, the pediatrician suspects child abuse and recommends further investigation before the child is discharged.

A Perspective from a Pediatrician

Clinical Background[14,15]

The estimated incidence of femur fractures in the United States in the one-year age group is 33 per 100,000 children. Clinicians evaluating femur fractures in this age group use the history, physical examination, and radiographs to make a reasonable determination between accidental and non-accidental injury.

Walking or running increases the likelihood of a femur fracture from tripping and falling. Therefore the index of suspicion for abuse in a non-ambulatory child is higher. The description of the mechanism of injury from the family or caretaker must be plausible and there should be no inconsistencies in the story over time or between different family members. Delay in seeking medical care and a history of previous injuries raises the index of suspicion. It is essential to ask about other factors in the history that are known to increase the risk of child abuse. These include child-related factors (medical fragility, special needs, behavior problems, a non-biologic relationship to the caretaker), social factors (isolation, domestic and intimate partner violence, poverty, unemployment), and caretaker factors (substance abuse, mental health problems, a criminal history, and inappropriate expectations for child behavior and supervision).

The physical examination must include observation of the quality and appropriateness of the interaction between the child and caregiver. Note should be made of other physical findings that might indicate the possibility of abuse/neglect such as bruises and other skin lesions or scars, soft tissue swelling, presence of soft or hard callus, poor hygiene, and indications of infrequent diaper changes. Radiographic data contribute to making an assessment of the risk of non-accidental femur fracture. Sub-trochanteric and metaphyseal fractures are more highly associated with abuse than longshaft fractures, but are not pathognomonic. The decision to proceed with further evaluation is based on whether there is a reasonable history for the femoral fracture, appropriate timing in seeking medical care, and no evidence of additional trauma or neglect. If further evaluation is warranted, a skeletal survey or scintigraphy (bone scan) and radiographs of any area with specific clinical findings should be done.

In summary, when evaluating a child with a femur fracture all the elements described have to be considered and, unless the physician is confident that the fracture is accidental, an immediate report must be made to child protective services.

Professionalism Considerations[15,16]

In this scenario the professionalism issues revolve around the following four questions:

- Did the orthopedist not consider child abuse?
- Did the orthopedist lack the knowledge to make a correct decision after thinking of child abuse as a possibility?
- Did the orthopedist not act on the suspicion of child abuse because this was the child of a neighbor?
- Is the pediatrician wrong in suspecting child abuse?

Orthopedic surgeons – whether they are in general or pediatric practice – should routinely evaluate all injuries in children to determine whether they are accidental or non-accidental. They should have the knowledge and skills to perform this task and, if they are unsure, readily consult with colleagues who are more knowledgeable or experienced. However, if no consultant is available the physician must file a report with child protective services.

Telling a family that he/she is filing a report of suspected child abuse is anxiety provoking for a physician. Reactions by the parents/caregivers to the news of the report and the need for additional investigation may range from acceptance and appreciation to denials, attempts to leave, and, rarely, violence. It is essential that the physician not be swayed from his/her legal (and moral) duty to report a suspicion of child abuse because of fear of how the family may respond. Equally important, it is critical to recognize and eliminate from the decision-making process factors that negatively influence sound clinical judgment. Examples of influencing factors include knowing the family (as is the case in this scenario), making a judgment about the family from superficial impressions of appearance, and erroneously believing that a nice family would not abuse their child.

Opinion

As a physician, you are the advocate for the child and you are required by law to report suspected child abuse. Keeping this in the forefront of your mind is the key to handling these difficult situations. Most medical education programs today offer communications skills training related to child abuse using role-play or standardized patients. This training makes it easier to discuss suspected child abuse with a family for the first time in the real clinical setting.

The duty to report supersedes the professional confidentiality inherent in the doctor–patient relationship. Physicians are protected from legal liability when they report in good faith. It is not the physician's job to "prove" or to "be certain" that abuse has occurred before reporting. Instead, reporting puts in motion the process that ensures that an abused child will be protected from further harm or finds the case "unfounded."

Approaching the family in a non-accusatory manner, demonstrating support and empathy while explaining that the overriding concern is for the safety and welfare of the child usually defuses a negative response from the family. It is crucial to explain your legal obligation to report and also what will happen after the report is filed; for example, representatives of child protective services and perhaps the police will speak with the family as part of the investigation.

Throughout my career in pediatrics when I have seen injuries, rashes, and so forth, I have always asked myself "could this be a result of abuse?" I hope that this approach has allowed me to identify most, if not all, the cases of child abuse that have presented in my practice.

J. Lindsey Lane, M.D.
Associate Professor of Pediatrics
Jefferson Medical College

A Perspective from a Medical Director of a Child Abuse Program

The physician who identifies or comes in contact with a child with a suspicious injury has four major professional responsibilities: to the child as a patient, to the child's family, to the child's referring or primary physician, and to society. Medical professionalism requires a primary focus on patient welfare. Any physician providing medical care for a child has an ethical responsibility to the child's family; however, the primary responsibility is to ensure the welfare of the child patient.

The orthopedist in this case may face a conflict involving his/her professional responsibilities as a physician with his/her personal relationship as a neighbor to the parents of the child. Physicians are sometimes met with the professional challenge of providing appropriate medical care for individuals who are friends or colleagues. This challenge is magnified when the physician with the personal relationship with the family is providing medical care for a child with possible or suspected abuse. Personal bias related to the physician's education, experiences, attitudes, and beliefs affects recognition of abuse.[17–19] The most difficult cases to recognize are those children with parents who have characteristics much like the physicians conducting the evaluations. Adding a personal relationship to these other apparent biases further interferes with an objective approach.

It is stressful for both the physician and the family to approach the evaluation of suspected abuse. Avoiding this stress, however, may place the child's welfare at further risk by not identifying ongoing abuse.[18] The physician must recognize that the primary responsibility is providing appropriate care for the injured patient. Part of that responsibility is to understand how the child became injured and preventing subsequent injury. Estimates of the risk of repeat injury from abuse in a previously abused child are as high as 35 percent.[19] The physician must consider the possibility that the child may have been abused either while in the care of someone else or while in the parents' care. If the child has been injured through an act or an omission by the child's parents or other "substitute" caretakers, addressing the act or omission is necessary to prevent future injury.

In the United States, all fifty states have laws that require health care providers to report suspected child abuse to child protective services agencies so they can conduct investigations and make interventions when appropriate.[19] In many cases of suspected abuse, the final diagnosis is made through a collaborative effort of medical professionals and community agencies.[20] The cornerstone of statewide systems to evaluate suspected child maltreatment, treatment for families with abuse histories, and child abuse prevention programs is the appropriate recognition of the abused child and appropriate recognition of injuries that are truly unintentional. Problems in recognition are often caused by a false or misleading history misdirecting the diagnostic process, a process often shaped by the history.[17] Lack of recognition can result in not properly reporting the incident to child protective service agencies. Problems in reporting can also be traced to physician bias and physician beliefs that reporting requires a high probability of abuse or that child protective service systems will make things worse.

Abuse must be considered in the differential diagnosis of all childhood trauma. An injury pattern is rarely specific for abuse or accident without careful consideration of the explanation provided. Accidental injury is very common and both inflicted and accidental injuries may be seen simultaneously in a child. As a general consideration, the more severe the injury and/or the younger the child, the more extensive is the need for diagnostic testing for additional injuries and a consideration of possible abuse.[19] If a lack of appropriate supervision or exposure to a high-risk situation was responsible, at minimum the physician should address child safety and "accident prevention" with the parents. Familial and social risk factors should be considered. However, the single most important consideration in suspected abuse is whether the history provided adequately explains the type, location, and severity of the injuries found on examination, radiographic imaging, and laboratory testing.

What is not clear from the scenario is whether the pediatric team was being consulted for asthma management, to help evaluate for possible abuse, or for some other reason. But the reason for the consultation does not change the pediatrician's responsibility to the patient welfare and should not alter the medical recommendations or conclusions. It may, however, affect how the pediatrician approaches the family and the orthopedist. The pediatrician must recognize a responsibility to consider the possibility of abuse in any injured child, conduct a careful and comprehensive evaluation, assess the explanation provided for the injury, and determine whether there is a reasonable suspicion that the injury may have been caused by abuse.[18–20] As a consultant to the orthopedist, the pediatrician should discuss the findings and concerns with the orthopedist, but the pediatrician must assume responsibility when there is a reasonable suspicion of abuse and report the suspicion to a child protective services agency.

Allan DeJong, M.D.
Medical Director, Children at Risk Evaluation (CARE) Program
Alfred I. duPont Hospital for Children, Wilmington, Delaware

PATIENT WELFARE – PSYCHIATRY

Mrs. Gold is a sixty-nine-year-old retired widow who lives independently and is competent to make her own financial and medical decisions. Mrs. Gold has been experiencing a severe episode of major depressive disorder and her symptoms have not responded to several trials of antidepressant medications. Consequently her psychiatrist, Dr. Smith, has recommended a course of electroconvulsive therapy (ECT). Mrs. Gold has agreed to receive ECT but her children call Dr. Smith to discuss their opposition to this plan.

A Perspective from a Psychiatrist

Clinical Background
ECT has been an efficacious psychiatric treatment for more than sixty years. Meta-analyses and double-blind random assignment studies have

consistently demonstrated the therapeutic benefits of ECT in reducing depressive symptoms and improving patients' quality of life.[21,22] Because of its greater efficacy and more rapid onset of action relative to antidepressants, ECT is particularly valuable in treating patients whose symptoms have not responded to medications or whose depression is life threatening (due to suicidal risk or limited oral intake).[21] Nevertheless, many misconceptions about ECT persist.[23]

In contrast to portrayals of ECT in television and film, the ECT procedure[21] is not a dramatic one. Patients are given a short-acting intravenous anesthetic medication (typically a barbiturate) and a medication to minimize muscle contractions (typically succinylcholine). Once the patient is asleep, an ECT stimulus lasting several seconds is given via two electrodes that are positioned on the patient's head. The induced electrical seizure typically lasts for thirty to sixty seconds and is accompanied by a minimal amount of bodily movement. Within about five minutes, the patient gradually awakens from anesthesia.

As with all medical procedures, ECT has potential side effects as well as therapeutic benefits.[21] The most common side effects are headache, muscle aches, and nausea or vomiting. During the ECT-induced seizure, patients may exhibit alterations in blood pressure, heart rate or cardiac rhythm that are detected with routine monitoring and generally resolve spontaneously. Rarely, more serious pulmonary or cardiovascular complications can ensue, with a mortality rate that appears comparable to that of anesthesia alone. Memory difficulties may also occur around the time of ECT but typically improve once the ECT treatments are completed. However, a small number of individuals report longer lasting (or even permanent) gaps in memory. Each of these potential therapeutic benefits and side effects of ECT are reviewed with the patient as part of the informed consent process.

Professionalism Considerations

Across medical settings and specialties, disagreements about recommended treatments are commonly observed between patients and families or among family members. As typified by this clinical scenario, the clinical decision making and informed consent processes associated with ECT are often particularly complex. Most families have realistic concerns about the potential benefits and side effects of ECT for their family member. In addition, individual family members may have specific biases about psychiatric treatments, including ECT, because of their own experiences or belief systems. The persisting stigma and misunderstandings about ECT among lay people (as well as in the medical community)[23] also make it difficult for patients and families to obtain accurate information to assist with their decision making.

Communicating with family members is important regardless of whether they agree or disagree with the recommendation for ECT.[21,24] Particularly, given the repeated nature and side effects of ECT treatments, families will often need to provide the patient with pragmatic assistance (e.g., transportation supervision if ECT is associated with confusion). In addition, family disagreements about treatment may jeopardize the patients' emotional support network, magnify patients' level of stress, and exacerbate patients' symptoms. Although some clinicians are reluctant to speak with family members because of concerns about confidentiality, most patients are in favor of family involvement. With patient consent and in emergency situations, family contact is permissible.[25] Generally, conversations with family members include obtaining information about the patient's history, hearing family observations that are relevant to diagnosis or treatment, and providing the family with information and education about mental illness and its treatment.

Whenever a procedure such as ECT is contemplated, it is important to consider whether the patient has the decisional capacity to provide informed consent. To give consent, patients must understand the procedure that is being recommended, apply reasoning in considering the consequences of the recommended treatment or therapeutic alternatives, accurately appreciate the way in which this information applies to them, and be able to make a logical treatment choice based on this understanding, appreciation, and reasoning about the procedure.[25] Although psychiatric illness, in and of itself, does not change the presumption that an individual is competent, a patient's ability to appreciate the consequences of a particular decision may be shaped by specific mental symptoms. Thus, cognitive deficits (e.g., due to dementia or associated with depression) can impair the ability to recall and understand information about the procedure, suicidal ideas can affect perceptions of mortality risks, and the ambivalence and indecision that often occurs with depression can limit patients' ability to make a choice about treatment. If a patient lacks decisional capacity, substituted consent (possibly by a family member) or a judicial hearing will be necessary, with the exact requirements varying from state to state. However, for many patients, educational interventions can be used to improve decisional capacity and most individuals are able to provide informed consent.[25]

Opinion

Upon receiving a phone call from Mrs. Gold's children, the first step is to obtain Mrs. Gold's permission to speak with her family members. In doing so, it is helpful to specifically delineate information that Mrs. Gold would or would not want shared with her family. Such a discussion can also provide insight into the patient's relationship with the family and background information about family experiences that may influence their opinions of ECT.

Assuming that Mrs. Gold gives permission for Dr. Smith to speak with her children, the next step is determining whether this is best achieved by phone or with an in-person meeting, either with the family alone or with Mrs. Gold and the family together. During discussion with the family, it is usually best to begin with open-ended questions about their concerns.

Dr. Smith will also want to provide information about ECT, including the potential benefits and risks of ECT as compared to other therapeutic options, and the specific details of the procedure. After the meeting, Dr. Smith should speak with Mrs. Gold to review the meeting discussion and address any additional questions. Assuming that Mrs. Gold continues to agree with ECT and that she has the decisional capacity to provide informed consent, ECT can be initiated as planned.

Laura J. Fochtmann, M.D.
Professor of Psychiatry and Behavioral Science
Stony Brook University School of Medicine

A Perspective from an Attorney and Ethicist

What should the physician do when his or her competent informed patient wants to proceed with treatment that family members object to?

The patient, Mrs. Gold, is competent to decide to undergo this treatment, and has given consent. But before ECT begins, her psychiatrist, Dr. Smith, hears from Mrs. Gold's family members that they oppose the treatment plan, which they have learned of from the patient. So, we know that the patient has discussed the proposed treatment with family members, but we do not know the nature of the patient's relationship with her family, or if the physician had any prior interactions with family members. Should Dr. Smith even be talking to the family members?

The physician must strike a balance between respecting patient autonomy, preferences, and values, while acting in the patient's best interests and making patient welfare the first priority.[26] He or she should assume in the absence of evidence to the contrary that the family has the patient's welfare at heart, too, and recognize family members' role and concern for the patient. First, Dr. Smith should discuss with Mrs. Gold whether it is acceptable for him to talk to family members about her care. Confidentiality and respect for patient privacy are key to patient–physician relationships and the trust necessary to sustain them. In addition to ethical obligations, physicians must be aware of state and federal confidentiality requirements, including the Health Insurance Portability and Accountability Act of 1996 (HIPAA) Privacy Rule. Patients will not speak candidly about their health problems and care if wishes about privacy are not respected. Sometimes family or friends of a patient want to talk to a physician but ask them not to reveal to the patient that they are doing so or what they have said to the physician. The physician is not required to keep such secrets and must act in the patient's best interests.[27]

Assuming discussion with family members is acceptable to the patient, the physician might explore what the family actually knows about the diagnosis and prognosis, and what troubles family members about the treatment plan. Fictional accounts of ECT, such as the portrayal of the procedure in the film *One Flew over the Cuckoo's Nest*, have often been downright scary. ECT is controversial in the eyes of the public, and many people are skeptical of its effectiveness, probably believing it is a relic of the past. Family members may not be aware of ECT's acceptance in the medical community and when its use is indicated. They may also be worried about side effects or know things that the doctor does not (for example, if the patient is just going along with the plan because she doesn't want to be seen as "difficult").

While patient autonomy should be respected and the competent patient should be empowered by the physician to make informed health care decisions, consensus building among family members to at least understand the physician's recommendation and the patient's preference is desirable. It is, after all, the family who likely knows the patient best, and will live with the consequences of her health care decisions. In fact, in some cultures and families, health care decision making is a family role embraced by the patient.

Even so, families sometimes have difficulty being heard. Although its focus is on families with active caregiving roles, one article has noted that in practice and in the medical literature, there is a tendency "to equate families with trouble."[28] Also, "physicians often assume that conflict is undesirable and destructive,"[29] says another article, written in the context of end-of-life-care decision making. The authors recognize, however, that "conflict handled well can be productive, and the clarity that results can lead to greater family, patient, and clinician satisfaction."[29] Discussions based on the shared interest of physician and family members for enhancing the patient's welfare can clarify treatment goals (and on what evidence they are based). Furthermore, discussions will help build consensus, or at least signal to the family members that they have been heard and respected.[29]

The physician's primary duty is to the patient and her welfare. Ultimately, Dr. Smith should respect the treatment preferences of this competent, informed patient. Working with the family, when the patient desires this, requires strong communication, a process which takes time, but is probably time well spent. Family members often have a role to play in the patient's health care too.

Lois Snyder, J.D.
Director, Center for Ethics and Professionalism
American College of Physicians

PATIENT WELFARE – SURGERY

A general surgeon working in a community hospital learns he is HIV positive six months after a needle stick injury. He is uncertain whether to disclose this information to anyone who may report his diagnosis to the hospital where he works.

A Perspective from an Infectious Disease Physician

Clinical Background

What is the risk of this surgeon transmitting his HIV infection to his patients? While there are many case reports and clusters of patients acquiring HBV (hepatitis B virus) and HCV (hepatitis C virus) from infected clinicians, there have been remarkably few documented cases of HIV transmission from clinician to patient. Since the recognition of the HIV epidemic in 1981, there have been only eight patients proven to have become infected from a health care worker, most of whom were not infected from an HIV-positive surgeon.[30] These occurrences have been so rare that the true risk of a patient acquiring HIV from an infected surgeon is unknown, and retrospective epidemiological studies have been unable to implicate HIV-infected surgeons in the transmission of their infection to their patients.[30] Thus, it is unclear how much of an infectious risk this surgeon poses to his patients.

Professionalism Considerations

Primum non nocere. Above all, do no harm. This maxim of nonmaleficence, the basis for the physician–patient relationship, is surely one of the oldest ethical principles to guide medical practice.[31] Can this principle help this unfortunate surgeon make his difficult decision?

Decision making in ethics, as decision making in the rest of medicine, should be evidence-based and informed by empiric scientific data as much as possible. Knowledge of the risk of transmitting bloodborne pathogens – especially HIV – is germane to this case. Since the early 1980s, when HIV was recognized to be the cause of the acquired immunodeficiency syndrome (AIDS), medical professionals have regarded HIV as a potential occupational hazard. Operating room personnel are recognized to be at particularly high risk for occupational injuries that expose them to their patients' pathogens, and a variety of strategies for preventing or mitigating these injuries have been developed and become routine in surgical practice.[32] Efforts have lead to a reduction in on-the-job transmission of HIV, HBV, HCV, and other bloodborne infections.

What are the consequences of this physician disclosing his infection to his colleagues or to his patients? The American College of Surgeons' *Code of Professional Conduct* reminds practitioners that trust is integral to the practice of surgery, and that disclosure to patients of their therapeutic options and risks is a professional obligation.[33] But if this surgeon is otherwise physically, mentally, and intellectually competent, and if public health and infectious disease experts cannot clearly define or calculate the risk that he might pose to his patients, will his patients be well served if they are routinely informed of his HIV serostatus? For comparison, most physicians would not feel morally obligated to disclose to their patients other personal medical conditions (e.g., diabetes, cancer) or family issues (e.g., marital discord) that might profoundly affect the physician's own life, but would not necessarily affect their professional work. And who in his hospital will the surgeon be able to trust with this personal medical information and help him decide whether or how it will affect his practice? After all, he is now a patient with a chronic disease, and like all patients he enjoys legal and ethical protections and deserves to have his medical information held in a confidential manner.

Opinion

The complexities of this surgeon's dilemma have been problematic to professional societies and legislative bodies. In fact, there are few published guidelines that can be used to determine the right action in this case.[34] One expert committee has developed "a list of exposure-prone procedures and a decision chart that indicates under what conditions infected physicians can practice beyond the need for disclosure."[30] I agree with these guidelines, which stipulate that this general surgeon would be counseled to avoid participation in surgical procedures that have been assessed as particularly risky (e.g., cardiothoracic surgery; orthopedic procedures), but would be allowed some latitude to continue medical practice, especially if his HIV infection is well controlled. Further, I agree with this committee's conclusion that routine disclosure "is unnecessary, ineffective, and inappropriate" in guiding the physician's practice.[30]

The tenets of professionalism include a call for physicians to serve the greater needs of society. With an increasing need to retain skilled surgeons in the workforce,[35] this physician provides a community service by continuing his practice, even if limited. Perhaps the most urgent professional injunction that this surgeon must heed is to seek and be adherent with expert medical care for his HIV infection. It is imperative that he find an experienced and knowledgeable clinician with whom he can establish a trusting doctor–patient relationship, who can guide him with his collegial relationships, and longitudinally assess his ability to continue professional activities. With appropriate education and treatment he will likely "do no harm," stay healthy, and remain a valued member of his profession and his community.

Ira K. Schwartz, M.D.
Associate Dean of Medical Education and Student Affairs
Director of Admissions
Emory University School of Medicine

A Perspective from an Expert on Physician Disability

The physician who encounters a patient with a non-curable disease or disability faces a direct challenge to his/her sense of professional mastery. Such disabilities may be interpreted as a failure of medicine.[36] But if the individual with the disability is also a physician he/she confronts a special paradox, being in a high status social role (doctor) while simultaneously being in a low status role (patient). The cognitive dissonance that results from this concurrence of social roles helps to explain the reluctance of the physician-patient to disclose his illness or limitations if at all possible.[37,38] "Invisible" disabilities such as those which may be produced by HIV disease, cardiopulmonary disease, chronic pain, or milder degrees of hearing and visual impairments may allow the affected physician to pass as able-bodied. Severe neuromusculoskeletal diseases such as spinal cord injury, stroke, or multijoint arthritis are, by their nature, more immediately visible and cannot be concealed from medical peers or patients.

I have had to deal with these issues of self-disclosure during my own career as my lifelong visual impairment progressed to functional blindness. From that personal experience, I have concluded that the primary criterion for disclosing disability is whether it has any potentially negative implications for the patient under treatment. As a physiatrist, I primarily see patients with neuromusculoskeletal problems as local as lower back pain or as generalized as quadriplegia. The overwhelming majority of these patients can be examined and managed by me without the need for functional vision, given the easy access to computer technology and secretarial staff. If there is a skin lesion, it passes out of my powers of observation (though an educated hypothesis can be made), and referral to a sighted colleague or other specialist is the immediate action taken.

The most important characteristic required by any physician with significant functional impairment is unimpaired judgment. This implies a clear awareness of the limits of one's own clinical competence. We all have our limits or else there would be no need for more than forty medical and surgical subspecialties. In such circumstances excess hubris can be far more disabling than any motor or sensory limitation. The decision to limit one's practice or even to terminate it due to disability should begin with the affected physician's thoughtful assessment of the effects of disability on clinical practice. Many factors need to be considered: for example, motor or sensory deficits loom far larger for a surgeon than for a medical specialist or psychiatrist; group or hospital practice settings can give access to other clinicians and support staff that facilitate compensatory strategies, and specific procedures can be referred to colleagues if their performance is affected by a disability.

What should a physician with a disability such as visual impairment say to the patient? Do you shake hands and start the interview by informing the patient that you are blind, visually impaired, or something in that vein? This seems no more necessary than telling the patient that you have a bad headache/stomach ache, or that you are in a foul mood because you had a major argument with your spouse just before coming into the office. These daily experiences can certainly color the physician–patient interaction, but I would like to think that if the pain or the argument was bad enough to compromise clinical ability the physician would not engage in any patient care at that time. The same should hold true for more permanent disabilities. I would not presume to work as a dermatologist, ophthalmologist, or surgeon given my vision loss, but it has only minimal effect on my daily practice as a hospital-based academic physiatrist. I do not think that the physician with a disability needs to keep the disability a secret, but it only needs to be directly addressed if its presence may negatively impact patient care.

An HIV-positive physician whose practice does not involve invasive procedures (for example, a psychiatrist or medical specialist whose diagnostic and therapeutic practice does not entail increased risk of a needle stick) should not need to disclose his/her HIV status. For the HIV-positive physician whose practice does involve invasive care it should not be forgotten that a physician's own illness or disability may provide a unique window into their patients' world which can heighten the practitioner's empathy for the disability experience.

Stanley F. Wainapel, M.D., M.P.H.
Clinical Director, Department of Rehabilitation Medicine,
Montefiore Medical Center
Professor of Clinical Rehabilitation Medicine,
Albert Einstein College of Medicine

PATIENT WELFARE – EMERGENCY MEDICINE

*A sixty-seven-year-old ill-appearing man was sent to the emergency depart-
ment from his primary care physician's office with a fever and cough that he
had had for the past three days. He presented to his physician's office late in the
afternoon and, because his physician did not have access to appropriate studies or treatment modalities, was sent to the ED after an initial evaluation. He
had previously felt well, and had no past notable medical history. In the
emergency department, his initial blood pressure was 96/44 and improved to
104/60 with one liter of normal saline. His other vitals included a temperature
of 100.4, heart rate of 124, which decreased to 110 with intravenous fluids
(IVF), a respiratory rate of 26, and pulse oximetry of 90 percent. Significant
laboratory results included a white blood cell count of 16,600 per cubic milli-
meter with 92 percent neutrophils, and creatinine of 1.8 mg/dL. The chest
radiograph demonstrated a consolidation in the right middle lobe.*

*The patient stated that he felt better after initial treatment of IVF, antipy-
retics, and antibiotics. The emergency physician called the patient's primary
care doctor and recommended that the patient be admitted. The primary care
physician, who had seen the patient earlier in the day and sent him to the ED,
asked the emergency physician not to admit the patient but rather to discharge
the patient from the emergency room, to continue him on the oral antibiotic,
and tell him to follow up in the office within two days.*

A Perspective from a General Internist

Clinical Background

At the turn of the century Sir William Osler described pneumonia as "the
captain of the men of death," as it accounted for an estimated 5 million
deaths per year. The development of antimicrobial therapy has dramatically
reduced this, but pneumonia remains a major health issue today.

Over the last thirty years there have been over a hundred studies looking at
the prognosis of community-acquired pneumonia.[39] Most of these studies
were to identify patients at high risk, so that appropriate attention, including
intensive care unit admission, could be employed.[40] A recent study looking at
hospitalization of nursing home residents has demonstrated increased costs
without benefit of decreased morbidity and mortality[41] associated with hospitalization compared with non-hospitalization.

Given the recognition of scarce resources, measures to identify individuals
who can safely receive care at home, rather than be hospitalized, have been
identified.[42] Authors of the PORT (Pneumonia Patient Outcomes Research
Team) identified that the absence of certain clinical findings, such as systolic

hypotension, tachypnea, or laboratory findings, such as acidemia, or hypo-
natremia may safely predict a patient who can successfully be treated in
a non-hospital setting.[42]

Professionalism Considerations

This case touches on multiple issues of professionalism, including patient
welfare, honesty with patients, commitment to a just distribution of finite
resources, and managing conflicts of interest. The latter, managing conflicts
of interest, can be addressed first. The ED physician may feel that the
patient's best interest is in hospitalization, but that may be borne out of fear
of litigation based upon lack of post-discharge follow-up. Utilizing a conflict
resolution strategy[43] with the patient's best interests as the ultimate goal
should help to resolve this issue. In this model, one separates the people
from the problem, focuses on common interests, and considers options that
will satisfy all parties. Clearly both physicians have the patient's best interest
at heart, with the goal of safe, effective treatment of the patient's pneumonia.
Setting this as the goal allows the exploration of different options for treatment and disposition, allows a patient-centered approach, and eliminates
physician-centric perspectives. Using this approach generates care options
that include inpatient and outpatient care, and allows discussion of these
options from a patient-centered point of view.

Whether or not this patient should receive a hospital bed when there are
"sicker" patients is a more difficult issue. Although dogma states that we
should not ration health care resources at the bedside, the medical literature
suggest otherwise.[44] The central tenets of professionalism – nonmaleficence,
autonomy, beneficence, and justice – insist that physicians put patients first.
Not providing appropriate care, such as hospitalization if necessary, because
of the theoretical needs of others places a patient's physician in the role of
public health provider, not primary physician and advocate. Although at
times these roles may overlap, in this particular situation they are conflicting.
Doing what is best for this individual patient, or beneficence, requires that
other concerns be subjugated to the patient's best interests.

More importantly, and in line with honesty with patients, a study looking at
disclosure of information about rationing of care to patients found a substantial majority of patients in favor of physicians explicitly providing information[45] regardless of the outcome of the decision. The older model of
paternalism in medical decision making, as well as the more recent consum-
erist model, both fail in this setting, as decision making should be a shared
physician–patient responsibility. To fully understand the implications of
these shared decisions, patients need to be provided with all appropriate
information in a manner that they can comprehend. The role of both

physicians in this setting is to convey this information without bias, in a manner that is understandable to the patient.

All health care decisions should ultimately be made with an orientation to the patient's welfare. In this scenario, this perhaps is the "easiest" professionalism issue, although couching this decision in the realm of evidence-based medicine is still fraught with difficulty. The interpretation of clinical data[46] and development of a differential diagnosis is not simple, and is only the first step in the application of the evidence-based medicine guidelines mentioned previously. Applying the PORT[42] criteria, generated from population-based studies may miss the subtle nuance of each individual patient, information that the patient's primary physician may well have, and allow him or her to make a more tailored decision in this patient's care.

Opinion

The patient's primary care physician has to balance the evidence available in the medical literature with the validity of applying it to this particular patient. The patient's clinical status after ED triage and initial management suggests that he can be safely treated at home. Recognition of potential conflicts between the patient's general internist and the emergency medicine physician caring for the patient, and the ethical pitfalls that arise out of this, is paramount in the appropriate management of this patient.

Lawrence Kaplan, M.D.
Professor of Medicine
Assistant Dean for Clinical Education
Temple University School of Medicine

A Perspective from an Emergency Physician

Conflict resolution and risk stratification are integral to the practice of emergency medicine. Frequently, the assessment of risk and level of risk that a physician is willing to assume for a given patient leads to conflict between the emergency physician and physician potentially admitting that patient. Risk, in this case, can be thought of as the odds of that patient dying or being permanently disabled from the disease process that brought him or her to the emergency department. In many cases, this risk can be quantified using clinical decision rules such as the Pneumonia Severity Index derived from the Pneumonia Patient Outcomes Research Team (PORT). By adding numerical values assigned to various demographic factors, co-morbid conditions, physical examination findings, and laboratory results, a PORT score is calculated. The PORT score puts a patient into one of five different risk classes. The creators of the decision rule concluded that patients in risk classes I and II can be safely treated as outpatients, while class IV or V patients require hospital admission. For patients in risk class III, where the mortality rate ranges from 0.9 to 2.8 percent, recommendations vary. In the original PORT article, Fine et al. suggested "brief inpatient observation" for class III patients.[42] A subsequent article that Fine co-authored recommended outpatient treatment for class III patients,[47] and an informal survey of online PORT score calculators reveals that most recommend "outpatient or inpatient treatment depending on clinical judgment."[48,49]

Clinical decision rules are very helpful, but can't always be applied uniformly. Such a rule or guideline should be thought of as an adjunct to clinical experience and not a calculator that will always spit out the correct conclusion if you just enter the available objective data. Medical societies which create guidelines for the management of community acquired pneumonia such as the Infectious Diseases Society of America, American Thoracic Society,[50] and American College of Emergency Physicians[51] have recognized the limitations of objective admission criteria and have concluded that a physician's clinical judgment should supersede strict application of these scoring systems. As these groups indicate, risk is difficult to assess, and risk stratification cannot be completely objective.[52] There is also no universal agreement on what amount of risk is acceptable when discharging a patient home from the emergency department.

When there is conflict regarding the disposition of a patient, two physicians with roughly the same set of data, but different conclusions, must ultimately come to an agreement. Ideally, these discussions should be collegial. Often, new information is introduced which changes the opinion of one of the physicians. This information might include previously unknown medical history, social factors, results of a prior workup, unexpected lab results, strong feelings on the part of the patient, the availability of early follow-up, or conclusions drawn from medical literature relative to the case.

Based on the available data, our hypothetical patient with pneumonia has sepsis. A reanalysis of PORT patients in a subsequent study revealed that pneumonia patients with severe sepsis have a mortality rate of 13 percent regardless of risk class.[53] We don't have the arterial blood gas results necessary to determine whether our patient meets the definition of severe sepsis used in this article, but given his level of hypoxia measured by pulse oximetry, it is quite likely that he would. Additionally, utilizing an alternative, and perhaps superior, clinical decision rule, CURB-65, with the incomplete data that we do have, would confer a mortality of 9 percent on our patient, leading to a recommendation to "consider hospital supervised treatment."[54] Our patient also has renal dysfunction that is likely due to hypovolemia and hypoperfusion of his kidneys. We are missing his blood urea nitrogen level, but can confidently infer from his elevated creatinine that it would be greater than the CURB-65 cutoff, putting him in a group with a mortality of 22 percent, where the proposed treatment options are "manage in hospital as severe pneumonia" and "assess for ICU admission."[54] Sharing this information with the admitting physician would likely preclude the need for a lengthy discussion, and result in mutual agreement on inpatient admission.

At times, a solution or compromise does not arise from a simple exchange of information. When conversations regarding disposition evolve into disagreements, professionalism becomes paramount. Above all, both physicians should walk away from these disagreements with their dignity intact. As soon as one of the participants becomes disrespectful or dismissive, the conversation will quickly deteriorate and the common goal of doing what is best for the patient becomes subservient to the more ego-satisfying goal of winning a heated argument. Acknowledging the validity of the other physician's position, while calmly and clearly stating your own is a good way to show respect for a peer. Certainly, there are times when a physician must advocate passionately for his or her patient, but this should be more of a last resort, when diplomacy fails.

This "sixty-seven-year-old ill-appearing man" with sepsis and hypoxia from lobar pneumonia requires admission to a monitored bed for treatment with oxygen, intravenous fluids, and intravenous antibiotics. While sole reliance on a clinical decision rule might indicate otherwise, the vast majority of physicians would agree with this statement. It is important to remain professional while resolving conflicts of interest, but for our hypothetical patient, the only acceptable dispositions are either an inpatient admission or a discharge from the emergency department against medical advice (provided he clearly understands the risks of leaving a monitored setting, is capable of making medical decisions, and still refuses to be hospitalized). There are instances where compromise is reasonable or even preferable during discussions of disposition, but when using clinical judgment one should always err on the side of patient safety. Typically, hospital admission is a safer alternative to discharge home. In this case, it is the clear choice.

H. Edward Seibert, M.D.
Assistant Residency Director, Department of Emergency Medicine
Jefferson Medical College

SUMMARY – PRINCIPLE OF PRIMACY OF PATIENT WELFARE

Background

The primacy of patient welfare stands with patient autonomy and social justice as one of the pillars of professionalism.[26] In this section, the origins and evolution of the principle of patient welfare will be described. Also, the challenges now faced by the medical profession in fulfilling society's expectation that this principle will guide the patient–physician relationship will be explored.

The principle of patient welfare is based on a dedication to serving the interest of the patient. "Altruism contributes to the trust that is central to the physician–patient relationship."[26] Patient welfare derives from both the "individual" trust between each patient and physician and the "collective" public trust that is built between society and the medical profession as a whole.

Physicians are simultaneously healers and professionals. These roles have different origins, traditions, and links to patient welfare. The role of the healer, long recognized by society, arises from third-century Hippocratic tradition and has always been intuitively understood. The Hippocratic Oath is the earliest expression of a beneficence model of moral responsibility in medicine.[55] It acknowledges physicians' special knowledge and skills, as well as a commitment to using those skills to benefit patients. In addition, the physician is enjoined from doing harm unless the treatment, on balance, benefits the patient. In contrast, medicine as a profession has its origins in the guilds of the Middle Ages. Professionals are granted autonomy, status, prestige, and significant rewards in return for moral and altruistic behavior. "This formed the basis of the social contract between medicine and society, and functioned relatively well as long as both the profession and society were reasonably homogeneous and shared many values."[56]

The concept of a social contract was proposed by Hobbes, Locke, and Rousseau over three hundred years ago.[57] They suggested that it was based on a reciprocal set of rights and privileges. As care of patients has become more complex and the role of the physician more multifaceted, the expectations of both patient and physician have evolved. In addition to morality and altruism, the expectations of physicians by society in the twenty-first century include assured competence, accountability, transparency, objective advice, and promotion of the public good. In turn, physicians expect that society will expand their prerogatives, to include self-regulation, a value-driven and adequately funded health care system, a role in public policy, and a shared responsibility for health. Regardless of the specifics at various points in time, trust is fundamental to this relationship. "Society must trust individual physicians and physicians must believe that society will meet its reasonable expectations."[58]

Paul Starr noted in 1982 that the contract needed to be revised to cope with the growing tensions between the medical profession and society.[59] The social agenda of the 1960s and 1970s had a significant impact on the social contract as medicine emerged to consume a large portion of the wealth of the

United States and many other Western nations. It was a time when traditional values and all sources of authority, including medicine, were viewed with an increasing skepticism. There were complaints that the profession was exploiting its position to advance physicians' own self-interest rather than the needs of society in general and their patients in particular. There was concern that medicine had failed to self-regulate and that its institutions were more committed to serving their own members than to serving society. Medicine was accused of failing to meet some of its central obligations under the social contract. Medicine's response was defensive, lending further support to the criticism.[56]

It was also during this period of time that government and the private sector were taking increasing control of the business of medicine, specifically, who and what would be covered by third party payers. As this was recognized by the public, when blame for a less than ideal medical system was meted out, medicine was held less responsible than once would have been the case, since it was no longer viewed as holding a monopoly over health care. A positive, if unintended consequence of this loss of control, was that medicine was perceived as being more objective when it offered commentary on the state of the health care system.

Fortunately, society still has great respect and dependence on the role of the physician as healer. Patients still want to have a relationship of trust with their physicians.

> It is paradoxical that … while the profession has actually lost power, and in particular the ability to control its market, there appears to be the opportunity to rebuild trust. The public wishes physicians, not corporations or the state, to make major decisions regarding their health and health care. Also, physicians want to regain the power to make such decisions. For the first time in decades there appears to be a confluence between what the public wants and what the medical profession wants.[60]

This was illustrated in the debate about health care in the 2008 presidential election.[61,62]

It is important to note that there are some objections to the description of the relationship between medicine and society as a "contract" as put forth in the Physician Charter.[26] One objection is that the term "contract" implies a written formal agreement that is enforceable by law and has a lack of trust. Moreover, contracts are written with a legal tone, often in the third person.[63] From this perspective, a comparison between a contract and an oath leaves the contract wanting.

As doctors begin their careers in medicine, they are inducted with an oath, often the Hippocratic Oath. Oaths, in contradistinction to contracts, are always in the first person, and ask that the newly formed professional openly affirm a commitment to the profession, to patients, and to oneself. An oath is a solemn promise that makes physicians a part of a moral community.[64] It sets the profession apart in committing to something beyond self-interest. It is also a reminder of the continuity of the profession. As Swick et al. write: [63]

> We perceive the major difference between the Charter and the Hippocratic Oath to be the contractual nature of the Charter as opposed to the older, more cove-nantal model for the physician-patient relationship ... If a contract connotes a relationship of distrust, a covenant connotes a relationship of trust, even though both reflect a degree of commitment ... In a covenantal model, the physician's task is not to meet the minimum standards stipulated by a contract but rather to be worthy of trust, not to behave in a certain manner because one is constrained to do so but because one feels a genuine commitment to the values of an oath.

Although physicians of today share the core values espoused in the Hippocratic Oath with the healers of the past, the practice of medicine has changed dramatically in the last forty years. Physicians and their patients need to acknowledge these changes and openly discuss the impact that this has had on them and our profession. It should be expected that professionalism will continuously evolve as the health care system, societal needs and expectations, and each physician's needs and expectations change.

While the collective values of the profession evolve with changes in the wider society, individual physicians develop their professional values as they progress through the hierarchical career stages of medical school, residency, fellowship training, and then practice. All physicians have not had the same experiences, though. The medical profession is more diverse now than ever before. The demographic spread of the profession now includes recent graduates and physicians who trained fifty years ago. With each succeeding medical school class, the diversity of values and personal goals has also grown, reflecting the broader background from which the graduates come. It seems inevitable that this would result in significant generational differences in professional values. One area of tension has centered on the concept of altruism and physicians' quality of life. While there is an inherent conflict in the concept of altruism between self-interest and the patient's interests, some physicians in practice have viewed the younger generation's emphasis on the importance of quality of life issues as a perceived lack of commitment, particularly time commitment, to patient care. Although there are many similarities across the generations of physicians, the differences cannot be ignored if there is to be a continued identification with the profession. As Irvine notes, "medicine's professional values must be constantly negotiated with a changing society and with a changing cohort of members. For such negotiations to take place responsibly, however, new generations of physicians must learn professionalism."[65]

Keeping up with new medical information has always challenged physicians to be lifelong learners. In our electronic age, much more information is now also available to patients. This presents a new challenge to physicians as an increasing number of patients come to see their physician with their own medical suggestions and want to be more involved with decisions about their care. "Medicine is in transition from a predominantly doctor oriented culture to a patient centered culture of professional values founded on the principle of patient autonomy."[66] This is a change in the dynamic of the patient–physician relationship to which physicians trained in an earlier time need to adjust.

The patient–physician relationship is necessarily a fiduciary one, in which the imbalance of power between the two individuals requires a high level of trust.[67] This idea of fiduciary professionalism was first described by the eighteenth-century Scottish physician John Gregory.[67] He delineated three key elements: (1) physicians must accept the intellectual discipline of science to assure that their practice will be free of bias; (2) the primary consideration of the physician should be the protection and promotion of the patient's health; and (3) physicians should keep all forms of self-interest, economic and otherwise, systematically secondary.

Review of the Cases and Commentaries

As insurers and the government are increasingly involved in decisions regarding the care of patients, Gregory's second point – protecting and promoting the patient's health – has become more problematic. This is nicely illustrated in the adult primary care case of Spandorfer and Gordin on approved drug therapies, as well the commentary by Ecker and Campbell regarding the obstetric care of a high-risk patient. A poorly designed plan of care advocated by an insurer can lead to inappropriate use of tests, treatments, or procedures. It is very difficult for the physician when a program promotes and measures one action, but the patient's condition requires another. Physicians have a societal obligation to work to change any such system to keep the patient's need foremost. Hendrickson describes this process very compellingly: "Physicians must retain within the profession a sense of responsibility for critically evaluating new initiatives . . . and for constantly seeking the best ways to support each other in providing the highest-quality care to their patients and their communities."[67]

In describing the primacy of patient welfare, the Physician Charter notes, specifically, that "market forces, societal pressures, and administrative exigencies must not compromise this principle."[26] Counterbalancing these external influences must be the physician's commitment to altruism, a commitment that is central to the physician–patient relationship. Physicians are required in the course of the practice of medicine to ask very personal questions and to carry out invasive procedures. This can only be carried out in an atmosphere of trust and this trust will only be given if the patient believes that the physician is placing the patient's interest before their own.[58]

Although the concept of altruism is most often discussed as influencing how the physician will directly deal with his or her patients, there is also a more personal aspect for the physician. This is illustrated in the commentaries by Eaton and McFadden (see Chapter 2) about a first year medical student who has been ill but has not sought medical attention. One must have self-awareness and recognize one's own biases to be capable of looking out for the best interests of one's patients. How a physician reacts to his or her own vulnerability will no doubt affect the way that a patient in need is viewed. There is little doubt that the ill or stressed physician is not as likely to be sympathetic, caring, or attentive to patient needs. Doctors are human, with human foibles, including the susceptibility to illness and stress. If we want to be partners with our patients, and do the best job for them that we can, we need to recognize, and deal with, our own problems.

Self-awareness is one of the many areas of professional behavior that physicians must be careful to model for medical students and residents. Trainees will not learn that they should attend to their own well-being if they don't see their mentors behaving this way. Medical students and residents need to have opportunities to reflect on the link between their own well-being and their ability to sustain the capacity to truly care for others. The tension between the explicit and tacit values that students see encourages students to "objectify their patients and devalue their sensitivity."[68] All physicians need to develop and maintain their self-awareness to connect with, and respond to, their patients' experiences.

This theme is echoed in the case of the sleep-deprived student thoughtfully analyzed by Gould and Cook (see Chapter 2), but there are other themes that this case also illustrates. Patients want to be able to trust that their doctors are competent and caring. One of the assumptions made when physicians were granted privileges associated with a profession was that they would self-regulate quality. When the evidence became clear that a tired doctor, especially one still in training, was more likely to make mistakes, trying to minimize errors related to sleep deprivation became crucial. It has not been easy, in part because of the generational differences in expectations between doctors of different ages who are trained at different times. The message that being tired is to be expected and worked through is a part of the hidden curriculum.

Younger physicians are sometimes criticized by their older colleagues as unprofessional for taking into consideration personal lifestyle and balance in making career choices. The complaint is that they lack the intrinsic values necessary for the medical profession. The recent enactment of work hour regulations by the Accreditation Council for Graduate Medical Education has created a generational conflict. Smith points out that "baby boomer physicians, who 'thrived' in the old system, blame residents and students for the new regulations. They fail to acknowledge that society is deeply concerned about the harmful effects of long work hours and fatigue on making life and death decisions."[69] The risk is that physicians will blame residents for being less dedicated than they were/are. Smith also adds that "professionalism must be defined by the essential qualities (embrace being a physician, caring and altruistic, honesty and integrity, team player, strive for excellence, accept the duty for serving patients and society, courage and heroism) of a physician regardless of hours worked." Medical educators must stress that it is excellence that should be rewarded, not endurance.

In a social contract, there are rights and responsibilities for both physicians and the society as a whole. A large part of the tension that physicians now feel is due, in part, to what they perceive as their loss of autonomy. Autonomy was supposed to be one of those privileges granted to physicians in the social contract in exchange for their compassionate, high-quality care. As corporations and insurers have reined in the options in the physicians' armamentarium by restricting what they will pay for, physicians have sometimes felt that the only way that they could fight back was with deception. This is a counterproductive tactic, though, putting the physician on the slippery slope of not always being truthful. And such tactics may potentially open the door for charges of dishonesty. This is a time when doctors should take a stand for what they feel is in the best interest of their patients and recapture the trust that the public so desperately wants to place in their physicians. Although "deception may be a symptom of a flawed system, in which physicians are asked to implement financing policies that conflict with their primary obligation to the patient,"[70] it is a better course to work to change the system than to risk the good name of the profession. Such a course, once discovered, also invites increased oversight, and further compromises the autonomy of the physician. These points are also nicely exemplified in the case discussion by Spandorfer and Gordin on approved drug therapies, as well the commentary by Ecker and Campbell regarding the obstetric care of a high-risk patient.

Spandorfer and Gordin's case also illustrates an area of overlap between the principles of patient welfare and social justice. Physicians cannot ignore the cost of the diagnostic tests and treatment that they prescribe. It is a new age of accountability and given the huge amounts of money spent on health care, lack of attention to such factors opens the door to outside, non-provider intervention. Caution is advised, however. Cohen and Gabriel write,

> We should welcome the introduction of good business practices from the world of commerce. Such practices are essential if we wish to optimize the effectiveness of the care we provide, increase its safety, reduce its variability, and expand its reach. Where commercialism has no place, and professionalism must prevail, is in the value-laden domain of social justice and the sacred domain of the doctor-patient relationship.[71]

It would be preferable for the physician, if he or she really believes that the insurance company's algorithm for care is inappropriate, to work with them to change the recommendation.

The child abuse case, sensitively discussed by Lane and DeJong, has similarities to the case of the ill medical student, in that it asks that physicians to know themselves and their biases, their weaknesses and strengths. Patients assume that physicians will have the patient's best interest as their most important guide in making medical decisions. To maintain trust, this expectation must be met, even in situations that make the physician uncomfortable. Aristotle described the virtue of practical wisdom, or phronesis, as the capacity of deliberation and judgment and discernment in difficult moral situations.[72]

Teaching students this capacity is one of the jobs of a mentor. Aristotle also maintained that we learn by practice and the best way to learn virtue is to model a virtuous person. DeRosa[73] lists six virtues entailed by a professional commitment and the outcomes that actualize that commitment: (1) fidelity to trust; (2) benevolence; (3) intellectual honesty; (4) courage; (5) compassion; and (6) truthfulness. Making sure that a patient receives the care that they need sometimes requires all of these virtues, especially courage.

The second principle described in the Physician Charter,[26] patient autonomy, is a principle invoked in the case of the woman with depression carefully considered by Fochtman and Snyder. The principle of autonomy gives the patient the authority to make decisions about his or her own treatment as long as the care is appropriate and is in keeping with ethical practice. It also assumes that the patient is competent to make a decision about their care. Patients are able to exert their autonomy when their physician is honest with them and gives them enough information about their condition that they are able to make an informed decision about their treatment. Just as a physician expects that their autonomy be respected, so should they hold patient autonomy as a trust to be upheld whenever possible.

The case of the physician who has contracted an HIV infection, with insights by Schwartz and Wainapel, broadly illustrates nonmaleficence, the principle generally associated with the maxim primum non nocere, "above all, do no harm." If a physician has a condition that will put his patients at risk, he must disclose at the very least, and avoid (clinical) situations that put his patients at risk. This requires self-awareness of when this is appropriate and the conviction to do the right thing, even if the physician loses some of his or her prerogatives in the process. As Huddle concludes, "the bread and butter of morality in medicine is not in the 'hard cases' where the right way forward is difficult to see; it is acting rightly when the right path is clear before us but other pressing needs and desires pull us away from that path in the midst of day-to-day medical routine, under the often burdensome stresses of contemporary medical practice."[74] It is difficult to think of a moral principle that could be invoked to justify a physician's nondisclosure when faced with a high risk situation.

The case of the ill patient who presents to the emergency room for treatment when his own physician was not available, and the reflective discussion by Siebert and Kaplan, outlines a number of tensions that physicians may feel when they are caring for patients that may include factors such as the setting in which they practice and who pays them. In describing the primacy of patient welfare, the Physician Charter notes, specifically, that "market forces, societal pressures, and administrative exigencies must not compromise this principle."[26] The physician's commitment to altruism must act as a counter-balance against these external influences.

Conclusion

The concept of patient welfare has implications for the physician, the individual patient, and society at large. The commitments of each to the other are not static. They change as society and the role of the physician evolves. This chapter has described the evolution of some of the expectations inherent in a social contract. It also makes some suggestions about how future actions of members of the profession of medicine can help to shape the ongoing transformation of the physician–patient relationship.

Clara Callahan, M.D.
Lillian H. Brent Dean for Students
Jefferson Medical College

REFERENCES

1. Lanza FL. A guideline for the treatment and prevention of NSAID-induced ulcers. members of the ad hoc committee on practice parameters of the American College of Gastroenterology. *Am J Gastroenterol.* 1998;**93**(11):2037–2046.

2. Simon LS, Hatoum HT, Bittman RM, Archambault WT, Polisson RP. Risk factors for serious nonsteroidal-induced gastrointestinal complications: Regression analysis of the MUCOSA trial. *Fam Med.* 1996;**28**(3):204–210.

3. Feldman M, McMahon AT. Do cyclooxygenase-2 inhibitors provide benefits similar to those of traditional nonsteroidal anti-inflammatory drugs, with less gastrointestinal toxicity? *Ann Intern Med.* 2000;**132**(2):134–143.

4. The Kaiser Family Foundation and Health Research and Educational Trust. Health care marketplace project. 2006.

5. Fischer MA, Schneeweiss S, Avorn J, Solomon DH. Medicaid prior-authorization programs and the use of cyclooxygenase-2 inhibitors. *N Engl J Med.* 2004;**351**(21):2187–2194.

6. Roughead EE, Zhang F, Ross-Degnan D, Soumerai S. Differential effect of early or late implementation of prior authorization policies on the use of COX II inhibitors. *Med Care.* 2006;**44**(4):378–382.

7. Smith C, Cowan C, Heffler S, Catlin A. National health spending in 2004: Recent slowdown led by prescription drug spending. *Health Aff (Millwood).* 2006;**25**(1):186–196.

8. Heffler S, Smith S, Keehan S, Borger C, Clemens MK, Truffer C.U.S. Health spending projections for 2004–2014. *Health Aff (Millwood).* 2005;Suppl Web Exclusives:W5–74-W5–85.

9. Cox ER, Motheral B, Frisse M, Behm A, Mager D. Prescribing COX-2s for patients new to cyclo-oxygenase inhibition therapy. *Am J Manag Care.* 2003;**9**(11):735–742.

10. *Assessment of Risk Factors for Preterm Birth. ACOG Practice Bulletin #31.* Washington, D.C.: American College of Obstetricians and Gynecologists; 2001.

11. Iams JD, Goldenberg RL, Meis PJ, et al. The length of the cervix and the risk of spontaneous premature delivery. National institute of child health and human development maternal fetal medicine unit network. *N Engl J Med.* 1996;**334**(9):567–572.

12. Berghella V, Odibo AO, To MS, Rust OA, Althuisius SM. Cerclage for short cervix on ultrasonography: Meta-analysis of trials using individual patient-level data. *Obstet Gynecol.* 2005;**106**(1):181–189.

13. Sosa C, Althabe F, Belizan J, Bergel E. Bed rest in singleton pregnancies for preventing preterm birth. *Cochrane Database Syst Rev.* 2004;(1)(1):CD003581.

14. Thomas SA, Rosenfield NS, Leventhal JM, Markowitz RI. Long-bone fractures in young children: Distinguishing accidental injuries from child abuse. *Pediatrics.* 1991;**88**(3):471–476.

15. Ludwig S. Child abuse. In: Fleisher GR, Ludwis S, Henretig FM, Ruddy RM, Silverman BK, eds. *Textbook of Pediatric Emergency Medicine.* 5th ed. Philadelphia, PA: Lippincott, Williams, and Wilkins; 2005.

16. McDonald KC. Child abuse: Approach and management. *Am Fam Physician.* 2007;**75**(2):221–228.

17. Leventhal JM. The challenges of recognizing child abuse: Seeing is believing. *JAMA.* 1999;**281**(7):657–659.

18. Sirotnak AP, Grigsby T, Krugman RD. Physical abuse of children. *Pediatr Rev.* 2004;**25**(8):264–277.

19. Kellogg ND, American Academy of Pediatrics Committee on Child Abuse and Neglect. Evaluation of suspected child physical abuse. *Pediatrics*. 2007;**119**(6): 1232–1241.

20. Hudson M, Kaplan R. Clinical response to child abuse. *Pediatr Clin North Am*. 2006;**53**(1):27–39, v.

21. American Psychiatric Association. *Practice of Electroconvulsive Therapy: Recommendations for Treatment, Training and Privileging*. 2nd ed. American Psychiatric Press; 2001.

22. Greenhalgh J, Knight C, Hind D, Beverley C, Walters S. Clinical and cost-effectiveness of electroconvulsive therapy for depressive illness, schizophrenia, catatonia and mania: Systematic reviews and economic modelling studies. *Health Technol Assess*. 2005;**9**(9):1–156, iii–iv.

23. Dowman J, Patel A, Rajput K. Electroconvulsive therapy: Attitudes and misconceptions. *J ECT*. 2005;**21**(2):84–87.

24. Marshall T, Solomon P. Professionals' responsibilities in releasing information to families of adults with mental illness. *Psychiatr Serv*. 2003;**54**(12):1622–1628.

25. Lapid MI, Rummans TA, Pankratz VS, Appelbaum PS. Decisional capacity of depressed elderly to consent to electroconvulsive therapy. *J Geriatr Psychiatry Neurol*. 2004;**17**(1):42–46.

26. ABIM Foundation. American Board of Internal Medicine, ACP-ASIM Foundation. American College of Physicians-American Society of Internal Medicine, European Federation of Internal Medicine. Medical professionalism in the new millennium: A physician charter. *Ann Intern Med*. 2002;**136**(3):243–246.

27. Snyder L, Leffler C, Ethics and Human Rights Committee, American College of Physicians. Ethics manual: Fifth edition. *Ann Intern Med*. 2005;**142**(7):560–582.

28. Levine C, Zuckerman C. The trouble with families: Toward an ethic of accommodation. *Ann Intern Med*. 1999;**130**(2):148–152.

29. Back AL, Arnold RM. Dealing with conflict in caring for the seriously ill: "It was just out of the question". *JAMA*. 2005;**293**(11):1374–1381.

30. Reitsma AM, Closen ML, Cunningham M, et al. Infected physicians and invasive procedures: Safe practice management. *Clin Infect Dis*. 2005;**40**(11):1665–1672.

31. Beauchamp TL, Childress JF. Nonmaleficence. In: *Principles of Biomedical Ethics*. 5th ed. New York: Oxford Univ Press; 2001:113–117.

32. Berguer R, Heller PJ. Strategies for preventing sharps injuries in the operating room. *Surg Clin North Am*. 2005;**85**(6):1299–305, xiii.

33. ACS Task Force on Professionalism. Code of professional conduct. *J Am Coll Surg*. 2004;**199**(5):734–735.

34. Russi M.HIV and AIDS in the workplace. *J Occup Environ Med*. 2002;**44**(6): 495–502.

35. Esposito TJ, Rotondo M, Barie PS, Reilly P, Pasquale MD. Making the case for a paradigm shift in trauma surgery. *J Am Coll Surg*. 2006;**202**(4):655–667.

36. Wainapel SF. The physically disabled physician. *JAMA*. 1987;**257**(21):2935–2938.

37. Wainapel SF. A clash of cultures: Reflections of a physician with a disability. *Lancet*. 1999;**354**(9180):763–764.

38. Lewis SB. The physically handicapped physician. In: **Callan JP,** ed. *The Physician: A Professional Under Stress.* Norwalk, CT: Appleton-Century-Crofts; 1983:318–326.

39. Fine MJ, Smith MA, Carson CA, et al. Prognosis and outcomes of patients with community-acquired pneumonia: A meta-analysis. *JAMA.* 1996;**275**(2):134–141.

40. Farr BM. Prognosis and decisions in pneumonia. *N Engl J Med.* 1997;**336**(4): 288–289.

41. Kruse RL, Mehr DR, Boles KE, et al. Does hospitalization impact survival after lower respiratory infection in nursing home residents? *Med Care.* 2004;**42**(9): 860–870.

42. Fine MJ, Auble TE, Yealy DM, et al. A prediction rule to identify low-risk patients with community-acquired pneumonia. *N Engl J Med.* 1997;**336**(4):243– 250.

43. Fisher R, Ury W. Getting to yes: Negotiating agreement without giving in. 1981.

44. Hurst SA, Slowther AM, Forde R, et al. Prevalence and determinants of physician bedside rationing: Data from Europe. *J Gen Intern Med.* 2006;**21**(11):1138–1143.

45. Schwappach DL, Koeck CM. Preferences for disclosure: The case for bedside rationing. *Soc Sci Med.* 2004;**59**(9):1891–1897.

46. Metlay JP, Kapoor WN, Fine MJ. Does this patient have community-acquired pneumonia? Diagnosing pneumonia by history and physical examination. *JAMA.* 1997;**278**(17):1440–1445.

47. Metlay JP, Fine MJ. Testing strategies in the initial management of patients with community-acquired pneumonia. *Ann Intern Med.* 2003;**138**(2):109–118.

48. http://www.mdcalc.com. Accessed August 21, 2008.

49. U.S. Department of Health and Human Services Web site. http://www.pda. ahrq.gove. Accessed August 21, 2008.

50. Mandell LA, Wunderink RG, Anzueto A, et al. Infectious diseases society of America/American Thoracic Society consensus guidelines on the management of community-acquired pneumonia in adults. *Clin Infect Dis.* 2007;**44** Suppl. 2:S27–72.

51. American College of Emergency Physicians. Clinical policy for the management and risk stratification of community-acquired pneumonia in adults in the emergency department. *Ann Emerg Med.* 2001;**38**(1):107–113.

52. Arnold FW, Ramirez JA, McDonald LC, Xia EL. Hospitalization for community-acquired pneumonia: The pneumonia severity index vs clinical judgment. *Chest.* 2003;**124**(1):121–124.

53. Dremsizov T, Clermont G, Kellum JA, Kalassian KG, Fine MJ, Angus DC. Severe sepsis in community-acquired pneumonia: When does it happen, and do systemic inflammatory response syndrome criteria help predict course? *Chest.* 2006;**129**(4):968–978.

54. Lim WS, van der Eerden MM, Laing R, et al. Defining community acquired pneumonia severity on presentation to hospital: An international derivation and validation study. *Thorax.* 2003;**58**(5):377–382.

55. Beauchamp TL, McCullough LB. *Medical Ethics: The Moral Responsibilities of Physicians.* Englewood Cliffs, NJ: Prentice-Hall, Inc; 1984.

56. Cruess SR, Cruess RL. Professionalism: A contract between medicine and society. *CMAJ*. 2000;**162**(5):668–669.

57. Gough JW. *The Social Contract: A Critical Study of Its Development*. Oxford, England: The Clarendon Press; 1957.

58. Cruess SR. Professionalism and medicine's social contract with society. *Clin Orthop Relat Res*.2006;**449**:170–176.

59. Starr P. *The Social Transformation of American Medicine*. New York: Basic Books; 1984.

60. Cruess RL, Cruess SR, Johnston SE. Renewing professionalism: An opportunity for medicine. *Acad Med*. 1999;**74**(8):878–884.

61. Blendon RJ, Altman DE, Benson JM, et al. Voters and health reform in the 2008 presidential election. *N Engl J Med*. 2008;**359**(19):2050–2061.

62. Obama B. Modern health care for all Americans. *N Engl J Med*. 2008;**359**(15): 1537–1541.

63. Swick HM, Bryan CS, Longo LD. Beyond the physician charter: Reflections on medical professionalism. *Perspect Biol Med*. 2006;**49**(2):263–275.

64. Pellegrino ED. The medical profession as a moral community. *Bull N Y Acad Med*. 1990;**66**(3):221–232.

65. Irvine D. The performance of doctors. I: Professionalism and self regulation in a changing world. *BMJ*. 1997;**314**(7093):1540–1542.

66. Johnston S. See one, do one, teach one: Developing professionalism across the generations. *Clin Orthop Relat Res*. 2006;**449**:186–192.

67. Hendrickson MA. Pay for performance and medical professionalism. *Qual Manag Health Care*. 2008;**17**(1):9–18.

68. Coulehan J. Viewpoint: Today's professionalism: Engaging the mind but not the heart. *Acad Med*. 2005;**80**(10):892–898.

69. Smith LG. Medical professionalism and the generation gap. *Am J Med*. 2005; **118**(4):439–442.

70. Bogardus ST Jr, Geist DE, Bradley EH. Physicians' interactions with third-party payers: Is deception necessary? *Arch Intern Med*. 2004;**164**(17):1841–1844.

71. Cohen JJ, Gabriel BA. "Not just another business": Medicine's struggle to preserve professionalism in a commercialized world. *Obstet Gynecol*. 2002;**100**(1):168–169.

72. Barnes J, ed. *The Complete Works of Aristotle: The Revised Oxford Translation*. Princeton, NJ: Bollingen; 1984; No. 2.

73. DeRosa GP. Professionalism and virtues. *Clin Orthop Relat Res*.2006;**449**:28–33.

74. Huddle TS, Accreditation Council for Graduate Medical Education (ACGME). Viewpoint: Teaching professionalism: Is medical morality a competency? *Acad Med*. 2005;**80**(10):885–891.

Principle of Patient Autonomy

Cases and Commentaries

An eighty-seven-year-old man wants prostate cancer screening despite his family physician's recommendation that such screening is not warranted. He has not had any change in urinary symptoms over the past five years. His past medical history is significant for chronic atrial fibrillation, hypertension, and advanced osteoarthritis. His medications include warfarin, diltiazem and acetaminophen. He has no family history of prostate cancer.

A Perspective from a General Internist

Clinical Background

Screening for prostate cancer is done through palpation during a digital rectal examination (DRE) and measurement of the level of prostate specific antigen (PSA) in blood serum. Digital rectal examination allows for palpation of only a portion of the prostate gland. PSA measurement is used to augment the digital rectal examination in screening. PSA levels are known to rise as the prostate volume increases, even in the absence of cancer. The recommendations for initiation and frequency of prostate cancer screening are controversial. The presence of new urinary or sexual symptoms should prompt an evaluation to exclude the presence of prostate cancer.

Further testing for prostate cancer takes place if the DRE is abnormal with marked asymmetry, presence of a nodule or nodules, or a hard consistency. PSA levels that are within the normal range but rise more rapidly than expected are also an indication for further testing. A PSA level outside of the normal range in the absence of prostate infection leads to further testing as well.

The additional testing might include transrectal ultrasound of the prostate with prostate biopsy. If prostate cancer is diagnosed, a staging evaluation with a computerized tomogram of the abdomen and pelvis is done. Disease felt to be localized to the prostate can be treated with surgical excision (prostatectomy either through transabdominal or laparoscopic/robotic method), external beam radiation, or radiation seed implantation.

Prostate biopsies can have false negative results due to sampling error. Risks of biopsy include pain, bleeding, infection, and nerve damage. The risks of treatment for prostate cancer include those of biopsy, but also erectile dysfunction and urinary incontinence, and, in the case of radiation, gastrointestinal side effects.

Professionalism Considerations

It is expected that physicians will work with patients to prevent disease and promote early detection to decrease morbidity and mortality. Many cancer screenings – such as colonoscopy for colon cancer – show a survival benefit in early detection. The benefits of screening for prostate cancer in elderly men are less clear. The reasons for the lack of clarity include the facts that most of these cancers are slow growing and the patient is more likely to die from conditions other than prostate cancer. Also the morbidity from the evaluation and treatment process is not insignificant.

Physicians have an obligation to provide informed consent to the patient[1] and to follow the patient's wishes if the patient has capacity and their wishes are reasonable. Even if the patient's wishes are not what the physician would choose, they should be followed. In the situation described, the physician should explain the process of prostate cancer screening and discuss the scenarios regarding abnormal findings. After this is done, the physician should review the further diagnostic studies and the treatment options that the patient may face. At this time, one would need to be sure that the patient has capacity and understands the implications of proceeding with screening. Cultural sensitivity about perceptions when discussing PSA testing is important.[2]

It is also important for the physician to understand why the patient wants the screening. Some patients may state that they would want to be diagnosed and treated as aggressively as possible while others may simply want to know "the likelihood they have cancer" for their own piece of mind and may have no intention of pursuing treatment. The patient's reasoning for screening/testing may indicate gaps in knowledge that the physician should address.

The physician is well aware that if the patient has an elevated PSA, many tests, treatments, and potential complications might very well follow. The patient would also need to know all of this information. In this case, the patient's atrial fibrillation and anticoagulation would add a complexity and risk to the process, for if biopsies were indicated, stopping the anticoagulation and administering interim anticoagulation would be needed.

Opinion

Before proceeding with DRE and PSA measurement, the physician should review with the patient the fact that the absence of new urinary symptoms lowers the probability that aggressive prostate cancer exists in this elderly man. Noting that 25 per cent of men in their seventies will have an elevated PSA is important information to share.[3] Description of the additional steps that would be needed to obtain a biopsy – given his atrial fibrillation and anticoagulation – should follow, along with treatment issues previously outlined. The lack of clarity that early detection has a benefit in mortality should also be emphasized.[4] It is appropriate for the physician to verbalize his/her opinion about the utility of the screening. The physician can recommend against screening if that is his/her belief, while reinforcing that the physician will continue to provide care, guide, and refer as indicated. The physician should not refuse to do the testing if this is the patient's ultimate wish.

David Lambert, M.D.
Senior Associate Dean for Medical Student Education
University of Rochester School of Medicine and Dentistry

A Perspective from a Bioethicist

This case presents a conflict between clinical judgment about what is in the patient's best interest and patient autonomy, or the freedom to make one's own decisions regarding medical care. In general, patients do have the right to make their own decisions about medical care. However, there are a few key exceptions that limit that right. Respecting patient autonomy is just one professional commitment. It is tempered by other commitments, including providing quality care and acting in the patient's best interest (patient welfare). If a patient is making a decision that the physician believes is life threatening, either for the patient or others, the physician can and should intervene.[5] Serious conflicts arise when a patient disagrees with the physician about what is in the patient's best interest. Judgments about patient welfare are always a matter of values and interpretation, not objective evidence alone. For example, some cancer patients legitimately opt out of surgery or further treatment even if it means shortening their lives in favor of enhancing the quality of life they have remaining.

One further condition for respecting patient autonomy is assuring that patients are making choices that are voluntary and with full understanding of the issues. Rather than taking patient preferences at face value, they should be explored. In this current case, we do not yet know what the patient understands about prostate cancer screening and the likelihood that he will benefit from it. Culturally, we are inundated with messages about the importance of cancer screening and prevention.[6] It is understandable that a gentleman would come into a clinical visit with a preference for screening. Indeed, select screening patterns suggest that the majority of men receive PSA testing[7] and, in one population-based survey, 67 percent of men over eighty-five believed their physician recommended screening.[8] As Dr. Lambert describes in his commentary, the physician should be up-front with the patient about the real likelihood of having an elevated PSA at age eighty-seven and the potential for complications from doing the follow-up tests.

The physician may feel that he is actually jeopardizing patient welfare or misusing resources if he goes along with the patient's preference to screen. The U.S. Preventive Services Task Force guidelines promote informed decision making and support men making their own choices in the case of prostate cancer screening, largely because the evidence does not provide clear direction.[9]

The guidelines do suggest an appropriate stopping point for screening, stating that men with less than ten years of life expectancy are the least likely to benefit. Is it important for this man to understand his overall prognosis? It has been argued that honest conversations with patients about what to expect with their illnesses are difficult for physicians emotionally and practically and because prognosis is difficult to predict.[10] Clinical probabilities do not specifically predict a single individual's life expectancy as many patient stories affirm.[11] The physician's obligation in this case could be more focused on the need to assure the patient is making an informed decision to move forward with screening, rather than having an obligation to not administer an inappropriate test. This physician faces the communication challenge of maintaining a good relationship with the patient while being honest with him and striving to achieve best practices.

The crux of this dialogue is to assure that the patient is making an informed choice. A good starting point for that discussion is to understand the patient's position – what is his perception of his current health status and his prospects for the future? What expectations or concerns does he have regarding prostate cancer and prostate cancer screening? If the decision-making discussion can start with an exploration, the physician is in a much better position to meet the patient appropriately, and either rectify misunderstandings or affirm appropriate concerns and offer guidance for alternative ways of holding those fears at bay.[12]

Once the patient's position is better understood, the physician can share his or her thinking with the patient in a process Howard Brody describes as "transparency."[13] Rather than needing to give an exhaustive analysis of the existing data and current controversies with testing, the physician need only provide enough access to what is informing his or her thinking about the preferred decision to not screen at this time. By sharing one's thinking, the physician can be honest with the patient without being confrontational. After checking in again – "Does what I am saying make sense to you? What are you thinking about now, given what I have just said?" – the physician can ask for a decision from the patient, which may even be to simply postpone the test for now until he has had more of a chance to consider his options and the implications of his choices. Offering postponement of the decision as one of the alternatives can be helpful. With this as an option, the patient is less likely to feel this is a forced choice situation. Realistically, this patient will be returning to see the physician soon enough for monitoring of his other chronic conditions allowing an opportunity for further discussion.

In summary, this case presents what appears to be a classic conflict between patient autonomy and the duty to provide quality of care. However, on closer examination, I argue that this case should be viewed as an opportunity to be honest with the patient and have a forthcoming and exploratory discussion with him about what his hopes and fears are for the remaining years of his life. While not easy, and certainly not done in the space of a ten- or fifteen-minute visit, these conversations are worth having and we all (family members, friends, and professional contacts) would do well to create the opportunities for them.

Kelly Fryer-Edwards, Ph.D.
Associate Professor
Department of Bioethics and Humanities
University of Washington School of Medicine

PATIENT AUTONOMY – ONCOLOGY

A forty-nine-year-old woman with stage 2 breast cancer (3 cm tumor with no lymph node involvement) and a lumpectomy two months ago wants to discontinue all treatment (radiation, chemotherapy) for her cancer and begin "alternative medicine" treatments in Mexico.

A Perspective from a Family and Palliative Care Physician

Clinical Background

The choices and decision making faced by a forty-nine-year-old woman with stage 2 breast cancer are complex and often bewildering.[14] In this vignette, the patient has already made decisions regarding diagnosis and staging surgery, lumpectomy, mastectomy, sentinel node dissection or axillary lymph node dissection; radiation therapy, and adjuvant therapy which may include chemotherapy, hormonal therapy, or monoclonal antibodies depending on tumor type.

These treatment options are not without significant side effects. Healing from surgery entails pain and discomfort, some disfigurement of the breast, and the possibility of lymphedema. Following radiation, the breast tissue may be somewhat firmer than non-irradiated tissue. Systemic adjuvant therapy, especially chemotherapy, has frequent side effects including nausea, vomiting, hair loss, fatigue and menstrual irregularities, to name a few.

Beyond these physical side effects, women in treatment for breast cancer may experience many other effects. Dealing with the uncertainty of the outcomes is by itself very stressful. The woman and her whole family are affected. The energy for caring for children may be affected; decisions around what to tell the children are challenging. Effects on her sexuality and the relationship with her partner may also be issues. The American Cancer Society (ACS) has recognized the challenges that women in this situation face and much more effort has recently gone into supportive care for women in treatment. The ACS also recognizes that many women seek complementary care "along with mainstream medical care" or alternative "instead of standard medical treatments" at this time.[15]

Professionalism Considerations

As a physician, when your patient wants to discontinue standard medical therapy, one usually begins by asking, "Why?" We know that reasons women may give include difficulty with the side effects of treatment or mistrust of Western medicine or their practitioner.[16] It is an opportunity for the physician to reflect on how supportive he/she and the team have been. Conceivably this could be a cry for help, "You're not listening to me and I really need to get your attention." Each concern needs to be sensitively explored with the patient. Statements such as "I am really committed to providing the best care to you. Could you help me understand why you are making this decision?" may be helpful openers. A physician could even acknowledge, "Sometimes our patients want to stop treatment because they feel unsupported. Is there anything we could do to make you feel better?"

Once it is established that there are no reversible factors in the patient's decision, a physician must consider whether the patient is making an informed refusal of treatment. This process entails revisiting the patient's understanding and appreciation of the risks and benefits of the treatment you are offering. This may also be an opportunity to review whether other less toxic treatments might be offered instead.

The ACS suggests some questions that patients may consider in making their decisions about alternative therapy that may identify dangerous treatments:

- Is the treatment based on an unproven theory?
- Does the treatment promise a cure for all cancers?
- Do the promoters tell you not to use regular medical treatment?
- Is the treatment or drug a secret that only certain people can give?
- Does the treatment require that you travel to another country?
- Do the promoters attack the medical or scientific establishment?[15]

In discussing these questions, we may unearth a significant difference in values. Our medical culture values rationality in decision making and views the scientific paradigm as paramount. Not all of our patients share these values. Some patients may find comfort in anecdotal accounts of success and find our detached statistics difficult to fathom and frankly overwhelming. While we may present information in different ways – on paper, with words, with graphs, online – we do tend to insist that patients accept our values. Some patients however prefer to follow advice from a trusted friend, or a relative with a "miracle cure."

The challenge then becomes how to support a patient with a "nonscientific" viewpoint. Supporting patient autonomy includes supporting decisions that we may consider unwise or different than our own. It may be tempting to fall into a more paternalistic role, to argue strongly against the patient's wishes or use fear to coerce the patient into changing her mind. It may even be difficult not to feel angry towards the patient.

One way through these challenges is to move away from trying to get the patient to see the situation through our eyes, and to truly see it from the patient's perspective. This struggle will likely be seen by the patient as a sign of our caring. This caring goes far in building trust in the doctor–patient relationship, which is built on so much more than our expertise. With trust, the patient may reconsider what we have to say. If the patient only feels that we are reacting to having our authority and viewpoint challenged, she may not be as sympathetic.

Opinion

Supporting a patient who is making a decision to stop traditional therapy, which offers an evidence-based and potentially good outcome, for alternative therapy, which has little or no evidence base, is difficult. Our patient may be making a decision irrationally. In such a case, using more rationality is unlikely to be helpful. I believe that forming a partnership with the patient to meet her needs is more likely to result in the patient listening to the physician's view. A good option is to offer to monitor her progress and resume care if she does not meet with success. The public are clear that they prefer their health practitioners to work together and are interested in "integrative health" where they don't have to choose one approach over another.[17] They may also prefer to make decisions we don't agree with.

Monica Branigan M.D., MHSc (Bioethics)
Family Physician in Palliative Care
St Joseph's Health Center, Toronto, Canada

A Perspective from a Medical Humanities Scholar

This case is notable in that there is, strictly, no doctor here at all. The case describes the patient and her decision making – or, to be exact, what she wants. It leaves the reader to infer or imagine a place for the physician. This absence is especially significant where the central problem is a patient's apparent desire to remove allopathic medicine, and by implication its practitioner, from her life. The case raises questions about appropriate professional deportment in the face of an implicit rejection of the values of the profession itself.

The case raises the difficult but not uncommon predicament of acknowledging, evaluating, and helping manage patients' use of non-allopathic therapeutic paradigms. More fundamentally, though, it also leads us to explore the implications of respecting patient autonomy: At what point must the physician reassert professional authority? What happens when a patient's apparently autonomous choice is to make the physician disappear? How does this affect the patient's identity as patient and the doctor's identity as doctor?

But before we allow the physician to be erased by the patient's disclosure that she wants to become the patient of a different kind of medicine, we (and the physician) must be careful to establish the precise motivation behind her announcement.

The case tells us a little about the patient. She is middle-aged and female. Her cancer at diagnosis was somewhat advanced, but not hopelessly so. She consented to and underwent surgery, a relatively conservative lumpectomy and not a mastectomy. The word "discontinue" suggests she has begun radiation and chemotherapy but now wants to stop. We must speculate – as will her physician – about what has made her change her mind. We wonder about earlier conversations. How were her diagnosis and her treatment options presented to her? Did her doctor minimize the suffering and inconvenience that would ensue? Did the patient begin the treatment assuming no viable alternative, all the while fearing there was little hope of benefit? How much trust did she feel when she made earlier decisions? Was the information on which she based her initial decisions appropriately tailored to her particular life situation and values, as well as to the type and stage of her cancer? And what has changed since then?

Answers to these questions will help clarify the meaning of her present decision – if it is in fact a decision at all. Is she simply putting him on notice that she is leaving or is she asking for advice, support, reassurance, or permission to explore other modalities while continuing as his patient? She may fear that seeking alternative treatment constitutes some unforgiveable infidelity to the medicine in which she has, till now, placed her faith. In the face of a potentially lethal disease, questions of faith and belief, which some may see as superstitious, are not irrelevant. The patient's life may be at stake. The information and values underpinning her autonomy as a patient have never needed as much reinforcement and support as they do now.

The physician, then, must take great care not to jump to conclusions about her motivation and intentions, even if he feels defensive in the face of this most radical challenge patient autonomy can pose to a physician's sense of professional authority. The patient, faltering in her own will to tolerate a taxing course of treatment, may be presenting the Mexican alternative not as an announcement but as a test of the doctor's faith. His response, then, requires a fine balance between respect for her right to self-determination and confidence in the authority of the medical paradigm in which he practices.

The physician needs to find a way to respect the patient even though he may feel that she is expressing disrespect for his work, ingratitude for his help, even infidelity to this patient–physician relationship. He must avoid belittling or trivializing her interest in alternatives, but he must also retain the authority of his own professional expertise. He must tread the line between paternalism and resignation.

This is not a simple matter. Expansive openness to alternatives can lead to profound and dangerous contradictions in the rationales behind treatment. Patient autonomy is based in informed consent, and being informed assumes (perhaps optimistically) a degree of understanding and acceptance of the fundamental scientific and philosophical assumptions underlying the treatment consented to. Some have argued that belief – "buying into" the meaning of the treatment – can make a difference to its efficacy and tolerability. A loosely open-minded physician, who simply encourages her to continue radiation or chemotherapy while she expands her search, without his involvement, for cure or relief to other health care paradigms, might in fact further diminish the patient's flagging confidence in her current course of treatment.

The professional test here is that of fidelity – and therefore attention – to the patient even in the face of this apparent vote of no confidence. The physician needs to begin by inviting the patient to provide a detailed account of the story that underlies her announcement. Setting aside defensiveness, the physician must listen for her reasons and her beliefs. By presenting her plans, perhaps as an ultimatum to her doctor, the patient may be exercising her right to autonomy at a time when the cancer and its current treatment have made her feel disempowered and trapped. To take her at her word without exploring further may be a kind of abandonment, for there is more at stake here than treating the disease. The physician must be a precise and insightful interpreter of the patient's words – and also of what she has not (yet) put into words. Then he must collaborate with her in plotting out the next part of her story, whether or not he will be included as a character in it. In this way his authority as a physician will no longer be tied to her compliance as a patient, but instead to her autonomy as a person.

Catherine Belling, Ph.D.
Assistant Professor, Medical Humanities and Bioethics
Northwestern University Feinberg School of Medicine

PATIENT AUTONOMY – NEPHROLOGY

An eighty-three-year-old widow with known progressive renal failure and depression, who signed a living will several years ago stipulating that she does not desire dialysis or other aggressive interventions at the end of life, is admitted in uremic coma. The patient's only child comes from another state and demands that dialysis be started.

A Perspective from a Hospitalist

Clinical Background

Uremic coma is the advanced stage of metabolic encephalopathy associated with renal insufficiency. Early symptoms of uremic encephalopathy often include memory disturbance, agitation, and confusion. As azotemia worsens, these symptoms progress to the profound alteration in consciousness classified as coma.

We know that this patient has progressive kidney disease. The encephalopathy likely indicates her renal function has now declined to levels associated with end stage renal disease. Alternatively, this patient may have suffered a new renal insult, with acute renal failure superimposed on her chronic renal disorder. In either case, the encephalopathy is a marker for significant renal dysfunction, and the only successful treatment at this time would be initiation of dialysis. Indeed, uremic encephalopathy is one of the absolute indications for the initiation of dialysis.[18]

Professionalism Considerations

Before instituting any therapy, one must consider the risks and benefits specific to the individual patient, as well as the impact of the therapy on the patient's quality of life. Moreover, this information must be presented to the patient as she makes decisions about the planned treatment. The immediate benefit of dialysis in this case would be the amelioration of the encephalopathy. However, balanced with this must be the fact that dialysis is one of the most demanding therapies of any offered by modern medicine. An important change in lifestyle associated with dialysis relates to the multiple treatment sessions per week. Older patients typically choose hemodialysis, which is scheduled for three to five hours, three times per week. Consideration of a treatment's impact on quality of life should also include expected symptoms associated with that therapy. For dialysis patients common symptoms include pain, fatigue, and sleep disturbance.[19]

It is also important to review the expected prognosis with a patient. Comprehensive statistics for patients with kidney disease are available, and these statistics can be striking for patients who are considering dialysis. Based on 2004 data, a woman her age would spend an average of sixteen days in the hospital per year in addition to the regular outpatient dialysis treatments. The survival statistics are quite sobering in this patient's demographic group. A 2003 study found the one year survival rate for a dialysis patient eighty years old or more to be 59.2 percent. The five year survival rate for this group is only 8.4 percent.[20]

Thus, the decision to begin dialysis, based only on absolute and relative indications, is not always a straightforward one. This step must be made in concert with an informed patient. Age, other medical conditions, and quality of life are necessary factors to consider in the decision-making process. It is probable that this patient was presented these facts when she decided to forgo dialysis in her advanced directive.

The issue here is the conflict between this patient's prior wishes to decline dialysis and her daughter's current demands that this therapy be started. Can a patient's closest living relative overrule an advanced directive when the patient is not able to voice her current preferences?

The ethical principle central to this dilemma is the respect for patient autonomy. This encompasses "a person's right to hold views, make choices and take actions based on personal values and beliefs."[21] An important aspect of patient autonomy is the process of informed consent or informed refusal. The latter applies to this case. In denying future dialysis in her advanced directive, the patient has used her right of informed refusal. And by preparing an advanced directive, the patient has exercised her autonomy and provided an answer to the question of whether or not she would want dialysis.

As the closest living relative, the patient's daughter would be legally granted status as a substitute decision maker to assist in making decisions of consent or refusal for the patient. However, there are important criteria that guide substitute decision making. One, that the patient must currently lack the capacity to make a medical decision, is met in this case. A second important stipulation is that the patient's wishes for a given medical decision are unknown. Here, the patient's advanced directive states her wishes regarding dialysis, and so this specific decision does not need to be made in consultation with a substitute.

It is important to address the daughter's emotional well-being as one assists in such an ethically charged situation. Indeed, acknowledging her feelings and concerns will be as helpful as any other action. Many families also benefit from consultation with pastoral care services as they face a loved one's terminal illness and discuss end-of-life decisions. The patient's daughter should be offered this option.

This physician must also explain the ethical conflict that would ensue if dialysis was begun in a kind, non-judgmental manner. It would be useful to review the advanced directive and reinforce that the patient herself asked not to have this invasive therapy. As part of this process, it is equally important for one to explore the reasons why the daughter is requesting that dialysis be started. This discussion will help the health care team better assist the daughter in coping. If the daughter still demands this treatment, an important option would be to consult with the ethics committee of the institution for further guidance.

Opinion

It is not ethically appropriate to begin dialysis for this patient. The patient's daughter cannot overrule the patient's previously stated wishes. She cannot be a surrogate for this important decision, since the decision has already been made directly by the patient. In ethical terms, overruling the advanced directive would be a violation of this patient's right to refuse treatment and her autonomy.

John Caruso, M.D.
Associate Professor of Medicine, Assistant Dean for Graduate
Medical Education and Affiliations
Jefferson Medical College

A Perspective from a Bioethicist

At the level of rules and principles, the ethics of this case are simple: We should act in accordance with the patient's informed preferences, as best we can determine them. And failing that, we should do what will benefit her the most, or at least inflict the least harm and suffering.

Of course, this answer hides a host of complexities. Does a statement made several years ago, in other medical, psychological and social circumstances, apply now? Did her refusal of dialysis apply only to the "end of life?" Assuming this, how confident are we that her current medical condition qualifies? And what about this daughter? Why is she asking that dialysis be started? Is she thinking dialysis can stave off death indefinitely or only hoping for a chance to say goodbye? What does she think her mother would want, and what reasons does she have for thinking it?

Different answers to these questions will lead us toward different decisions about what to do. A plan of action is required but just as important is how we decide what to do, and what professional and personal qualities and virtues we bring to the task. Thinking she is most concerned with her own needs, we might respond to the daughter's request in a brusque and imperious way, drawing a firm line, and refusing to consider anything other than what the living will clearly stipulates.

This response lacks compassion. We have to be open to the possibility that it is really the daughter's grief and fear of losing her mother at the root of this request; we will see beyond her words only if we have genuine concern for her as a fellow human being. We need to be moved by her grief, to console her and to be gentle with her, even if we're convinced that we should not do as she asks.

It's this compassion, not standing on the principle of substituted judgment, which will lead us to frame the decision in a way that acknowledges the daughter's need, rather than confronts it. "I know you love your mother, and don't want her to die. We don't want her to die either. But we're at the point where there's little we can do to stop her dying that's not going to make her last days worse for her. I don't want that for her, and I don't think you do either."

The imperious response carries another vice, as well – the moral certainty that comes from a lack of imagination, about many things. What are the daughter's needs that are driving this demand? Hatred and revenge, love and need for amends, hope for a few last words, emotional dependence?

These aren't equal and each needs to be handled in a different way in order to get to the right decision. What's more, we need the imagination to see that the daughter is most likely not motivated only by her own needs. Most people's motives are not so one-dimensional. She likely cares about her mother, and does not want her to suffer yet can't bear the thought of losing her. Recognizing and exploring this ambivalence will help us find a path to agreement.

Finally, we need the imagination to understand the reasoning beyond the patient's words that she does "not desire dialysis." Was she concerned or even fearful of side effects, poor quality of life or futility? Each of these reasons could lead to different decisions about whether the use of dialysis now is consistent with her preferences, not just with her literal words. We must strive to honor the values and goals of the patient, even with her words right in front of us.

Exercising our moral imagination in all these ways helps us maintain some humility. The world, the ethical world included, is a complicated place. Maybe her daughter is right; or at least we can imagine circumstances in which she would be right. Then we can approach her with respect, as a moral equal. Even if in the end we disagree, we understand how easy it is to get it wrong.

Acting in an ethical way is more than knowing the ethical principles or rules that apply. It requires us to be compassionate, imaginative, and humble. Only then will we be able not just to do the right thing, but to do it in the right way, and with the right spirit.

Thomas Tomlinson, Ph.D.
Professor and Director, Center for Ethics and Humanities in
the Life Sciences
Michigan State University

PATIENT AUTONOMY – PEDIATRICS

A sixteen-year-old child with muscular dystrophy is admitted for evaluation and management of pneumonia associated with respiratory distress. Two similar hospitalizations have resulted in prolonged intubations. As the patient's pulmonary status deteriorates, the child announces that he would rather die than be intubated. The parents appear teary eyed and distraught by his wishes.

A Perspective from a Pediatrician

Clinical Background

The muscular dystrophies are a group of disorders characterized by progressive muscle degeneration. Multiple types exist, each distinguishable by its own unique genetic defect and inheritance pattern. The presentation, age of onset, and rate of progression may differ significantly between the various types.

Duchenne muscular dystrophy is the most commonly encountered muscular dystrophy, occurring in one in 3,600 male infants. Muscles deteriorate slowly over the first few years of life often resulting in a delay in diagnosis until two to three years of age. Early findings include development of limb/girdle hypotonia, delayed motor milestones, a waddling gait, scoliosis, and calf hypertrophy. By seven, most children can no longer walk. Weakness of the bulbar muscles makes eating and speaking difficult. Diaphragmatic and intercostal involvement results in poor cough, frequent pneumonias, and respiratory insufficiency. Cardiomyopathy is common. On average, death ensues by age eighteen as a result of acute respiratory or cardiac failure. Currently there is no treatment to reverse or halt the progression of this disorder.

Recent advances in management of muscular dystrophy have permitted survival into the second decade of life. For patients without chronic respiratory insufficiency, improved critical care management has resulted in survival rates of 90 percent for acute respiratory failure from pneumonia.[22] Advances in therapy to improve pulmonary toilet and utilization of chronic mechanical ventilation have made significant impact.[23,24] In one recent study, severely disabled patients reported a perceived quality of life similar to unaffected controls regardless of their level of disability.[25]

Professionalism Considerations

Since most pediatric patients are not legally or intellectually able to make their own medical decisions, pediatricians need to help parents decide what care is in the best interest of their child. With time the child may be able to voice an opinion. In order to try to respect this opinion, the parent and physician should offer choices, if indeed safe and equal choices are available. In many instances, however, choice about medical care is not possible.

In this case, the patient has a chronic, terminal illness. He has been living with severe disability for some time, and has experienced the unpleasantness of being ventilated for acute respiratory failure on two previous occasions. He can relate to his parents how upset he would be if he had to experience this ordeal again. Although he should know that his disease is fatal, his level of maturity may not allow him to understand the true meaning of withholding treatment in this situation. As a minor, he is not legally allowed to supersede his parent's decisions. In this situation, helping his parents make a decision about further treatment based on probable outcomes, the likelihood of worsening disability, expected level of discomfort, and the psychological well-being of their son is the responsibility of the treating pediatrician.

This patient has a life-ending disease about which his parents should have been previously educated. They should already be aware of the expected outcomes, and should know that they may have to make some tough decisions. The deteriorating nature of their son's condition could be a sign that worse times are ahead.

If appropriate counseling about advanced medical strategies has been previously introduced, they should already have some idea about the use of assistive respiratory devices to prolong his life. Evidence has shown that these non-invasive devices are safe, painless, and quite effective at maintaining health. More invasive forms of therapy requiring tracheotomy are also available and effective. These devices are now commonplace and parents can be easily trained to manage them at home with little difficulty. Although these modalities are available, they are in no means required, and families need to consider their possible benefits to decide what is in the best interest of their child. The best time to introduce these concepts to families is before a crisis occurs.

Opinion

In this case, the parents need to be told that the likelihood of their son surviving this episode of pneumonia is quite good. In fact, with proper therapy it is expected that he would survive. Improved sedation strategies may be available to make his time on the respirator more comfortable. It would be expected that upon successful treatment of the pneumonia he will regain his previous state of health. As such, if the only reason that the parents would withhold treatment is that their child doesn't want to be on a ventilator, my personal opinion would be to convince them otherwise. As pediatricians, we do things that children don't like every day. It would be no more correct to withhold therapy in this case than to withhold vaccines because they hurt, or not look into a child's ear because it may make him cry.

In certain other situations, not initiating care may be best. For example, if it was anticipated that the patient would need to begin chronic ventilator management, or if it was not expected that the child would make a reasonable recovery, discussion about not initiating care may be in order. If this child already had chronic respiratory failure, and if the parents and child have previously discussed the issue and decided that they would not wish to elevate care beyond simple means, then this may be the time to prepare for the child's death. The child, parents, and pediatrician should work together to develop an understanding of the technologies available to sustain life and their threshold in utilizing those means.

Paul J. Bellino III, M.D.
Janet Weis Children's Hospital, Geisinger Medical Center
Danville, Pennsylvania

A Perspective from a Pediatric Psychologist

First, let us acknowledge the medical, ethical, and existential challenges of the situation.[26,27] Here is a patient with a progressive neuromuscular disorder that will foreshorten his life expectancy. Muscular dystrophy is a formidable foe, especially in the context of a society that values youth and vibrancy, health and long life, and expects medical brilliance and vanquishment of disease. At the heart of this case lies the fragile balance of integrating restorative medicine and palliative care for the patient and his family, and the ethics and burden of escalating technology.[28–30]

Our sixteen-year old patient is indeed an adolescent, not a child. Some, including the patient himself, might view him as a young man. For the sake of clarity, let us assume that our patient has Duchenne muscular dystrophy and is of normal intelligence. He has lived with the disease for his entire life and has experienced two similar hospitalizations for respiratory distress that required prolonged intubation. When he declares that he would rather die than be intubated again, we must acknowledge that he is coming from a place of first-hand, intimate, lived experience. It behooves us to elicit, listen to, and understand the patient's point of view. Through this process we bring forth and clarify the patient's perspective, decision-making capacity, and wishes that are so vital to moving forward. Although parents in most cases retain legal authority to make decisions about their teenager's medical care, this fact does not and should not restrict parents and practitioners from involving youngsters in discussions and decisions about their care in a manner consistent with their cognitive and emotional maturity.[26,27]

There are several important questions. How emergent is the situation? Is immediate intubation required? Does the team believe that this is an acute reversible process? If so, does the patient understand this? In the largest study to date documenting the outcome of patients with neuromuscular disease admitted to the pediatric intensive care unit (PICU), most recovered without the need for prolonged invasive ventilation. The authors of this study recommend that patients be provided with acute respiratory support in anticipation that they are likely to recover.[30] That said, repeat hospitalizations and the use of non-invasive home-based ventilation were common, with the prospect of chronic respiratory failure. Ideally, in our patient's situation, it would be possible to institute measures short of intubation to improve his comfort and respiratory status and to enable us to better assess the patient's perspective, decision-making capacity, and health care values. Since the patient is able to communicate clearly and coherently now, we need to take advantage of this window of opportunity.

It is likely that issues of disease progression and decision making have been previously broached, given the patient's condition, recent prolonged critical care hospitalizations, and the standard of integrating palliative care into chronic care.[27,29] Are there any previous conversations and understandings from which to draw upon and guide us now? Does the patient have a realistic view of his future course should acute treatment not be pursued? How does he envision his life and what is he hoping for? Has he known other patients who have more advanced disease and who are technology dependent? If at all possible, the patient should have the opportunity to share his views and concerns in the presence of his family as well as independently, because it may be difficult for him to be forthcoming about his needs and wishes in the midst of his family's anguish. Who has provided care and established trust, and who may have insight into the patient's and family's underlying health care values and may be in a good position to counsel and advise the patient, his family, and the team?[28] Perhaps there is a community pediatrician, pulmonologist, home health nurse, respiratory therapist, social worker, psychologist, or chaplain who can enlighten the process? Inclusion of psychosocial staff in family meetings has been associated with better synchrony between staff and family recognition that end of life is at hand, better symptom management, and earlier referral to hospice care in the pediatric oncology population.[31]

Clearly, the teary-eyed distraught parents need attention and care, and the opportunity to sort through the situation and decisions at hand. Hearing their son state that he would rather die than be intubated is likely to be very upsetting and may unleash deep fear, grief, and guilt. They may struggle and feel overwhelmed with the decision to pursue immediate critical care for their son against his stated wishes. Or, they may be able to step back and reflect on whether repeat intubation is right for their son. The realities of the disease, reconfigured parental role as a result of the disease, uncertain prognosis and the pressure of past treatment success conspire to make parental decision making complex.[31] Several factors influence parental decision making at end of life including the perceived quality of the child's life, the likelihood of getting better, perceptions of the child's pain or suffering, what parents believe the child wants, religious and spiritual beliefs, and advice from family and practitioners.[32]

Acute care providers often do not have the luxury of time.[31] The team would do well to provide a calm and non-anxious presence, to institute measures short of intubation to ensure the patient's comfort, and, if possible, to enlist the help of practitioners who know the patient and family well. Ultimately, this team's job, as impossible as it may seem, is to educate, support, and advise patients and their families to find the ever-changing balance of restorative and palliative interventions that maximize quality of life and help mitigate physical and emotional suffering.[29] Indeed, each patient's voice needs and deserves to be heard loudly and clearly throughout this delicate process.

Elaine C. Meyer, Ph.D., R.N.
Director, Program to Enhance Relational and
Communication Skills (PERCS)
Director, Institute for Professionalism and Ethical Practice,
Children's Hospital Boston
Associate Professor of Psychology
Harvard Medical School

PATIENT AUTONOMY – PSYCHIATRY

A thirty-year-old schizophrenic man sees his psychiatrist and tells him that he wants to stop the antipsychotic medication that he had been on the past twelve years. The patient works as a taxi cab driver.

A Perspective from a Psychiatrist

Clinical Background

Adherence to an antipsychotic regimen is critical to the maintenance of re-mission in schizophrenia. Without medication, 60–70 percent of patients will relapse within the first year and almost 90 percent will relapse within two years.[33] Unfortunately, most patients find the experience of taking an anti-psychotic medication dysphoric.

This dysphoria is related in part to a general non-specific subjective expe-rience, and in part to specific side effects. Recently developed antipsychotic medications are well known to cause dramatic weight gain, while older an-tipsychotic medications cause a variety of movement-related side effects, such as dystonia, parkinsonian symptoms and tardive dyskinesia. Some patients also experience akathesia, an intense restlessness that responds poorly to adjunctive medication management. So it is not surprising that the taxi driver wishes to discontinue medication.

On the other hand, stopping medication may lead to an acute psychotic episode, which can be exquisitely painful. Cherished goals may be lost. As the patient's thoughts become disorganized, the ability to maintain a job, hous-ing, and even personal hygiene and nutrition may deteriorate. If paranoia develops, the patient may experience the terrifying belief that others are plotting against his life. He may hear voices criticizing him, and invading his privacy by remarking on his every behavior. No physician who has ever seen a patient in acute psychosis will take medication discontinuation lightly.

Professionalism Considerations

When working with a patient who is not following treatment recommenda-tions, the approach of many physicians is to educate and exhort the patient. If this is not successful, the physician often disengages, with a shrug of the shoulders and a reduced commitment to problem solving. This is an under-standable reaction, but not likely to lead to a satisfying outcome for either patient or doctor.

A genuine commitment to patient autonomy requires the physician to take an active role in supporting the patient in directing his or her own care. This requires the physician to actively elicit patient concerns, communicate in clear terms, assess the patient's understanding, screen for poor decision-making capacity, and sometimes to support the patient in making the best of a choice that the physician disagrees with.

In this case, there are some signs that things have been going very well in the doctor–patient relationship. Rather than simply stopping his medication, this patient comes to the doctor to discuss his plans. Apparently the physician has previously communicated interest in the patient's experiences and opinions about treatment. The patient does not anticipate being shamed by the doctor, and does not expect the doctor to be offended by his questions.

This psychiatrist needs to learn why the patient wants to stop the medication. Perhaps there is a side effect that if well managed will be more acceptable to the patient. Perhaps the patient has misconceptions about the medication that can be addressed by education. Perhaps an irrational concern about the medication is a first indication of relapse, and additional supports should be called into play.

The doctor should assess the patient's understanding of his diagnosis and of the risks of discontinuing medication. This should include asking the patient to describe his understanding to the doctor. Simply relating the facts and asking the patient, "Do you understand?" may fail to uncover important deficits in understanding. Genuine autonomy requires a well-informed patient who is able to reason clearly.

If the patient has reasonable concerns about continuing medication, has been stable for a significant period of time, and has a good back-up plan in case of deterioration, the patient and the psychiatrist may be able to reach an agreement about how to proceed. Unfortunately, schizophrenia often affects the capacity for insight. Patients may be unaware of their deficits, or they may have irrational explanations for their symptoms. It is not unusual for a psychotic patient who is suffering a great deal to deny that anything is wrong with him or her, and to refuse treatment. This places the physician in a very uncomfortable position. The principles of patient welfare and patient autonomy come into conflict.

In general, society in the United States balances this conflict by permitting mentally ill patients to refuse treatment unless they pose an imminent threat to themselves or others.[34] Jurisdictions vary regarding what qualifies as an imminent threat, what treatments may be imposed, and how government oversees involuntary treatment. The greater the impingement on autonomy, the greater the justification for limiting it must be. Former and current patients have spoken persuasively to legislators and regulators about the harmful effects of forced treatment.

On the other hand, many mental health advocates feel that the current balance favors autonomy too much. Severely mentally ill patients who are not threatening themselves or others are permitted to refuse treatment. Some wander the streets, vulnerable to abuse and with inadequate food and clothing. Some seclude themselves in their rooms, where family members must watch in distress as a loved one refuses to eat or bathe. These scenarios lead many family members and mental health workers to feel that concern for patient welfare should override concern for autonomy. Widely publicized dramatic episodes of violence often lead to calls for broader powers to compel treatment, although few mentally ill patients will ever commit an act of significant violence.

Opinion

If I were the treating psychiatrist for this patient, I would recheck the accuracy of the diagnosis and the appropriateness of the medication regimen and work with the patient to reach a treatment plan that had a reasonable chance of averting relapse. If we could not come to an agreement, and the patient persisted in wanting to discontinue medication, I would help the patient make plans for what we would do if he became psychotic, with consideration of both his welfare and the welfare of his family and the public.

Working as a taxi driver, this patient is often alone with members of the public. Although most psychotic individuals are not violent, there is some increased risk of perpetration of violence. I would monitor him carefully for signs of increasing hostility. It is less obvious but equally important to monitor him for vulnerability to victimization in this isolated job. Mentally ill patients are more likely to be victims than perpetrators of violence.[35] If I saw indicators of increasing risk, I would insist that he restart his medication, or take other measures to protect the patient and the public.

I would also have to consider what I could effectively manage in my work setting. As a solo practitioner with an office-based practice, I would not be well equipped to manage psychosis. I would refer if necessary. I am usually willing to work with patients who refuse my recommendations, but supporting patient autonomy does not mean agreeing to do more than I can realistically do.

Kimberly Best, M.D.
Director of the Division of Psychiatric Education
Albert Einstein Medical Center, Philadelphia, PA

A Perspective from a Mental Health Patient and Advocate

I am a person living with a mental illness who, like the cab driver, makes difficult decisions about my own mental health care. My response to this case study is drawn primarily from reflections on my own experience of living with a psychiatric disorder.

As someone diagnosed with mental illness for over twelve years, there have been multiple times I stopped taking medication without the input of friends, family, or a doctor. Needless to say, these periods were riddled by failure and instability. I was making decisions in a vacuum, completely alone. In order to get better I had to move beyond my comfort zone and reach out to others for help. Over time I have begun to realize my privilege in doing so, as I gained access to five key resources that many others do not receive when they reach out in the same way. These five resources constitute my "golden web" of recovery.

1. A health care professional familiar with my medical history
2. Excellent education about treatment options
3. Supportive family and/or peers
4. Financial means to afford the best treatment
5. Understanding of recovery as leading to quality of life – not only suppression of symptoms.

In thinking about the cab driver I wonder whether he has access to such a web. With what tools has he been equipped to make decisions? Does his family receive him with compassion and offer support? Can he afford the medication he needs? Does he have access to a professional with knowledge of his personal history? If so, does that professional offer him more than one treatment option? Does the professional direct his care in a way that leads towards quality of life, not only the suppression of symptoms? Does the professional educate him about medications and their side effects? Is the cab driver's input into his treatment plan valued?

Without my golden web it would have been easy to fall, to lose hope, and to stop pursuing treatment. It would also have been easy to persist on a medication that was not a good match for my body and to settle for a life of lesser quality than what I now have.

Psychiatric medications are strong and can have severe side effects. For instance, one medication I took was very successful in controlling my recurrent delusions and paranoia. However, it caused me to gain over forty pounds and led to a risk of developing diabetes. Another medication I was prescribed caused me fatigue so severe I was unable to drive. Yet another had sexual side effects that interfered with having a healthy relationship. The pills, in essence, became bitter to swallow. They complicated an already complicated life. At times it seemed hard to distinguish which was worse, the disease or the medications. However, over time and with persistence my doctor and I found an effective mix. My social/community network helped me gain coping skills to fill in gaps that still existed, since with mental illness there is no cure yet.

Unlike so many people with mental illness seeking treatment, I am lucky enough to have a doctor who offers me options, and who expects me to experience more in my life than an absence of symptoms. I have adequate time with the doctor – forty-five minutes at each of the visits – to relate my most recent thoughts, moods, symptoms, and side effects. There is a thoughtful study of my concerns and a heartfelt wish to help me get better. My family is ever present, cheering me on during the most difficult times – like when my clothing size swelled from a size 8 to a size 16. They have assisted me monetarily when I could not work. In turn, I have ceased making decisions in a vacuum.

Where does this leave the cab driver? Is he making his decision in a vacuum as I once did – thinking he can solve any problem on his own? Or is there something more beneath the surface of this story that we cannot see because it was not told? In other words, where is the golden web?

Sarah O'Brien
National Alliance on Mental Illness, Arlington, VA

SUMMARY – PRINCIPLE OF PATIENT AUTONOMY

Background

In contrast to the principle of patient welfare that has roots in antiquity, patient autonomy emerged as a tenet of professionalism only recently. Prior to this, most major medical decisions were made by physicians, with good intentions but without full participation of the patient. In the latter half of the twentieth century, major increases in public and private research funding catalyzed biomedical research that, in turn, began the technological transformations of medical practice. In this setting of unprecedented growth in the power of the medical establishment and the potency of medical interventions, the call for attention to the person – to patient's rights and primacy as decision makers – emerged.

"Bioethics was born out of a crisis of imperialism in biomedical research and medical treatment."[36] Respect for autonomy – "the duty to protect and foster a patient's free, uncoerced choices" joined the long-standing principles of beneficence (the duty to promote good and act in the patient's best interests) and nonmaleficence (the duty to do no harm).[37]

The patient's rights of self-decision can also be viewed as one example of the rights of self-determination codified by Anglo-American law. It is not a coincidence that scholarly attention to patient autonomy grew in concert with the women's and civil rights movements. Early bioethics scholarship focused on "assuring that the paternalistic doctor stays dead and buried."[38] That kind of overstatement is matched by excesses in the name of autonomy that leave the physician a mere technical advisor. So, how has the definition of patient autonomy actually evolved over the past forty years and, most important, how can we get it right?

The evolution and complexities of autonomy in the patient care setting has been analyzed in elegant detail by Carl Schneider.[39] He presents two very different theoretical models of patient autonomy, representing the extremes, as a starting point for clarity: mandatory and optional autonomy. They are briefly described here.

The mandatory model, also called "independent choice,"[39] places emphasis on the patient's duty to make medical decisions. In this model, individuals are obliged to be self-governing, to not burden others with their decisions and owe it to themselves to make their own choices. The physician's role is to provide information, ascertain that the patient understands this information, and "at least encourage if not require the patient to make diagnostic and therapeutic decisions."[40]

The optional model, in contrast, proposes that patients are entitled to make medical decisions but not required to do so. In this model, it is recognized that individual and situational barriers exist to full autonomy. It is again the physician's role to educate the patient, and to try to remove or at least minimize barriers to making decisions. Yet it is accepted that a patient may not want to exercise full autonomy and may want to share decision making. This is akin to the model, described by Quill and Brody, of enhanced autonomy, wherein decision-making power is tailored to the person making the decision. "There is active listening, honest sharing of perspectives, suspension of judgment and genuine concern for the needs of the patient . . . The assumptions, values and perspectives of both parties are fully explored."[41] In a call to re-affirm our contract with society, the Physician Charter on Professionalism states: "Physicians must have respect for patient autonomy. Physicians must be honest with their patients and empower them to make informed decisions about their treatment."[42]

Using the enhanced autonomy model, we can look critically at patient autonomy in the "real world" of patient and physician. It is important to add that medical decision making takes place in the context of a health care bureaucracy; drug formularies, practice guidelines, insurance protocols, the interests of the physician, the institution, payers, and other potential conflicts of interest also impact the process. Now more than ever, we must respect our patients as people and strive to provide patient-centered care in the multitude of micro-systems that comprise our often chaotic health care system. As challenging as this is, taking time to really listen to our patients and to effectively communicate our medical expertise is of paramount importance.

The process of securing informed consent is fundamental to patient autonomy. Informed consent implements and protects the patient's choices and is based on respect for autonomy. The principles of beneficence, nonmaleficence, and justice also provide an ethical foundation for the consent process. An informed patient can more fully be engaged in, and take responsibility for, his or her health care.

The consent of the patient allows the physician to provide care. Without consent, the unauthorized touching of a person is considered battery, even if the goal is to provide medical treatment. Most often, especially in the setting of the hospital, patients provide written or oral consent for a particular test or procedure. This is known as expressed consent. In many medical encounters, however, consent can be implied or presumed when the patient presents to a physician for evaluation and care. In medical emergencies, consent to treatment to sustain life or restore health is implied unless it is known that the patient would refuse the care.[43]

The doctrine of informed consent focuses on the content and process of consent. The physician should provide enough information to allow a patient to make an informed decision about whether and how to proceed about a proposed test, procedure, or other treatment. The information should include the physician's recommendation. The patient (or his or her surrogate where appropriate) should be adequately informed about the nature of the medical condition; the objectives of treatment and possible outcomes; the alternatives to treatment; and risks of the proposed treatment. Physicians should be sensitive and respectful in their disclosure of all relevant medical information to patients.[44] The patient's decision should be voluntary and uncoerced. All states have statutes or case law requiring and setting standards for informed consent.

Written patient information or outside resources such as articles and Web sites may assist patients in better understanding their options. Communication techniques such as having the patient explain information back to the physician may also enhance comprehension and decision making. The patient should have ample opportunity to ask questions in making an informed decision about whether to proceed with or to decline a test, procedure, or other care.

Adult patients are considered competent to make decisions about medical care unless declared incompetent by a court. Frequently in clinical practice, physicians and family members make decisions for patients who lack decision-making capacity without a formal competency hearing in court. Decision-making capacity is defined as the ability to receive and express information and to make a choice based on that information and the individual's values. This clinical approach is ethically acceptable if the physician has carefully determined that the patient is capable of understanding the nature of the proposed treatment, the alternatives to it, and the risks, benefits, and consequences of it. However, assessing patient understanding can be difficult. The capacity to express a particular goal or wish can exist without the ability to make more complex decisions. Higher proof of capacity should be required by the physician as the seriousness of the consequences of the decision increases.[37]

An appropriate surrogate should make decisions when a patient lacks decision-making capacity. Decisions should be made based on the patient's preferences. Surrogate decision making recognizes the principle that the patient's rights and wishes should not be lost when the individual can no longer speak for him or herself. Some patients have appointed a surrogate through a durable power of attorney for health care. When patients have not selected surrogates, family members often serve as surrogates. Some states have health care consent statutes that specify who and in what order of priority family members or close others can serve as surrogates. Physicians should be aware of legal requirements in their states for surrogate appointment and decision making.

The legal foundations of informed consent were established in cases involving treatment of patients, but the same principles apply to informed consent for research.

As shown in Figure 4.1, the medical decision-making process is facilitated by situations in which the patient and physician agree to proceed or not to proceed with an intervention. Patient autonomy dilemmas occur when there is a "mismatch" between the physician/medical team and the patient or patient proxy in a decision on a course of action. Note that in this figure, as with 2 × 2 tables created to describe sensitivity, specificity and predictive values of a diagnostic test, the "gold standard" is the patient/proxy choice at the top, the column legend. Ultimately, in the vast majority, although not all situations, the final choice belongs to the patient. The Physician Charter says that patient decisions are paramount, "as long as those decisions are in keeping with ethical practice and do not lead to demands for inappropriate care."[42] This is true for mundane decisions such as taking medication for hypertension as well as in decisions that require explicit informed consent. It may also mean that the patient decides that someone else should be the decision maker, such as a family member or members, or the physician.

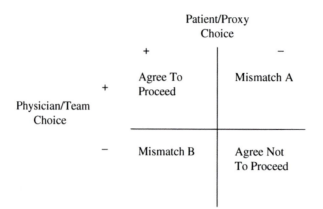

Figure 4.1. Medical Decision Making in 2 × 2 Format

Review of the Cases and Commentaries

This concept is a useful starting point for review of the patient autonomy cases. Both of the student-faculty commentaries are mismatches between students who wish to provide care and patients who do not want it. In the first, an elderly patient, tired with pneumonia, asks a second year student to return the next day to finish an assigned history and physical due that day (see Chapter 2). This interaction is, in a sense, a simulation of a patient–physician encounter. This data-gathering encounter has been specifically designed to benefit student learning. The medical student is not working with the patient's medical team and hence not officially linked to the official providers of care. However, time with a medical student, who brings a kind ear and companionship during the stress of a hospitalization, is of benefit to the patient. It is even possible that some piece of information from this encounter, appropriately directed, might improve this patient's care.

Medical ethics is often focused on the rights of the patient but patients also have ethical responsibilities. The eleven responsibilities cited in the AMA *Code of Ethics*[45] each emphasize aspects of collaboration between patients and their physicians and include the following statement: "Participation in medical education is to the mutual benefit of patients and the health care system. Patients are encouraged to participate in medical education by accepting care, under appropriate supervision, from medical students, residents, and other trainees." In fact, taken to the limit, patient acceptance of the participation of medical students and residents in their care is requisite to sustaining a population of competent physicians. Each person who allows medical students, residents, and other health professions students to participate in medical care is contributing to this social good.

This section of the code continues: "Consistent with the process of informed consent, the patient or the patient's surrogate decision maker is always free to refuse care from any member of the health care team." This ultimate right to refuse also applies to the second vignette, in which the educational setting shifts to the real world of the operating room (see the commentaries by Sade and King in Chapter 2). The fourth year student is a bona fide member of the patient's clinical team. The patient, who is scheduled for an elective surgery, explicitly tells the student and resident that he wants only the attending to do the operation. The student's dilemma is set up by the resident in stating that the attending and he will be doing the surgery and that the student will be observing. The dilemma comes to the fore when the attending, who was not present for the prior conversation, asks the student to assist with closure. This student, as in the first vignette, must weigh the respect for the patient's request against the perception that a clinical grade will suffer if the task is not performed. In both situations, as the commentaries describe, the patient's autonomy drives the appropriate response.

In both of these cases, better communication could have prevented these missed educational opportunities. Recruitment of appropriate patients for participation in the second year course should be done earlier the same day. Since clinical status and patient wishes may change, guidelines should also be provided to the second year students and preceptors to address acceptable alternatives when the patient refuses participation. As noted by Sade in Chapter 2, better preoperative communication, including definition of the roles of all involved, might have allayed the patient's concerns about student participation and would have at least prevented the awkward moment for the student in the operating room.

While it may seem that the eighty-seven-year-old man's request for prostate cancer screening is a very simple request, prostate cancer screening is a very complex issue (see Lambert's and Fryer-Edward's commentary in this chapter). This mismatch, between what this patient and what this physician think are best screening practices, pits hard, cold clinical probabilities against the power of personal experience.

The uncertainty about the effectiveness of prostate cancer screening is unfortunately unchanged since the U.S. Preventive Services Task Force first published evidence-based recommendations in 2002. The evidence is insufficient (category I) to recommend for or against routine screening for prostate cancer using prostate specific antigen (PSA) testing or digital rectal examination (DRE).[46] As noted in Lambert's commentary if early detection improves health outcomes at all, it is for men aged fifty to seventy and men over forty-five who are African-American or have a family history of a first-degree relative with prostate cancer.

This patient's personal experience with prostate cancer must be explored. The conversation should include thoughtful questioning about why he wants to be screened. Perhaps he knows someone who suffered or died from prostate or other cancers. Perhaps he heard very convincing anecdotes or testimonials about the benefits of prostate cancer screening from media coverage or an advocacy group. The ideas discussed in this dialogue will set the stage for honest, shared decision making.

The dilemmas in the next four cases involve treatment decisions. What the first three patients, with muscular dystrophy, schizophrenia, and breast cancer have in common is that they do not want treatment that the physician anticipates will have medical – in some cases life-saving – benefit.

For the sixteen-year-old with muscular dystrophy, as Bellino and Meyer have discussed, this patient, as a minor, cannot legally refuse intubation, as he is not yet legally vested with the right to make health care decisions. This exception to the ethical concept of patient autonomy derives from the principle that minors are not competent to provide voluntary and informed consent and that parents or guardians are better able to act in the best interests of a child[47] in the absence of abuse or neglect. However, research in decision making has shown that during the adolescent years minors are better able to weigh information and opinions and more capable of making their own judgments. The concept of adolescent assent, with engagement in discussion about the illness and seeking preferences regarding treatment, is proposed as an interim step toward full decision-making autonomy. Both the American Medical Association and the American Academy of Pediatrics[48] recognize the ethical duty to promote autonomy of minor patients by involving them in medical decision-making processes commensurate with their abilities. Yet neither offer clear guidelines on how to proceed when parents and adolescent patients disagree. Though physicians are encouraged to include minors in decisions and respect their autonomy, statutes permit parents to make almost all decisions on behalf of their children.[49] The primary exceptions to this are related to family planning and abuse.

For the schizophrenic man who tells his psychiatrist he wants to stop his medication, as noted by Best, the ethical dilemma is foremost between patient welfare and autonomy. Finding the optimal treatment plan, one that minimizes both the risks of psychosis and unpleasant side effects, is a delicate task well described by O'Brien. There is also subtext linked to mental competence and public health. There are circumstances that allow for involuntary treatment; these circumstances must meet standards for severe mental illness. This is defined, for example, in the Mental Health Act of Pennsylvania as "when capacity to exercise self-control, judgment and discretion in the conduct of affairs and social relations or to care for one's own personal needs is so lessened that one poses a clear and present danger of harm to others or to oneself."[50] This patient does not meet these criteria at this point in time and indeed, he has demonstrated good judgment in choosing to discuss his point of view.

The patient's occupation as a taxi driver raises special considerations. A physician has the responsibility to recognize impairments in patients' driving ability that pose a strong threat to public safety and which may need to be reported to the Department of Motor Vehicles.[51] The AMA guidelines specifically state that the driver must pose a clear risk, not a potential threat as in this case, to public safety for action to be considered. From both a personal and an occupational risk perspective, the importance of clear sensorium while driving must be factored into this patient's treatment planning.

The physician caring for a woman with breast cancer faces the issues of quality of care and patient welfare vying with patient autonomy, with her consideration of alternative medicine in Mexico instead of conventional treatment. As noted by Branigan and Belling, the reasons for this dramatic and life-threatening mid-treatment change of direction need thoughtful attention and thorough exploration. New use of alternative medicine has been associated with greater psychosocial distress and worse quality of life among women with stage 1 and stage 2 breast cancer.[52] In his extensive review of alternative cancer therapies, Ernst[53] has described the "life-cycle" of ineffective remedies. Anecdotal evidence, promoted by vendors and in the media, leads to interest in the conduct of rigorous clinical trials. When these turned out to be negative, proponents claim that the studies are flawed. These therapies then submerge into a medical subculture – the Mexico connection – and hopeful, sometimes desperate, cancer patients continue to seek them.

There are non-traditional therapies that have been shown to be effective as adjunctive treatment for breast cancer in randomized clinical trials. Electro-acupuncture, in combination with anti-emetic drugs, has been shown to further reduce nausea and vomiting in women receiving high-dose, highly emetic chemotherapy for breast cancer.[54] Although they did not improve clinical outcomes, relaxation techniques with guided imagery have been shown to improve quality of life measures in women with breast cancer.[55] A willingness to ask about use, to investigate the current status of alternative therapies, and to frankly discuss what is known about risks and benefits, enables the physician to align with patients who have interest in complementary and alternative medicine remedies. This approach may well avert the tragedy of such therapies replacing others with proven effectiveness.

In the last vignette in this chapter, an elderly woman who has had the foresight and taken the time to put her end-of-life choices into a living will is now comatose, and near death, due to renal failure. The medical basis of

ay well have been based on conversations with her physician
ɹring the years of her illness. The patient and her physician may
.ssed the demands of dialysis and prognosis in the very old. In
ɹom the United States Renal Data System, the one-year mortality
ɹnts aged eighty and older was 46 percent.[56] There is also an increased
ɹency of the usual complications in the elderly: hypotension during di-
ɹis, malnutrition, infection especially of vascular access sites, and gastro-
ɹtestinal bleeding.[57]

The legal basis of her decision is on the firm ground established by state
law, and by the Federal Patient Self-Determination Act of 1991. This Act
requires health care institutions to ask all adults admitted as inpatients
whether they have an advanced directive and to inform them of their right
to refuse treatment. Institutions failing to meet this standard risk losing
Medicare and Medicaid funds. The law has three primary purposes: (1) to
educate the public about state laws governing the refusal, withholding, and
withdrawal of treatment at the end of life; (2) to encourage wider use of
advance directives to prevent the uncertainty among doctors and family
members that often leads to prolonged treatment of the dying, and in some
cases to lengthy court battles; and (3) to reduce the costs of treatment at the
end of life by reducing unwanted and unnecessary intervention and the
perceived need for defensive medicine.[58] And, as noted by Meisel et al.,
end-of-life decision making when patients cannot speak for themselves is
not simple and may create fear of litigation. However, living wills do have
legal support in all fifty states either through legislation or case law.[59]

The real challenge here is to the interpersonal skills of this physician. If
a patient previously clearly expresses his or her wishes and is subsequently
incapable of making a decision, the family/surrogate should be told of the
patient's prior statements. It is not stated if the daughter was aware of her
mother's wishes and it is interesting that the daughter was not specifically
given durable power of attorney for health care. As next of kin, the daughter is
the default surrogate, but since there is a living will, she is very limited in her
right to contradict her mother's decision. For example, if she is able to convince the physician that her mother was depressed at the time the will was
written, its validity would come into question. This seems unlikely in this
case, but in fact we really do not know anything about the conversations or
relationship between this mother and daughter.

Conclusion

Which brings us full circle. Respect for autonomy is a fundamental ethical
obligation but autonomy alone is not the beginning and end of the ethical

analysis. Instead, resolution of ethical dilemmas often involves the weighing and balancing of conflicting principles, with careful consideration of all of the facts and physician recommendations coupled along with a healthy dose of good communication. Those who invoke patient autonomy as the key, or sometimes only, argument supporting a decision (such as in some cases of physician-assisted suicide) fail to consider the ethical, moral, and social heart of the matter they raise: autonomy for what? What are the purposes and consequences of such self-determination? As these cases illustrate, and real world experience reinforces, good patient care requires collaboration between patient (and/or family) and physician, and ethical analysis and decision making that reflects this alliance.

Susan L. Rattner, M.D., M.S.
Professor of Medicine
Professor of Family and Community Medicine
Jefferson Medical College

Lois Snyder, J.D.
Director, Center for Ethics and Professionalism
American College of Physicians

REFERENCES

1. Brawley OW. Prostate cancer screening: Clinical applications and challenges. *Urol Oncol.* 2004;**22**(4):353–357.
2. Chan EC, Haynes MC, O'Donnell FT, Bachino C, Vernon SW. Cultural sensitivity and informed decision making about prostate cancer screening. *J Community Health.* 2003;**28**(6):393–405.
3. Richie JP, Catalona WJ, Ahmann FR, et al. Effect of patient age on early detection of prostate cancer with serum prostate-specific antigen and digital rectal examination. *Urology.* 1993;**42**(4):365–374.
4. Concato J, Wells CK, Horwitz RI, et al. The effectiveness of screening for prostate cancer: A nested case-control study. *Arch Intern Med.* 2006;**166**(1):38–43.
5. Jonsen AR, Siegler M, Winslade WJ. *Clinicial Ethics: A Practical Approach to Ethical Decisions in Clinical Medicine.* 6th ed. New York: McGraw-Hill Medicinal; 2006.
6. Welch HG. Informed choice in cancer screening. *JAMA.* 2001;**285**(21):2776–2778.
7. Woolf SH, Chan EC, Harris R, et al. Promoting informed choice: Transforming health care to dispense knowledge for decision making. *Ann Intern Med.* 2005;**143**(4):293–300.
8. Gregory DJ, Chrischilles EA, Farris KB, Kohatsu ND, Lynch CF, Smith BJ. Decision-making for PSA screening: Avenues to modify screening rates. Poster Presentation and Abstract. CDC Cancer Conference. Atlanta, August 2007.
9. U.S. Preventive Services Task Force. Screening for prostate cancer: Recommendation and rationale. *Ann Intern Med.* 2002;**137**(11):915–916.

10. Christakis NA. Death foretold: Prophesy and prognosis in medical care. 2001.

11. Groopman J. *Anatomy of Hope: How People Prevail in the Face of Illness.* New York: Random House; 2005.

12. Steward M, Brown WW, McWhinney IRMcWilliams P. Patient-centered medicine: Transforming the clinical method. 2003.

13. Brody H. Transparency: Informed consent in primary care. *Hastings Cent Rep.* 1989;**19**(5):5–9.

14. National Comprehensive Cancer Network. http://www.nccn.org/patients/patient_gls/_english/_breast/4_stages.asp. Accessed July 24, 2008.

15. Complementary and Alternative Methods for Cancer Management. American Cancer Society Web site. http://www.cancer.org/docroot/ETO/content/ETO_5_1_Introduction.asp. Accessed July 9, 2008.

16. Hann D, Allen S, Ciambrone D, Shah A. Use of complementary therapies during chemotherapy: Influence of patients' satisfaction with treatment decision making and the treating oncologist. *Integr Cancer Ther.* 2006;**5**(3):224–231.

17. Snyderman R, Weil AT. Integrative medicine: Bringing medicine back to its roots. *Arch Intern Med.* 2002;**162**(4):395–397.

18. Hakim RM, Lazarus JM. Initiation of dialysis. *J Am Soc Nephrol.* 1995;**6**(5):1319–1328.

19. U.S. renal data system, USRDS 2006 annual data report: Atlas of end-stage renal disease in the United States; 2006.

20. Beauchamp TL, Childress JF. *Principles of Biomedical Ethics.* 5th ed. New York: Oxford University Press; 2001.

21. "Springing back" advance care planning in dialysis. *Am J Kidney Dis.* 1999;**33**(5):980–991.

22. Shaffner D. Neuromuscular disease and respiratory failure. In: Rogers MC, ed. *Textbook of Pediatric Intensive Care.* 3rd ed. Baltimore: Williams and Wilkins; 1996:235–261.

23. Jeppesen J, Green A, Steffensen BF, Rahbek J. The Duchenne muscular dystrophy population in Denmark, 1977–2001: Prevalence, incidence and survival in relation to the introduction of ventilator use. *Neuromuscul Disord.* 2003;**13**(10):804–812.

24. Eagle M, Baudouin SV, Chandler C, Giddings DR, Bullock R, Bushby K. Survival in Duchenne muscular dystrophy: Improvements in life expectancy since 1967 and the impact of home nocturnal ventilation. *Neuromuscul Disord.* 2002;**12**(10):926–929.

25. Kohler M, Clarenbach CF, Boni L, Brack T, Russi EW, Bloch KE. Quality of life, physical disability, and respiratory impairment in Duchenne muscular dystrophy. *Am J Respir Crit Care Med.* 2005;**172**(8):1032–1036.

26. Burns JP, Truog RD. Ethical controversies in pediatric critical care. *New Horiz.* 1997;**5**(1):72–84.

27. Institute of Medicine, Field MJ, Behrman RE, eds. *When Children Die: Improving Palliative Care and End-of-Life Care for Children.* Washington, D.C.: National Academies Press; 2003.

28. Hilton T, Orr RD, Perkin RM, Ashwal S. End of life care in Duchenne muscular dystrophy. *Pediatr Neurol.* 1993;**9**(3):165–177.

29. Klick JC, Ballantine A. Providing care in chronic disease: The ever-changing balance of integrating palliative and restorative medicine. *Pediatr Clin North Am.* 2007;**54**(5):799–812, xii.

30. Yates K, Festa M, Gillis J, Waters K, North K. Outcome of children with neuromuscular disease admitted to paediatric intensive care. *Arch Dis Child.* 2004;**89**(2):170–175.

31. Graham RJ, Robinson WM. Integrating palliative care into chronic care for children with severe neurodevelopmental disabilities. *J Dev Behav Pediatr.* 2005;**26**(5):361–365.

32. Meyer EC, Burns JP, Griffith JL, Truog RD. Parental perspectives on end-of-life care in the pediatric intensive care unit. *Crit Care Med.* 2002;**30**(1):226–231.

33. Lehman AF, Lieberman JA, Dixon LB, et al. Practice guideline for the treatment of patients with schizophrenia, second edition. *Am J Psychiatry.* 2004;**161** (2 Suppl):1–56.

34. Segal SP, Laurie TA, Segal MJ. Factors in the use of coercive retention in civil commitment evaluations in psychiatric emergency services. *Psychiatr Serv.* 2001;**52**(4):514–520.

35. Choe JY, Teplin LA, Abram KM. Perpetration of violence, violent victimization, and severe mental illness: Balancing public health concerns. *Psychiatr Serv.* 2008;**59**(2):153–164.

36. Rothman D. *Strangers at the Bedside: A History of How Law and Bioethics Transformed Medical Decision-Making.* Basic Books; 1991.

37. Snyder L, Leffler C, Ethics and Human Rights Committee, American College of Physicians. Ethics manual: Fifth edition. *Ann Intern Med.* 2005;**142**(7): 560–582.

38. Caplan A. Can autonomy be saved? In: *If I Were a Rich Man Could I Buy a Pancreas? and Other Essays on the Ethics of Health Care.* Indiana Univ Press; 1994.

39. Schneider C. *The Practice of Autonomy: Patients, Doctors, and Medical Decisions.* Oxford University Press; 1998.

40. Brody H. Autonomy revisited: Progress in medical ethics: Discussion paper. *J R Soc Med.* 1985;**78**(5):380–387.

41. Jones C. *Autonomy and Informed Consent in Medical Decision Making: Toward a New Self-Fulfilling Prophecy.* Washington and Lee Law Review; 1990.

42. ABIM Foundation. American Board of Internal Medicine, ACP-ASIM Foundation. American College of Physicians-American Society of Internal Medicine, European Federation of Internal Medicine. Medical professionalism in the new millennium: A physician charter. *Ann Intern Med.* 2002;**136**(3):243–246.

43. Quill TE, Brody H. Physician recommendations and patient autonomy: Finding a balance between physician power and patient choice. *Ann Intern Med.* 1996;**125**(9):763–769.

44. American Medical Association. Code of medical ethics opinion E-8.08 informed consent.

45. AMA Code of Ethics. Patient Responsibilities. Section E 10.02. AMA Policy Finder Web site. http://www.ama-assn.org/apps/pf_new/pf_online?f_n=browse&doc=policyfiles/HnE/E-10.02.HTM&&s_t=&st_p=&nth=1&prev_pol=policyfiles/HnE/E-9.132.HTM&nxt_pol=policyfiles/HnE/E-10.01.HTM&. Accessed August 7, 2008.

46. The guide to clinical preventative services 2007: Recommendations of the USPSTF:43–47.

47. Encyclopedia of Everyday Law: Treatment of Minor. ENotes 2008 Web site. http://www.enotes.com/everyday-law-encyclopedia. Accessed August 7, 2008.

48. Mercurio MR, Forman EN, Ladd RE, et al. American Academy of Pediatrics policy statements on bioethics: Summaries and commentaries: Part 3. *Pediatr Rev.* 2008;**29**(5):e28–34.

49. Kuther T. Adolescence: Medical Decision-making and Minors: Issues of Consent and Assent. BNET Today Web site. http://www.BNET.com. Accessed August 7, 2008.

50. Pennsylvania Statutes Annotated. Title 5. Mental Health. Chapter 15. Mental Health Procedures. Mental Health Act of Pennsylvania. http://www.treatmentadvocacycenter.org/LegalResources/StateLaws/Pennsylvaniastatute.htm. Accessed August 7, 2008.

51. AMA code of ethics. Section E-2.24 impaired drivers and their physicians.

52. Burstein HJ, Gelber S, Guadagnoli E, Weeks JC. Use of alternative medicine by women with early-stage breast cancer. *N Engl J Med.* 1999;**340**(22):1733–1739.

53. Ernst E. Complementary therapies for cancer. In: *UpToDate Desktop 16.1.* Waltham, MA: UpToDate; 2008.

54. Shen J, Wenger N, Glaspy J, et al. Electroacupuncture for control of myeloablative chemotherapy-induced emesis: A randomized controlled trial. *JAMA.* 2000;**284**(21):2755–2761.

55. Walker LG, Walker MB, Ogston K, et al. Psychological, clinical and pathological effects of relaxation training and guided imagery during primary chemotherapy. *Br J Cancer.* 1999;**80**(1–2):262–268.

56. Kurella M, Covinsky KE, Collins AJ, Chertow GM. Octogenarians and nonagenarians starting dialysis in the United States. *Ann Intern Med.* 2007;**146**(3):177–183.

57. Nuhad I. Complications of hemodialysis in the elderly. In: *UpToDate Desktop 16.1.* Waltham, MA: UpToDate; 2008.

58. Heitman E. The patient self-determination act and public assessment of end-of-life technology. *Abstr Int Soc Technol Assess Health Care Meet.* 1992:10.

59. Meisel A, Snyder L, Quill T, American College of Physicians – American Society of Internal Medicine End-of-Life Care Consensus Panel. Seven legal barriers to end-of-life care: Myths, realities, and grains of truth. *JAMA.* 2000;**284**(19):2495–2501.

5 Principle of Social Justice

Cases and Commentaries

"Justice is conscience, not a personal conscience, but the conscience of the whole of humanity. Those who clearly recognize the voice of their own conscience usually recognize also the voice of justice."

Alexander Solzhenitsyn

SOCIAL JUSTICE – CARDIOLOGY

A fifty-five-year-old woman complains that her husband is getting better care than she is for her coronary artery disease. They both have angina. She noted that her husband received a stress test, cardiac catheterization, and stent placement within three days after complaining of chest pain. She received the same treatment over a month period and only after she had repeatedly complained of chest pain to her internist.

A Perspective from a Cardiologist

Clinical Background[1]

While women are more likely to die from heart disease than any other cause, diagnostic approaches to their chest pain are often less aggressive than those for men. Twenty years ago it was reported that 40 percent of male patients with abnormal exercise radionuclide scans were referred for cardiac catheterization whereas only 4 percent of female patients were referred for testing.[2] In an analysis of patients who were entered in the CURE (Clopidogrel in Unstable Angina to Prevent Recurrent Events) trial, a study of patients treated for acute coronary syndrome, women were found to be less likely than men to receive coronary angiography (25.4 percent vs. 29.5 percent).[3] These gender-related differences in care are not limited to the United States. In a European survey of patients presenting to cardiologists with stable angina, women were less likely than men to receive cardiac exercise testing, less likely to receive coronary angiography even after adjustment for the results of their noninvasive test, and less likely to be referred for coronary artery revascularization. For those in whom significant coronary artery disease was diagnosed, women were less likely than men to receive secondary prevention therapies.[4]

Professionalism Considerations

The reasons for this gender specific health care disparity are multiple and complex and it is only within the past few years that they have come to light. Reasons include unsubstantiated medical beliefs leading to gender bias, gender-specific variations in the significance of presenting symptoms of heart disease, uncertainty about the diagnostic validity of stress tests in women, and gender-related differences in the agreement to undergo cardiac testing.

Coronary artery disease has long been considered a "man's disease." Women have been thought to be at lower risk of coronary artery disease, which may explain why less attention may be paid to symptoms of coronary artery disease in women when compared to men. While women with coronary artery disease often have their first cardiac event six to ten years later than men, this delay in disease presentation has contributed to a mistaken assumption that women are "protected" from coronary artery disease. When women are found to have coronary artery disease they are often at a more advanced stage than their male counterparts. Cardiovascular death rates are decreasing in men, but they remain constant in women.

Epidemiologic data suggests that chronic angina in women is less predictive of the presence of clinically significant coronary artery disease than in men. The Coronary Artery Surgery Study (CASS) demonstrated that 50 percent of women referred for coronary angiography to evaluate chest pain did not have significant coronary artery disease compared to only 17 percent of men.[5] This difference in symptom relationship to underlying coronary artery disease may explain why chest pain in women may be evaluated less aggressively than in men and may be the reason why the patient in our clinical vignette was evaluated with less urgency than her husband. Women, when presenting with cardiovascular disease, have a greater tendency to present with atypical chest pain or to complain of abdominal pain, dyspnea, nausea, and unexplained fatigue.[6]

The lower prevalence of clinically significant obstructive coronary artery disease in women results in a higher incidence of false positive exercise electrocardiogram stress tests compared to men. This lower diagnostic accuracy may add to the uncertainty of the chest pain evaluation in women. This may explain, in part, the findings of several researchers that a positive exercise test in women is often not followed up with subsequent testing.

Some have sought to attribute the differences in the intensity of evaluation and treatment of cardiovascular disease between women and men to a gender-related difference in agreeing to undergo cardiac testing. While one study has shown that elderly women are more likely than males to refuse coronary angiography another found that women were more willing than men to undergo these procedures.[7,8] Overall patient refusal to undergo cardiac evaluation is uncommon and is not explained on the basis of preference differences based on gender.

Data from a number of studies of pharmacologic treatment of acute coronary syndrome indicates that anti-platelets, beta-blockers, angiotensin-converting-enzyme inhibitors, and lipid-lowering therapies reduce the risks of future coronary artery vascular events by 25 percent for both women and men. While this benefit is undisputed, women have been demonstrated to be less likely than men to be prescribed anti-platelet and statin therapy at the time of their original angina assessment.

Regarding primary prevention strategies, there is evidence that a gender-related difference does exist for aspirin. A meta-analysis from the Women's Health Study as well as from trials involving a majority of men with no history of heart disease indicated that aspirin therapy reduces the risk of stroke but does not affect the occurrence of myocardial infarction in women. In contrast, for men, aspirin significantly reduces the risk of myocardial infarction with a non-significant increase in the risk of stroke. The reasons for this differential effect of aspirin are not clear but the findings of the research highlight the importance of an adequate representation of women in clinical trials as well as in applying data obtained from men in the care of women.[9]

Once women undergo coronary artery bypass surgery they are more likely to have a complex postoperative course, and are more likely to be readmitted with unstable angina or congestive heart failure. This may in part be a result of delayed diagnosis and referral for CABG when compared to men. Despite this difference in outcomes post coronary artery bypass surgery, survival was similar in men and women.[10] In addition, women who underwent coronary artery angioplasty with coronary artery stenting as treatment of acute coronary syndrome have been found to have benefit similar to that of men.[11]

Opinion

In this clinical scenario we are told of a woman with recently diagnosed angina whose evaluation was less aggressive than that of her husband. It is unclear whether her less aggressive evaluation was due to her clinical presentation suggesting non-cardiac chest pain, a more stable presentation than her husband's, over-zealous treatment of her husband which by contrast made the approach to her symptoms seem delayed, or a result of gender bias on the part of her physician for any one or more of the above reasons. Whatever the reason, it is essential that a woman presenting with anginal chest pain that may be angina undergo appropriate and timely evaluation and subsequent care.

Once coronary artery disease is diagnosed, medical and surgical therapies appear to have equivalent efficacy in both men and women. The key then is for the clinician to be aware that gender-based differences do exist in the evaluation and treatment of women with coronary artery disease. Hopefully an awareness of these differences will result in an equality of care.

Howard Weitz, M.D.
Professor of Medicine, Vice Chairman, Department of Medicine
Jefferson Medical College

A Perspective from a Sociologist

As much as the state of health care has improved in recent decades for both men and women, it is important to remember the long history of gender bias in medical care and how issues of unequal treatment linger today.[12,13] It is likely that you will interact with women – especially older women – who will have a personal history of having been treated in a manner different from men during a medical encounter. Studies, as outlined in Dr. Weitz commentary, have shown the disparity of care among men and women for cardiovascular disease – disparities that are increasingly recognized within the medical community.[14]

These studies show us that we must consider both the forms of gender bias that are operating and how these affect interactions with male and female patients during a medical encounter. Although paternalism has been in decline for many years, we continue to read media accounts describing how gender shapes our treatment and diagnosis of heart disease in a way that is detrimental to women.[15] Furthermore, until very recently, we constructed most of our knowledge about heart disease on research studies based solely on male subjects, with the corresponding viewpoint that heart disease was a male problem.[16] As a result of the focus on male subjects in research, the behavior and symptoms of men have been regarded as the norm, and the way that men presented symptoms of disease was extrapolated to women.[12] Yet, studies of various physical health problems have repeatedly demonstrated that men and women often exhibit different symptoms, thus triggering responses to disease that vary substantially by gender. Poorer care for women is often the result. Cardiac care is just one example of this. Research has shown that men and women exhibit different heart attack symptoms; chest pain is most common in men, but women often experience abdominal pain, fatigue, and nausea. Women also have a poorer survival rate after a heart attack.[17,18]

Recognition of the important differences in heart disease between men and women in recent years led to the National Institutes of Health (NIH) Women's Ischemia Syndrome Evaluation (WISE) study in 1996.[19] Findings from the WISE study indicate that up to three million women in the United States have been incorrectly labeled as "low risk" for heart attack because standard tests fail to catch their form of heart disease. Merz and colleagues summarize their findings from WISE as follows:

- "Traditional diagnostic tests that focus on identifying obstructive disease do not work as well in women compared to men."
- "The 'typical' female presentation of signs and symptoms of ischemic heart disease is more complex and multifactorial than that of men."
- "Although men and women face relatively similar traditional cardiac risk factor loads, there may be gender-specific differences in response to this atherosclerotic risk burden."

The differences cited in WISE create a substantial challenge to clinicians and highlight the need for understanding and awareness of gender differences in identification and management of heart disease. In the end, more research and better patient care is needed if gender bias in cardiac care is to be eliminated in the coming years.

Bridget K. Gorman, Ph.D.
Associate Professor, Department of Sociology, Rice University

SOCIAL JUSTICE – OBSTETRICS AND GYNECOLOGY

A twenty-two-year-old Latina has just undergone a right salpingectomy for a ruptured ectopic pregnancy. She presented to the ER (emergency room) in the middle of the night after suffering at home with abdominal pain. She was hemodynamically unstable. After the emergent gynecology consult was called, the patient explained she was hesitant to come to the ER since she has no insurance coverage. She is stable now, but received aggressive resuscitation for a two liter intra-abdominal blood loss. While breaking scrub after the case, the attending gynecologist says: "Too bad we couldn't take both of her tubes, it would have saved the tax payers money." She goes on to make further disparaging comments about Latinos and illegal Mexican immigrants. A resident gynecologist overhears these comments.

A Perspective from an Obstetrical and Gynecology Resident

Clinical Background

Ruptured ectopic pregnancy is the leading cause of pregnancy-related mortality in the first trimester.[20] While ectopic pregnancy occurs as a consequence of the blastocyst implanting somewhere other than the uterine endometrium, it most commonly occurs in the fallopian tube, with 75 percent of cases occurring in the ampullary portion.[21] As the pregnancy grows the tube can rupture, creating a surgical emergency. Ectopic pregnancy and, more importantly, ruptured ectopic pregnancy can have a confusing clinical presentation. When assessing a patient for first trimester bleeding and pain, 6–16 percent of the time they will have an ectopic pregnancy.[22]

The risk factors for ectopic pregnancy are varied and often overlap. In short, anything that has affected the tube, such as previous sterilization, pelvic inflammatory disease, in utero DES (diethylstilbestrol) exposure, as well as tubal reanastomosis, can increase the risk of ectopic pregnancy. Furthermore, infertility, multiple sexual partners, and previous genital infections also increase the risk of an ectopic pregnancy.[23]

The treatment of ectopic pregnancy has now broadened to include medical treatment with intra-muscular methotrexate or surgical treatment. With that noted, there is only one treatment for a ruptured ectopic pregnancy and that is definitive surgical management accompanied by aggressive resuscitation.

Professionalism Considerations

Rarely do issues of professionalism present themselves in such an egregious manner. No one would disagree that this attending surgeon has behaved inappropriately, allowing her cultural stereotypes and political views to dictate or even reflect on patient care. Many things could be behind such a comment. At best, it is a poorly chosen way to express her frustrations with the inequities in a health care system that would put someone in danger secondary to insurance concerns. At worst, it is this caregiver's true thoughts. Regardless of the motivation for the comment, the more nuanced issue of professionalism falls onto those who witness such a comment, in this case the resident obstetrician-gynecologist. For him or her, the issue is defining the limits of professional responsibility in light of complex circumstances, the majority of which are not in the resident's control.

The American College of Obstetrics and Gynecology has published a Code of Professional Conduct,[24] which is written not only to guide physicians in their roles as professionals, but to exemplify what a physician should aim toward and be held accountable for when falling short. The principle of justice is there invoked to avoid discrimination that is not illegal, but is immoral and unprofessional. The code, as a professional guide, addresses professional responsibility, imploring ob-gyn professionals to "strive to address through the appropriate procedures those physicians who demonstrate . . . unethical or illegal behavior."[24]

It is clear from a professional standard that there is an obligation in this situation. The resident present for the offending remarks needs to address the physician's conduct. This requirement is clear just as the manner in which it is to be implemented is murky. It is naïve to think that a resident and an attending are on equal footing in this situation. It is likewise naïve to think that the resident's concerns will be met with an enthusiastic response wherever and to whom they are brought. This is the crux of the conflict and is what makes being a professional difficult, while at the same time not diminishing the responsibility.

What is at stake? To defiantly tell the attending you think these comments are not only wrong but unethical may be your style, but unfortunately the medical system might make the consequences of such a comment onerous. Something is to be gained by looking at the classically Aristotelian definition of justice which when paraphrased implores us to treat equals equally and unequals unequally.[25] In this instance you are not equal with your attending; similarly our twenty-two-year-old patient does not have the same societal status and privilege as you and many others in society. Nonetheless, in both instances you are equal as moral agents participating in an imperfect, unequal system.

Opinion

Consequently, when unequal, in a system fraught with inequality, you act accordingly. Addressing the attending, asking her to explain what she meant in a non-threatening, non-judgmental manner is one option. Going to your program director, chief resident, or the attending's supervisor are also legitimate options. In each of those options you are recognizing your moral responsibility, while at the same time recognizing your limits. If just consideration of these options makes you uncomfortable, this is not surprising. It is better to be uncomfortable now, with time for reflection, than to find yourself meeting this challenge blindly and unprepared.

Throughout your medical career you will be faced with ethical decisions. For most people, ethical dilemmas are not as dramatic as the vignette. The real risk in ethical decisions with little drama is that against the backdrop of fatigue, power differentials, and time constraints, they can be ignored. As moments of personal definition are ignored, you no longer define yourself, but allow yourself to be defined. The sooner you can become attuned to quiet moments of definition, the sooner you can seize them as appropriately your own.

When surrounded by practitioners of high professional and moral fiber, all is well. When at a scrub sink, late at night, with an individual whose professionalism is grounded in intolerance, the potential loss is immeasurable.

Cynthia Brincat, M.D., Ph.D.
Department of Obstetrics and Gynecology,
University Michigan Health Systems

A Perspective from a Cultural Competency Advocate

It's always disconcerting when role models demonstrate behaviors and beliefs that are flagrantly inappropriate. We often assume that because people are in the healing professions, expressions of racism and callousness are not part of their vocabulary.

So it's tempting to dismiss this case as the unguarded ranting of one individual. But the current social context is powerful. Many Americans embrace the United States' tradition of open doors and integration, and enjoy the benefits of multiculturalism. For others, though, demographic trends trigger anxiety and anger, which is expressed and amplified at the neighborhood level, on the talk-show circuit, and in the national political discourse. Add to this the devastating medical and financial burden, caused by gaps in health insurance coverage, which causes patients to delay seeking care, and frustrates clinicians who have to deal with the consequences of financially strapped health care organizations.

The attending physician's outburst may also be a symptom of attitudes that prevail in the health care organization itself. Diversity – socioeconomic, ethnic, cultural, and linguistic – is a fact of life in the U.S. health care system of the twenty-first century. This diversity poses significant challenges to both individual staff and the organization itself, from communicating with limited English speakers to navigating cultural differences in how people respond to illness and treatment. If sensitivity and accommodation to these differences were valued by the organization, it's unlikely that the physician would have felt comfortable expressing her attitudes so freely.

In the worst-case scenario, we have to acknowledge that discrimination and racism still exist in health care. A growing literature base[26] documents patient perceptions and experiences of this, and describes entrenched disparities in health care access, treatment, and outcomes.[27] In the best of circumstances, health care organizations and training institutions are just beginning to prepare clinicians and staff to appropriately manage a patient population that may offer up a big-city stockbroker, an undocumented

Chinese immigrant, a Somali war refugee, and a troubled suburban teenager –
all in the same morning.

Accepting the challenge of speaking truth to power, as described in
Dr Brincat's commentary, is one response available to our resident. But it's
not the only one. If we accept that individuals both reflect and shape workplace attitudes, then the resident may look at this event as an eye-opening
opportunity for promoting change.

Cultural competence refers to the ability of individuals and organizations
to acknowledge and respond effectively to the cultural and linguistic differences posed by any person seeking services. Some clinicians care for diverse
populations and, with a curiosity born of concern, learn how to creatively
navigate these differences. A growing number of health care organizations –
as recognized, for example, by the Joint Commission,[28] NCQA (National
Committee for Quality Assurance),[29] and other accrediting bodies – are
investing leadership and resources in changing their organizations to meet
the needs of these diverse patients.

What can a health professional in training do? The first step is to learn more
about how to respond effectively to cultural diversity, with respect to both
individual skills and organizational change. Among many excellent resources
available are those produced by the American Medical Student Association,[30]
the Association of American Medical Colleges,[31] and the U.S. Department of
Health and Human Services Office of Minority Health.[32] The next step is to
investigate the demographics of the organization's service area. Where
do people come from? What languages do they speak? What is their
social, economic, and educational background? What can be learned from
the community organizations that represent and serve the represented
groups?

Next, have a look at the health care institution itself. Are there programs designed to bridge the linguistic and cultural differences between
the staff and the community? Are there trained medical interpreters on staff
or on contract, and are they used when needed? Are patient education programs for prenatal care, chronic disease management, smoking cessation,
and so forth, designed with the cultural values and social realities of the
community in mind? The National Standards for Culturally and Linguistically
Appropriate Services (CLAS) from the HHS Office of Minority Health offer
a good framework assessing the cultural competence of health care organizations.[33]

The process of looking at how a health care institution responds to linguistic and cultural issues is best done with colleagues. By asking questions of
staff, managers, and those in the community, you may find others who are
quietly concerned about the same issues. Perhaps they are the bilingual staff

that are called on to interpret, or the lab tech who doesn't know what to do when someone has misunderstood the pre-procedure fasting directions. Increasingly, managers concerned with quality improvement and patient safety are thinking about how to enhance data collection and target interventions to reduce outcome disparities between minorities and mainstream patient populations. The aim is to find a group of colleagues and cultural experts who can work together to raise awareness throughout the whole organization – through grand rounds that have a cultural component, short articles in staff newsletters, brown-bag lunch talks, or a formal training program.

Obviously, the offending physician of our case study may not be the first person on your committee. But by creating a working environment where diversity is acknowledged and respected, all staff – prejudices openly stated or denied – have the chance to learn another approach, and begin the process of change.

Julia Puebla Fortier
Director, Resources for Cross Cultural Health Care

SOCIAL JUSTICE – PEDIATRICS

A two-year-old African-American child returns to her pediatrician's office for further management of an elevated lead level. The mother, an executive banker, is disturbed because the front desk personnel continue to ask her for her Medicaid card despite the fact that she has private insurance. While waiting near the front desk, she observes that many white patients coming to the office are not asked for their Medicaid card.

A Perspective from a Pediatrician and Public Health Specialist

Clinical Background

Lead exposure has particular consequences for children under six and has been associated with behavior problems, lower IQ, anemia, renal disease and altered Vitamin D metabolism. The 2005 American Academy of Pediatrics (AAP) Policy Statement on lead exposure in children recommends that all children who are Medicaid-eligible should get routine lead level testing. Further, the policy statement suggests that most children with elevated lead levels are eligible for Medicaid.[34]

Before 1970, the primary source of lead was exposure to leaded gasoline fumes. Homes built along highways and busy roads often had lead deposits in their soil and play areas. Lead-contaminated dust can still be found today. With the removal of leaded gasoline, blood lead levels decreased in children by 40 percent between 1976 and 1980.[35] Lead poisoning was, however, still very prevalent in children and attention was refocused on the paint found in many homes, particularly in older, well-established residential communities. In the early 1900s, lead was added to paint because it made it more durable and, ironically, was used in the "best" homes. Before paint was reformulated without lead in 1977, almost all homes in America were painted with varying amounts of lead-based paint. Paints formulated in the 1940s have been found to contain as much as 50 percent lead.[36] Infants and toddlers, unaware of the potential lead exposure from flaking or peeling paint, are especially susceptible to placing paint chips in their mouths.

Professionalism Considerations

In this vignette, several assumptions are made by the front desk personnel that raise concern around confidentiality and race. Think about first impressions when a two-year-old African-American child returns for an elevated lead level test. Lead poisoning is often misinterpreted as a condition of the poor. It is clearly prejudicial for the office staff to assume that an African-American returning for a lead test is poor and/or on Medicaid.

Medical and lay communities alike are familiar with the principle of *primum non nocere*, or "first do no harm." This admonition refers not only to physical harm, but also to emotional and psychosocial harm. Pediatrics is a unique specialty because the health care of the patient is almost entirely dependent on the actions of a third party. We build a rapport with our patients' families in order to encourage parents to follow our recommendations for their children's care.

This mother's perception was that the office staff continued to ask about her Medicaid card because of her race. While it was clearly unprofessional of the staff to continue to ask despite the fact that she corrected them, there may not have been a racial motivation. However, for anyone in clinical medicine, the front desk is the face of one's practice. Attitudes, expressions, and comments of the front desk will reflect on patients' perceptions. Physicians may be unaware of how their staff is perceived by others. Nevertheless, they are assumed to be in tacit agreement with perceived prejudicial or racial attitudes, simply by failing to correct such behavior or by allowing such an individual to remain employed.

Regardless of the source of the lead contamination, the child in question will need monitoring of blood lead levels and may require more blood work and frequent visits for neurodevelopmental monitoring. If the mother feels resentment toward the office staff or perceives that she is being discriminated against, she may be unwilling to bring her child back for monitoring, which could ultimately lead to harm.

For any person who has worked hard to gain a position of high status, the implication that they possess a lesser status can be insulting. This is especially true for anyone who has had to overcome social or financial obstacles and racial prejudice to attain their current position. Making assumptions about a patient's social situation, regardless of the reasoning behind doing so, is likely to lead to resentment of the medical staff and may initiate miscommunication between the patient and the physician. It may even contribute to patient harm if the end result is a lapse in necessary testing or follow-up.

Opinion

The physician's first task would be to apologize to the mother for the perceived injustice on her part, and to tell the office staff to do the same. The second task would be to educate the office staff regarding the use of neutral terms and open-ended questions, such as "Do you have your insurance cards with you?" Using neutral language and apologizing if a misunderstanding occurs will often ensure that patients will feel respected and will ultimately get the medical care they need.

Erin Wright, M.D.
Cooper University Hospital, Camden, NJ

Walter Tsou, M.D., M.P.H.
Past President American Public Health Association
Center for Public Health Initiatives,
University of Pennsylvania

A Perspective from a Scholar on Medical Professionalism

For all its good intentions to educate physicians-in-training to give equitable and compassionate care to all people, medical education often misses the mark in one critical area: our unexamined prejudices. Too often we fail to acknowledge our human tendencies toward race- and class-based prejudices, toward heterosexism and religious intolerance, toward impatience with those who do not speak English. We fail to acknowledge the human propensity to diminish, belittle, scapegoat, or ignore other humans whose bodies, habits, and values do not resemble our own. It happens all the time across social class, educational level, and professions, including medicine. Doctors and nurses do it, in spite of taking pledges not to. And when we do acknowledge these tendencies, our response as medical educators has often been to try to "fix" them with so-called "competency" efforts that look something like this: Here's a group of people/patients who stand out because they're "different" from the unspoken norms of white, middle-class, able-bodied, heterosexual, Western, English-speaking, Judeo-Christians. Their characteristics (values, habits, orientations to health, illness, and dying, etc.) are X, Y, and Z. You must learn these and will be tested on these characteristics via a paper-and-pencil test or perhaps an OSCE (objective structured clinical examination). When you pass, you indicate "competency" and we don't have to worry about your attitudes and behaviors toward these "others" because you know their characteristics.[37]

Of course this is not the way humans operate, both those who seek to understand and those who seek to be understood. When we seek to understand, an awareness of and honesty about our biases, fears, reflexes, and defenses is a critical part of this never-finished process. Without such honesty, physicians are less likely to "arrive at an accurate diagnosis, prescribe appropriate treatment, and promote healing,"[38] and their patients are less likely to feel cared for and respected. Certainly the mother in this case did not feel respected in the waiting room, an essential part of the clinical environment for which the physician is responsible. She may also wonder about the quality of care her child is receiving in that very office.

Indeed, the often-cited report of the Institute of Medicine (IOM), *Unequal Treatment: Confronting Racial and Ethnic Disparities in Health Care* (2002), gives her plenty of reasons to question the care she receives. The report found that "a consistent body of research demonstrates significant variation in the rates of medical procedures by race, even when insurance status, income, age, and severity of conditions are comparable. This research indicates that U.S. racial and ethnic minorities are less likely to receive even routine medical procedures and experience a lower quality of health services."[39] Moreover, IOM committee member Thomas Inui, M.D., said that "the committee members were 'stunned' by a 'strong body of evidence' supporting the role that bias, stereotyping, prejudice, and clinical uncertainty on the part of health care providers play in perpetuating health care disparities."[40]

Do current educative efforts such as cultural competency courses reduce such health care disparities? Would a requirement that everyone involved in clinical medicine take such courses reduce the likelihood of the scenario involving the African-American mother and the Medicaid card? Perhaps, but it is unclear that such efforts ask any of us to examine our biases, stereotypes, and prejudices honestly; it is also unclear that such efforts ask us to work against these biases, stereotypes, and prejudices other than altering certain behaviors, speech patterns, and other overt attitudes toward persons of particular races, ethnic backgrounds, classes, religions, and sexual identities. That is, it is unclear that such efforts ask us to be permeable to authentic change because we come to realize our responses are disrespectful, unkind, and harmful to patients.

That said, how do we work toward authentic change? A first step would be to move discussions of cultural competency away from formulaic "characteristics" of nondominant groups. This is particularly important given that many academic medical centers, according to Inui, serve poor and minority populations from their immediate surroundings, and that often the only characteristics of these communities that medical students see are the negative circumstances that bring individuals to the hospital. Moreover, as Jeanette E. South-Paul notes, most patients cared for during medical training "are suffering from poor lifestyle choices, a lack of insurance and therefore a lack of access, and conditions that patients allow to get worse before they seek treatment. I don't think there is any way you can discount the resulting contribution of bias on continuing disparities in health care."[40]

These factors, along with cookbook approaches to cultural competency, contribute to the stereotypical assumptions made in the case in the vignette. We all must work toward better awareness of the perspectives, not merely characteristics, of nondominant groups, particularly those who have subordinate status relative to the dominant culture. Medical education – undergraduate, graduate, and continuing – must be developed that allows medical students and physicians to develop relationships with individuals and families whose so-called "differences" put them at a disadvantage for health-related services because of bias, stereotyping, and unequal distributions of wealth and power. Such relationships, however, involve more than context-stripped clinical encounters between doctors and patients. They involve, rather, an attempt to understand patients' lives at home and work, their attempts to access health care and other relevant services, their experience of being ill and the social causes of their suffering. With such a relational, context-driven orientation at play in clinical locations, patients are much less likely to encounter the kind of knee-jerk stereotyping described. They are, instead, far more likely to encounter the respect and compassion due to all patients in all their varieties, from all those contributing to their care.

Delese Wear, Ph.D.
Professor of Behavioral Sciences,
Northeastern Ohio Universities College of Medicine

SOCIAL JUSTICE – PSYCHIATRY

A psychiatrist declines to continue to care for a patient whom she has been following for bipolar disorder because the patient owes the physician several hundred dollars and has not paid the balance. The patient has been recently unemployed.

A Perspective from a Psychiatrist

There are many possibilities to consider. How old is the patient? How severe is his or her psychiatric condition and how much has it impacted his/her life and financial stability? Does the patient have insurance, savings, and other unpaid bills? How long has it taken to accumulate this balance? If the psychiatrist's fee is $200 a visit, then it might take only three or four visits for a balance of "several hundred dollars" to accrue. If he or she is a community clinic patient who is responsible for only $10–$15 as "co-pay," then it might have taken months or years to accumulate this balance. The question of how long it has taken to accrue this unpaid balance is important. It can shed light upon whether the psychiatrist has failed to be vigilant from the get-go (if the unpaid period is many months long) or is being unduly impatient in collecting money (if the unpaid period is only two or three visits). Although it is instructive to consider all the variables in such a vignette, in actual practice there is always more data available for consideration.

One can also read this vignette as a poem. One can sense that a dialectical tension between the physician's caring for a patient and safeguarding her own interests is being created here. We are being prompted to take this or that side. And, indeed, we are tempted to give in. One moment we are inclined to declare that the psychiatrist shows a lack of altruism by putting financial matters ahead of continuity of the patient's care. The next moment, we want to protest on behalf of the psychiatrist – after all, she has to put food on the family table – and pronounce the patient not holding up the other side of the bargain.

The vignette also highlights the built-in tension between medicine being a noble praxis of selfless devotion and a way of earning wages to sustain one's own life.[41] Medicine is both a "calling" and a profession and we are programmed to lean toward silent self-sacrifice. We snicker at the ostentatious lifestyle of the Beverly Hills cosmetic surgeon and admire the pediatrician who devoted his life to taking care of poor children in Africa. This is, however, a bit simplistic since this judgment is based upon caricature masquerading as reality. To find the psychiatrist unempathic and uncaring is to take a moralistic stance that overlooks the need to forge technical compromises and ignores the fact that the psychiatrist has to be "physicianly" toward her own self as well. Inordinate generosity leads to resentment and that is not good for patient care either. A balance has to be arrived at, one that can avoid the extremes of both clinical callousness and pathological altruism. To get to this balance, one requires an optimal mixture of experience, intuition, and knowledge of facts at hand. There are much larger questions, though, lurking in the background. Should the availability of medical care be a fundamental human right? Should practicing the "healing art" be conditional upon charging money? How is it that in this wealthy nation of ours there are so many people who cannot receive proper medical care? Should the world's richest, most powerful nation put greater premium upon taking care of its sick and suffering citizens?

Salman Akhtar, M.D.
Professor of Psychiatry and Human Behavior, Jefferson Medical College

A Perspective from a Public Health Expert

The fundamental unit and building block of any health care system should be the doctor–patient relationship. All efforts in financing care should be centered around the creation, maintenance, and preservation of this relationship. All other developed countries foster the doctor–patient relationship by providing some form of health insurance, even for their unemployed.

Unfortunately, the U.S. health care system is best characterized as a poorly constructed market-based system which determines access to care based on ability to pay. Private employers fund the majority of health services for people between the ages of eighteen and sixty-four who are working. In addition, others are able to obtain health care financing through government largesse linked to "membership" in politically acceptable categories. These groups include the elderly, the very poor, veterans, Native Americans, and people with certain diseases such as end-stage renal failure. Those who fit into such categories or have sufficient financial means are able to be covered with health insurance. All of the remaining (which now number over 45 million) are considered uninsured.[42]

Mental health patients also have multiple unique problems. Mental health patients are intensely vulnerable and often suspicious of others, including authority figures. Development of a trusting relationship can be difficult. To the extent that a bipolar patient has developed trust with his/her psychiatrist, loss of that relationship can be devastating and cause a major setback in care.

Second, ongoing psychiatric care necessitates a parallel discussion of treatment fees, beginning with the first visit and from time to time as necessary, so that there is a clear expectation from both patient and psychiatrist about payment.

Many mental health patients are caught in an insurance Catch-22. Those that are severely mentally disabled can qualify for Medicaid, if certified by a physician as disabled and unable to work. This requires access to a psychiatric evaluation, which is often difficult. Even if an individual is deemed mentally disabled and qualifies for Medicaid, he or she is subject to periodic re-certification and can be removed from Medicaid. Making this even worse, Medicaid typically pays less than most private insurance, severely limiting the number of psychiatrists willing to accept Medicaid payments. People with less severe illness who are unable to sustain employment are limited in their ability to get employer-sponsored health insurance.

Medicaid is a federal-state program, which means that under federal guidelines each state is free to set different eligibility standards and offer different benefits. As a result, prescription drug benefits vary from state to state as does access to medication. For mental health patients, the ability to obtain and afford psychotropic medications is essential for living.

Finally, an issue which remains politically difficult is parity in mental health reimbursements for psychiatrists and other mental health workers. In comparison to insurance payments to physicians who provide other health services (such as medical consultation or surgery) mental health reimbursements are usually less.

All of this is background to our current case. Our patient is recently unemployed, beginning an all too common spiral into loss of health insurance. Complicating the situation, our patient is already behind in payments and the psychiatrist is unwilling to continue care without some payment.

There are several considerations which should help determine the best action. Perhaps most important is the psychiatrist's judgment of the individual's mental health status. In someone actively mentally ill and in need of medications, termination of treatment cannot be recommended and is potentially illegal.[43] It is essential that the psychiatrist is able to separate her best clinical judgment from the patient's finances.

A more in-depth assessment needs to be made by the office staff to find a source of funding, including the likelihood of finding another job which carries benefits or the possibility of qualifying for Medicaid based on mental health disability. Another possibility is to develop a payment system which is affordable for the patient and acceptable for the office staff. Finding a guarantor of payment, such as a friend or family member, can be important.

Even if the patient is unable to afford payment and a guarantor is not found, a psychiatrist must continue treatment until the patient is stable or transferred to another care provider. Given the fragility of many mental health patients, one should not terminate treatment without some plan for follow-up care. Most communities have government-sponsored mental health centers which can provide competent follow-up, but transfer of mental health records and professional contact with the accepting psychiatrist is strongly advised.

The larger picture demands that we ask why psychiatrists and mental health patients are placed in this painfully awkward situation. All patients, but particularly mental health patients, need a safety net for financing their care. Our nation's lack of universal health care as an essential safety net for all patients is an embarrassment. Parity for mental health services is necessary to continue to attract medical students to the field of psychiatry. All of us should demand a system of financing health care which ensures quality, affordable health care for all Americans.

Walter Tsou, M.D., M.P.H.
Past President, American Public Health Association
Center for Public Health Initiatives, University of Pennsylvania

SOCIAL JUSTICE – SURGERY

A surgical waiting room contains many pamphlets from political campaigns urging the overhaul of medical malpractice. The pamphlets contain criticism of the local party candidate who does not support tort reform and solicits donations for the candidate who does. The patient, an attorney, is referred to this surgeon for evaluation of a rectal abscess. At the visit, the patient tells the surgeon of her unease about seeing political advertisements and brochures in the doctor's office and states she should probably be seeing a physician who is fully concerned about the patient's care and not as partisan.

A Perspective from a Surgeon and Ethics Committee Member

Clinical Background
A perirectal abscess represents an urgent surgical condition. This patient will require a procedure to drain the infection. It can be performed in the office or in the operating room, depending upon the location and size of the infection as well as other co-morbid conditions. Most perirectal abscesses result from an infection in glands located in the anal canal. The infection tunnels either between the internal and external sphincter (intersphincteric) or traverses both muscles and becomes a perirectal abscess (transsphincteric). Sometimes these abscesses will rupture spontaneously; however, most of the time surgical un-roofing is necessary.[44] If the abscess is small enough and located

on one side of the anus, office drainage with local anesthesia is commonly performed. If the abscess is very large, bilateral (horseshoe), or the patient has significant additional medical problems, it may be prudent to perform the procedure in a monitored setting. Antibiotics are not necessary unless the patient is immuno-compromised.[45]

Professionalism Considerations

Medical malpractice issues are a daily fact of life for all physicians. The manner in which we practice is influenced by fear of litigation in many situations, resulting in what is commonly called practicing "defensive medicine."

Never before have practitioners of medicine faced the current spiraling costs of professional liability coverage (medical malpractice insurance) nor has the impact on the profession ever been greater. Malpractice insurance costs have risen to such an extent in many states that some doctors have been forced to limit the scope of their practice or to move to other states that have tort reform and lower malpractice costs.[46] Data have shown states with caps on non-economic damages to have 12 percent more practicing physicians than those without.[47] Additionally the non-partisan Office of Technology Assessment has concluded that caps on damage awards were the only type of state tort reform that consistently showed significant results in reducing the cost of medical liability.[48]

With the physician being a cornerstone in the delivery of care, it is appropriate to examine the ethical responsibilities of the physician, not just in providing direct care in the traditional one-on-one model but in assuring ongoing access to the physician's services. Since 1847, the American Medical Association has codified the principles of medical ethics, developed primarily for the benefit of the patient and periodically revised, reflecting a succession of challenges and responsibilities. With competent and compassionate care paramount, two of the nine primary AMA principles are relevant to the current discussion:

- Principle 3. A physician shall respect the law and also recognize a responsibility to seek changes in those requirements which are contrary to the best interests of the patient.
- Principle 7. A physician shall recognize a responsibility to participate in those activities contributing to the improvement of the community and the betterment of public health.[49]

Taking the ethical guidelines from this leading organization a step further, the AMA specifically addresses many of the dilemmas faced by modern medicine as technology and circumstances continue to evolve. In the AMA's *Code of Medical Ethics*, section E10.018, titled "Physician Participation in Soliciting Contributions from Patients," addresses the current topic and specifically recommends that appropriate means includes "making information available in a reception area."[50] This statement, importantly, goes on to state that "physicians should avoid directly soliciting their own patients, especially at the time of a clinical encounter. They should reinforce the trust that is the foundation of the patient–physician relationship by being clear that the patients' welfare is the primary priority and that patients need not contribute in order to continue receiving the same quality of care."

Thus it appears that placing literature, including literature that requests political support and/or contributions, in the waiting room may be appropriate and in keeping with principles of medical ethics and duty to the patient. The presence of literature supporting a specific candidate who endorses tort reform allows patients to become more knowledgeable regarding this serious problem. Since this material also creates a situation whereby a patient may choose not to get appropriate medical attention, the physician should at minimum consider placing this information in a single, well-labeled location.

Opinion

This patient needs immediate drainage of the abscess. All other issues are secondary and it is the surgeon's responsibility to put the patient at ease as well as educate her as to the urgent and serious nature of her condition. Her physician should offer sincere regrets if she was upset with the literature in the waiting room and stress that the urgency of her medical problem is of more immediate importance. If there is not a "meeting of the minds" on this and the trust paramount to the doctor–patient relationship could not be forged, then it would be appropriate to recommend that the patient see another physician.

Gerald Isenberg, M.D.
Associate Professor of Surgery,
Jefferson Medical College
President, Association of Program Directors for Colon
and Rectal Surgery

Kenneth Mendel, M.D.
Clinical Associate Professor of Medicine,
Temple University School of Medicine
Founding member of Ethics Committee,
Crozer Chester Medical Center, Chester, PA

A Perspective from Medical Malpractice Plaintiff Attorneys

The relationship between doctor and patient is marked by a level of trust rarely found in other professions. This trust is the result of an age-old commitment by physicians to honor one basic creed: to place the interests of the patients they serve above all else. The ethical guidelines of the medical profession embody this creed. Principle 7 of the American Medical Association's *Code of Medical Ethics* states, "A physician shall, while caring for a patient, regard responsibility to the patient as paramount."[51] The *Code of Medical Ethics* similarly defines the patient–physician relationship as one that is "based on trust and gives rise to physicians' ethical obligations to place patients' welfare above their own self-interest and above obligations to other groups."[52]

For physicians, ensuring the patients' best interest remains paramount and requires a careful weighing of potential harms and benefits. For example, an oncologist knows chemotherapy causes numerous harmful side effects. The oncologist also believes that the benefit of eradicating cancer cells outweighs those side effects. Thus, the decision to prescribe chemotherapy serves the cancer patient's best interest.

In this case, the doctor has filled the waiting room with brochures that urge patients to support tort reform. Certainly, physicians are entitled to express their beliefs about political issues and personally advocate for change in law and policy.[53] By placing these tort reform brochures in the waiting room and urging patients to act, however, the doctor has exceeded the scope of personal advocacy. Rather, the doctor has thrust the tort reform debate directly into the physician–patient relationship. In so doing, the doctor has brought tort reform under the watchful eye of the obligation to regard his or her patients' welfare as paramount. Consequently, in order for this doctor's actions to be ethical and professional, the tort reform initiatives advocated in the brochures must be in the best interests of the patients who read them.

Like the decision to prescribe certain medication, determining whether tort reform is in the patient's best interest requires a weighing of harms and benefits to the patient. "Tort reform" refers to legislation that diminishes individuals' centuries-old right to seek accountability for wrongfully inflicted harms.[54] Medical malpractice tort reform laws commonly impose statutory limits on the compensation that injured patients can recover for non-monetary harms such as disfigurement, pain, and physical impairment.[55] These statutory limits apply regardless of the severity of the patient's injury. For many injured patients – especially children, the elderly, and others who earn little income – tort reform therefore means they are left with a severely limited, one-size-fits-all system of justice.[56] Thus, tort reform harms patients by forcing them to give up, either in whole or in part, their legal right to seek accountability and justice for harms caused by medical negligence.

What about the benefits to patients from tort reform? Perhaps this doctor believes that tort reform will lead to lower health care costs. The Congressional Budget Office, however, concluded that medical malpractice costs amount to only 2 percent of overall health care costs.[57] Maybe this doctor believes that medical liability is forcing doctors out of business and hindering patients' access to care. Yet recent studies show no empirical support for claims that doctors are fleeing certain locales because of liability concerns.[58] Finally, this doctor may believe tort reform will lower his or her liability insurance premiums. This consideration, however, should have no place in the weighing of patient harms and benefits as it concerns only the doctor's self-interest. Moreover, comprehensive studies show no correlation between tort reform laws and lower liability insurance rates.

In sum, the benefits to patients from tort reform pale in comparison to the significant harms. Consequently, by placing tort reform brochures in the waiting room and urging patients to act, this doctor has failed the physician's professional obligation to regard patients' interests as paramount. In so doing, the doctor's actions have undermined the profound and unique trust that defines the patient–physician relationship.

Kathleen Flynn Peterson, R.N., J.D.
Robins, Kaplan, Miller & Ciresi, Minneapolis, MN
Past President of the American Association for Justice

Thomas G. Sinas, J.D.
Robins, Kaplan, Miller & Ciresi, Minneapolis, MN

SOCIAL JUSTICE – NEUROLOGY

A seventy-two-year-old man with Parkinson's disease takes carbidopa-levodopa (Sinemet) and pramipexole (Mirapex). He asks his neurologist whether his pramipexole can be written in his wife's name, because he does not have a prescription plan and she does. His wife also sees the same neurologist. She has had a past history significant for a stroke and takes pramipexole for restless legs syndrome.

A Perspective from a Neurologist

Clinical Background

Parkinson's disease (PD) is a common neurodegenerative disease characterized by four cardinal clinical features: a 4–6 Hz rest tremor, bradykinesia, rigidity (cogwheeling), and postural instability. It affects approximately one in a hundred persons over age sixty-five although 10 percent of people with Parkinson's are diagnosed before age forty.[59]

Dopamine agonists (DAs) are approved as both monotherapy and adjunctive therapy to levodopa in the treatment of PD.[60] DAs have been demonstrated to delay the onset of motor complications compared to levodopa, and therefore play an increasingly important role in PD treatment, especially among younger patients.[61] In patients with more advanced disease, DAs are added to levodopa therapy to provide more constant dopaminergic stimulation.

Restless legs syndrome (RLS) is a subjective hyperkinetic disorder in which the patient experiences a restless sensation, often described as tingling or crawling, in their legs at night that improves with moving. The majority of RLS cases are idiopathic but there are several secondary causes including iron deficiency, pregnancy, and end-stage renal disease.

DAs are the treatment of choice in RLS.[62] In RLS, the dose typically is far less than that used to treat PD. Although the same side effects seen in PD (nausea, somnolence, compulsive behaviors) may be seen in RLS, side effects are less frequent because of the lower dosing.

Professionalism Considerations

With the rapid changes in health care in the United States, physicians increasingly face professional dilemmas arising from the costs of such care. In 2003, over one-third of uninsured adults did not fill a prescription for medication or pursue a recommended test or treatment because of cost.[63] In 2008, health care is a leading cause of personal bankruptcy: Americans now make a new bankruptcy filing every thirty seconds as a result of a health problem.[63] In light of these pressures, it is not surprising that a patient lacking prescription coverage would ask the physician to write a prescription in the name of an insured spouse.

Several arguments can be made in favor of writing such a prescription. The first is that the physician–patient relationship requires that the physician's primary duty is to act as an advocate for the patient and that this duty supersedes the interest of the insurance company that will pay for the prescription. The physician may feel compelled by the seeming unfairness of a health care system. Indeed, a 1999 study demonstrated that 57 percent of physicians surveyed were willing to use deception to get coronary bypass surgery for their patients where the physician felt it was medically indicated but not within the strict terms of the patient's insurance coverage.[64] Most of the surveyed physicians sanctioned their deception by arguing that their duty was to work as their patients' advocate within the rules of the third party payers until those rules compromise their patients' health.[64]

Another argument is that the benefits of misrepresentation are enormous.[65] If the patient does not have his pramipexole, he will experience worsening symptoms of Parkinsonism. Moreover, the lack of pramipexole may accelerate his development of motor complications. Fearing for her husband's health, the wife may forgo her doses of pramipexole so that her husband can take them. Yet, the typical dose of pramipexole for restless legs however is much less than that of Parkinson's disease. Therefore, the husband will be undertreated and the wife will be untreated. The end result is that both of your patients suffer.

A final argument is that the harm of misrepresentation is small.[65] Relative to an insurance company's assets, the cost of a prescription of more pramipexole than would be necessary to treat RLS is miniscule. Indeed, one author, arguing that it would be ethically acceptable to write a prescription for an uninsured patient in an insured relative's name characterizes such costs as "not even a blip on the insurance company's radar screen."[66]

On the other hand, numerous arguments exist for why the physician should not write the requested prescription. First, writing such a prescription undermines the physician–patient relationship. This relationship is based in part upon honesty. If the patient realizes that the doctor was willing to lie under one circumstance (even if to the patient's putative benefit) would the patient be able to trust the doctor to maintain confidences? Moreover, having committed a potential fraud on behalf of the patient, would the physician later fear that the patient might disclose that action to third parties such as a medical board or malpractice attorney?

What about the physician's relationship with the wife? If she is not aware of the deception, she could be harmed by inadvertently taking the amount of pramipexole meant for her husband, potentially resulting in an overdose or augmentation of her RLS. If she is aware of the deception and her insurance company challenged the amount prescribed as excessive for RLS, an investigation could reveal the deception and she could lose her insurance.

Furthermore, the benefits of the physician–patient relationship, such as privacy, exist because society sanctions the special nature of the relationship. Society grants these special privileges and protections but, in return, expects that these privileges will not be abused. Using the powers granted, such as writing prescriptions, in a fraudulent manner would lead to society limiting those benefits and establishing more intrusive oversight – further undermining the physician–patient relationship.

The next argument, inherent in the first, is that the patient is enlisting you in a fraud and potentially a crime. Federal law prohibits writing a prescription for anyone other than the intended patient. By writing the prescription in the wife's name in an amount necessary to treat her husband's PD, you are defrauding her insurance company. The dollar amount may be small, but this is legally considered fraud. If every physician engaged in similar behavior, the costs to the insurance companies could be significant. Ultimately, such fraudulent claims could result in increased premiums or even the loss of coverage as companies either went out of business or refused to write policies that covered prescriptions.

Finally, writing a prescription in the wife's name will do nothing to solve the larger problem of inequities in health care coverage. Indeed, such sub rosa tactics only perpetuate these inequities by encouraging the use of deception rather than confronting the fundamental problem of lack of prescription coverage.

Opinion

I would not write the prescription as requested. Although the physician–patient relationship is paramount, it is not without limitation. Here, the patient is asking you to engage in a fraud and possibly a crime. As noted, the implications of your potential action go far beyond a single prescription. As one author observed, "Advocacy without deception is consistent with a robust conception of the professional duty of fidelity to patients. But lying to health care payers to obtain preauthorization or payment crosses the line."[67]

Instead, I would urge the patient to review whether they have any non-essential expenses such as vacations that could be sacrificed instead of medication. If the husband were still unable to afford the medication, I would attempt to help him with other means of getting the medication, including samples, pharmaceutical assistance programs, local PD support networks, and social work. In the end, the patient may still not get the medication and may be angry. Nevertheless, if you explain your reasoning and concerns, most patients will understand and respect your position, especially if you try to help them obtain the medication through legitimate means.

Daniel Kremens, M.D., J.D.
Assistant Professor of Neurology, Jefferson Medical College

A Perspective from a Social Worker

This case raises interesting practical and ethical concerns for this family that are not uncommon in the field of medical social services these days. It would be quite easy for a physician to object flatly to writing a prescription in another person's name, since this is fraud. If this were a controlled substance, such as a narcotic, this discussion would go no further. Social workers find creative solutions on behalf of our clients. Somewhere in our training, we must have been told that if we fail to find a resolution for a client we are bad advocates! The task at hand is to find a way for this patient to receive his medications without diverting medication from his wife.

I would first determine if he is a veteran, as his age puts him in such a demographic. If so, he might be able to take advantage of low cost prescriptions through Veterans Affairs. The next option is to investigate state programs that help seniors pay for medication. To be eligible, an individual has to have a very low income, thereby disqualifying many. I would review the patient's insurance situation, and question why he does not have a pharmacy plan (assuming that he does have Medicare). The Medicare D program was quite confusing for seniors when it was introduced in 2006. I relied on a nonprofit insurance counseling agency that spoke to support groups and was willing to meet with patients individually to review all of their options. This is especially relevant since seniors, who don't sign up for a D plan, are penalized financially unless they have a better plan through an existing policy.

I would also suggest that when searching for a plan, he project his total pharmacy bill for the year and see if it is worth paying a higher premium to get more benefit. Carbidopa/levodopa is a relatively inexpensive medication, as it is made in many generic formulations. Pramipexole, however, is costly. He may be taking other medications as well. Mail order plans are often more cost effective as one can receive a three-month supply for the same co-payment as a one month supply.

Another avenue to check is the pharmaceutical company that makes pramipexole. Many companies have programs where patients can receive medications at a lower cost. For instance, Novartis has the Care Card, which is available to seniors who have Medicare but no prescription coverage. Unfortunately, with the advent of Medicare D many companies abolished patient assistance programs so it may not be a feasible alternative except for younger patients.

Marketing representatives from drug companies visit physicians' offices, frequently leaving not only branded items such as pens, but also medication samples. These samples are used to initiate treatment as well as assist those who have difficulty paying for prescriptions. This marketing is big business for companies and has come under public scrutiny. Medical organizations, academic health centers, and pharmaceutical companies have begun to address the ethics of the practice. One consequence of the trend to limit access of drug company representatives to practice sites is the loss of these samples.

Finally, there are programs such as the Free Medicine Foundation[68] and discount prescription cards that are widely accepted at most drugstore chains. These options are often for indigent seniors or those that are not Medicare eligible.

It is a dreadful task to inform a family, struggling to make ends meet, that there are no resources to help with the cost of medications. Hopefully, looking toward possible solutions through the government, private foundations, or pharmaceutical companies, assistance can be found.

Susan Reichwein, BASW
Program Coordinator
Parkinson's Disease and Movement Disorder Center,
University of Pennsylvania

SUMMARY – PRINCIPLE OF SOCIAL JUSTICE

Background

The goals of this section summary are to help students (1) understand the concept and impact of social justice in the context of health care, (2) apply the principles of social justice in the practice of medicine, and (3) use a conceptual framework to analyze the ethical and professional dilemmas contained in the cases presented and in future encounters.

The roots of contemporary social justice can be traced to ancient Greek philosophers such as Aristotle, who described the organizing principles that underlie modern society. Pivotal among these are the principles of liberty, equality, and the importance of each individual, concepts of justice and good, and the good person's aspiration to achieve the "good."

These principles and concepts govern the interactions among people, and the design of the basic structures of society, such as government and other institutions. The specific societal agreements surrounding concepts such as liberty, the right to vote, the importance placed on the autonomy and decision making of the individual, the rule of law and interpretation of justice in the context of a society, define the nature of that society. These principles and concepts are then functionally translated into laws, conventions, and standards of behavior in society.

The goal of a society so designed is to create a framework for interactions and cooperation among individuals, each of whom has unique skills, and whose life is enhanced through cooperation with others. This framework of interaction is governed by principles and rules that permit the resolution of disagreements, and the distribution of the "goods" produced by society.

Social justice can be defined conceptually, and be described in the form of the systems that deliver social justice within a society. Social justice is that set of circumstances of existence and distribution of "goods" that society believes are the right of each individual in that society to possess or experience. In the ideal state, the social justice systems include governmental and non-governmental institutions, professions, and individuals that assure each individual has at least those minimum circumstances and is in possession of those goods defined by a just society as required. When individuals or groups of individuals are found to be in a deficient position in relation to these circumstances or positions, society intervenes through its systems to remedy these deficiencies. This is a component of the social contract between the society and its citizens.

Many dimensions of the daily practice of medicine are governed by principles considered intrinsic to social justice. The providers of health care are a component of society's social justice system and are thus bound by social contract to our citizens. Current discussions and proposals to improve access to care and fair distribution of health care resources and to eradicate disparities in health care are all social justice issues. Furthermore, patient care delivery is also governed by guiding principles of professionalism that are grounded in social justice, including placing the patient's needs first, equal respect for each patient, and the physician's role as patient advocate.

In his pioneering work first published in 1957,[69] then revised[70,71] and restated,[72] John Rawls provides a modern conceptual framework for the theoretical construct of a just society. The role that the agreed upon principles of justice play is "to specify the fair terms of social cooperation" within the society.[73] These principles are used to specify the basic rights and duties, to regulate the benefits which arise from cooperation in society, and to allocate the burdens required to maintain society.[72]

In addressing the issues of equality, Rawls affirms the equality of all members of society as persons, and sets forth the principle that all have equal opportunity to achieve their potential. He recognizes, however, that while all persons are equal in their personhood and possess the same basic rights, liberties, and privileges, all persons are not equal in their innate capability or in the settings into which they are born. Thus, while an individual within society may possess the right to vote, the right to think as one desires, and the right to a job, one's life circumstances will vary based on the nature of those opportunities.

Society, according to Rawls and others,[74] is a mutual agreement on behalf of those within society to work together to maximize the benefit, the good, for all. In theory, the methods used to determine the distribution of the good derived from the efforts of those in society could differ. For instance, think about a society constructed to maximize the aggregate benefit with no consideration for the distribution of the good among those within society. In such a society, the work of many may be optimized to produce wealth for a few. The production of the goods may be maximized, but their distribution would be considered immensely "unfair" by those with little to show for their efforts. Examples of this construct are a feudal society or a society where slavery is employed.

Now imagine a society where the work of all is pooled, making use of the special skills of each member of society, and the goods distributed equally without regard to the contribution of the individual. The production of the goods may again be maximized, but their distribution may be considered immensely "unfair" by the high producers. Examples of this construct are a commune or a socialist society.

Using the concept of justice as fairness as a political philosophy, Rawls examines justice in the context of a democratic society. He outlines a principle, called the difference principle, which governs the just distribution of the goods produced by society, taking into account the differential productivity of those granted the gifts of intelligence, ability, and birthright, compared with the needs of those granted less intelligence, ability, and birthright. He proposes that the test of justice as fairness in the distribution of goods is that when there is an incremental good distributed to the most advantaged, there is an increase in the good distributed to the least advantaged in society. These increments need not be equal, but an improvement of the position of the most advantaged should be accompanied by an improvement in the position of the least advantaged.

This dimension of Rawls' proposition has stimulated a generation of thought, design, and debate regarding the concept of social justice in a democracy, and provides the conceptual basis for application theories and practical interventions. This includes providing an elegant and relevant framework for thought about the challenges facing American medicine and health care today. Are the fundamental rights of individuals as equals being recognized when it has been shown, independent of access to health care and insurance status, that delivery of certain services based on gender, race, or ethnicity are unequal?[75–78] By their very nature, given our current conceptualization of justice in the United States, are these disparities unjust and unfair?

Similarly, given the dramatic improvements in health care that have occurred over the past forty years, would Rawls judge that the difference principle has been applied correctly? Has the health care of our least advantaged citizens improved sufficiently in comparison with those who are most advantaged? This concept of justice as fairness offers a framework for examining two of the vignettes illustrating the principle of social justice which speak not only to barriers and bias in health care for the homeless and uninsured, but to the perpetuation of this bias.

Medical students, with supervision by a core of like-minded residents and faculty, provide one of few avenues to health care for the homeless. This care is important not only for the patients, but also for the students. Accordingly, effective July 1, 2008, the Liaison Committee on Medical Education standard IS-14-A was amended as follows: "Medical schools should make available sufficient opportunities for medical students to participate in service-learning activities, and should encourage and support student participation."[79] As described by Plumb and Pringle in Chapter 2, the refusal of some physicians to provide specialty services clashes with the ideals and classroom lessons about professionalism. In fact, this behavior enables a negative "hidden curriculum" that results in cognitive dissonance, and serves to build cynicism in some and elitism in others.

In their commentaries about the Latina with no insurance who presents late with severe bleeding due to an ectopic pregnancy, Brincat and Fortier in this chapter explore not only the impact poverty and ethnic bias has on health care, but also the hierarchical challenges of the medical education environment. The fear this patient experiences in seeking care collides with the callous, bigoted words of the faculty who proposes involuntary sterilization. This critical incident in the education of this resident challenges her medical, ethical, and professional essence. It is fair to say that Rawls would think that, for the patients who inspired these vignettes, we have failed to provide our least advantaged citizens with sufficiently comparable health care.

So how much improvement for the least advantaged is required in order to assess that distribution of improvement to the most advantaged is just? Since inequality in the distribution of goods is accepted in his construct, how unequal is still just? Here Powers and Faden propose a useful framework. In their treatise *Social Justice: The Moral Foundations of Public Health and Health Policy*,[80] they offer the premise that in a real-world, non-ideal setting, one must look at the consequences of the impact of unequal intellect, opportunities, and birthright, as well as the impact of society and its structures, on the individual in order to determine the practical issue of whether the individual is realizing justice in their daily life. They posit that a just society provides, at a minimum, for the "well-being" of each of their citizens. In this model of the social contract between citizens (of, in our case, the United States) and society, they identify six domains of personhood that must be examined in order to assure that the individual is in a state of well-being and that justice has been realized. These domains are:

1.   Health – Defined in the broad sense not only of access to health care services, but extended to the personal perception of health of the individual.

2. Personal Security – The ability to go about one's daily activities without fear of physical or emotional violence.

3. Reasoning – The ability and opportunity to reason and to apply that reasoning in life circumstances.

4. Respect – To be treated by others with respect and to have the opportunity, through life circumstances and the manner in which they are treated by others, to develop self-respect.

5. Attachment – The opportunity to form personal relationships; an essential element of human existence is the social nature of human beings.

6. Self-Determination – The right and opportunity to make decisions about one's own future.

Powers and Faden make the important observation that the dimensions of well-being interact, and that deficiencies in any one of these areas may have significant adverse consequences in any of the other essential domains.

What are the implications for physicians? One is obvious, and at the core of American medicine: The *health of the individual is one of the essential dimensions of well-being, and required of a society characterized by social justice.* Indeed, it is society's justice-based interest in the health of each individual that compels the contract between society and the profession of medicine and the other healing profession, nursing. This understanding that health is an essential component of well-being required for each member of society is also the reason that many professional organizations have argued for universal insurance coverage or at least catastrophic coverage for all citizens.

Of equal import is the observation by Powers and Faden that health is but one of the domains of personal well-being in a just society. The interactions of these determinants underscore the responsibility of the physician, along with other members of the health care team, to address these issues, whenever possible, in order to return the individual to health. Figure 5.1 presents a schematic representation of the responsibility of each physician, in interacting with the patient through the other five dimensions of well-being. Although these other dimensions may be less evident in the daily work of many physicians, on occasion the physician is the first or only person to identify one of these deficiencies, creating an opportunity for action.

Review of the Cases and Commentaries

Several of the vignettes in this section illustrate potential damage to a person's well-being that can come when health care is thwarted by negative interactions in other domains. In their commentaries about the two-year-old child

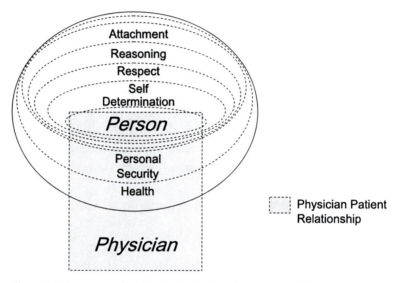

Figure 5.1. Domains of Well-Being Pertaining to Issues of Social Justice

with an elevated lead level, Wright, Tsou, and Wear highlight the interface between health and respect. The repeated requests to the child's mother, a banker who also is African-American, for a Medicaid card, raises the ugly specter of racial discrimination, although this may have been simply incompetence. This lack of respect sets the stage for diminished trust in the parent–patient–physician relationship and has the potential to compromise the health of her child.

The links between health and attachment frame the commentaries by Tsou and Akhtar about termination of psychiatric care for a bipolar patient who cannot pay for treatment and has lost this employment benefit. It is painfully clear that this loss of attachment threatens the health of this individual. He is one of the many millions of people who cannot gain or sustain access to care, which prevents development of the sustained productive patient–physician relationship so crucial to anyone living with chronic disease.

The patient with Parkinson's disease is struggling for self-determination when he requests that his physician write a prescription for him in his wife's name because she is the one with insurance coverage. In their commentaries, Kremens and Reichwein show empathy for this man and his struggle and seek an individual "work around" solution to serve justice for one, while refusing to violate the law. They re-affirm the principle that physicians, under ordinary circumstances in the United States, should not violate laws in their attempt to meet the health needs of a patient. They should use every opportunity at their disposal, including the involvement of a social worker and other members of the health care team, to craft a legal solution to the patient's needs.

It is altruism that is at the heart of the struggle explored by Rabinowitz and Eanes (in Chapter 2) in their probing commentaries about career choice. This student's calling to pursue medicine and commitment to rural family practice is pitted against the economic realities of medical student debt and unequal physician pay. According to the Association of American Medical Colleges, if this student finished medical school with the 2007 mean educational debt, she will graduate with $139,500 in loans to repay. As of 2006, the mean annual income of practitioners in ophthalmology was $300,000, in family medicine $170,000 and likely to be lower in rural areas.[81] There have been small market-driven increases in compensation due largely to the growing shortage in availability of primary care physicians.[82] The decisions made by medical students about career choice and residents about practice location and hours do raise serious concerns about access to care for all.[83]

An elegant example of the dynamic state of justice as fairness in society is explored by Weitz and Gorman in their commentaries about appropriate diagnostic and therapeutic intervention for coronary artery disease in women. It wasn't until the 1980s, led by the Coronary Artery Surgery Study and others that gender differences in the clinical presentations of coronary syndromes began to emerge. In 1986, new NIH guidelines called for inclusion of women in clinical trials, opening the doors to discovery. As late as 1990, prominent women in Congress, including Senator Olympia Snow, spoke to the need for better compliance with this mandate as women were still being excluded from studies of aging, heart disease and AIDS. Here, the issue of gender bias mixes with the boundaries of science and the time lag between discovery and standard of practice, resulting in unequal treatment based on gender to persist.

Connecting Social Justice, Professionalism, and the Individual Physician

The promise that each physician makes in public in reciting the Hippocratic Oath extends the contract between society and the profession to each individual physician and is implicit in every patient–physician interaction. It is the public promise to place the needs of patients above self-interest. As such, professionalism is the basis of the profession's contract with society.[84]

At an individual level, primacy of patient welfare is what Pellegrino[85] calls "effacement of self-interest," and others call altruism.[86] It involves doing the right thing for the right reason, even when not in the physician's own best interest. From this quiet, persistent, individual, and collective bravery flows all the other virtues and attributes of professionalism. Honesty, truth telling, integrity, compassion, respect, commitment to excellence and lifelong learning, all spring from that pledge that physicians make to put the needs of others above self.[87]

Trust is the mortar that unites the members of society with the profession, and effacement of self-interest is the cornerstone of the profession of medicine and its relationship with society.[88] It is through this relationship that physicians become agents of social justice, ministering to the sick and infirm to fulfill society's promise to all. It is through this relationship that, at a minimum, the six dimensions of well-being would be met at a level that would satisfy Rawls' theoretical difference principle, and would meet Powers and Faden's definition of well-being.

It is logical to ask: What should be the minimum level of the distribution of the good to the least advantaged in our society? More specifically, what would constitute a satisfactory minimum level of health and health care services? To these questions, we offer the following opinion. The definition of the minimum level of health and health care services for each member of our society is a dynamic and positively changing one, and is rightly governed by society through its political processes and the application of the principles of justice. Health care is not static; inexorably, it is moving forward.

As health care offers greater promise of cures and palliation while extending lifespan each year, so too must the promise to the least advantaged grow and expand. It is the ethos of physicians to provide as much as possible for their patients, regardless of their social or economic standing in society. At some juncture, a just society makes choices regarding both the distribution of the good (health care services), the availability or level of services to its citizens (services available to all), and how the burden of maintenance of this social structure will be allocated (economic sustainability). As discussed by Tsou in the psychiatry vignette in this chapter, our society has made this determination for subsets of the population: the very poor, the severely disabled, persons over the age of sixty-five and some less advantaged children. The rest of our citizens are still waiting.

Physicians are personally involved in the delivery of services required in order to maintain one or more of the six domains of well-being. Physicians must also be watchful of the interaction of health with the other dimensions of well-being, given their role and responsibility as agents of the profession, and the fulfillment of their personal and collective commitment to the members of society.

Medical students are the future of the profession of medicine. That future also holds the promise for taking action to construct a socially just health care system. Medical educators in alliance with students can be a force for changing and creating a better learning environment that takes advantage of countless opportunities to educate about social justice: informal conversations, formal discussions, defined curricula, blogs and webinars, grand rounds, public forums, conferences and national meetings, white coat and graduation ceremonies, and sponsored activities by the Alpha Omega Alpha Honor Medical Society and the Gold Humanism Honor Society. That environment also encompasses many individuals whom physicians interact with and learn from throughout their professional careers, for example patients, peers, colleagues in other professions, faculty, institutional and community leaders, the public, legislators, and policy-makers. As sociologist and civil rights leader W.E.B. Dubois reflected, "Education must not simply teach work – it must teach life."

An innovative platform for understanding social justice that incorporates advocacy and participation can empower medical students to take action and become doctors who adhere to a set of public roles and professional responsibilities as physician-citizens.[89] Successful advocacy requires clarity of purpose, good data, and effective strategies that are grounded upon promoting the skills and attitudes of good citizenship in medical education.[90] Examples of practical educational strategies to promote social justice across all learning environments in medicine include:

- Reviewing/revising the medical school's mission statement to ensure its relevance to social justice
- Stimulating recognition and discussion of the meaning and applicability of the social contract in health care and contemporary society
- Improving access to health care by documenting real-life experiences to better understand and educe fair distribution of health care resources in the context of rising health care costs
- Collaborating to improve systems of care by actively applying the principles of social justice and the essential domains of well-being in the practice of medicine
- Inspiring an institutional or outreach initiative addressing health care disparities to improve social justice in the community
- Motivating a local or national medical society to act on issues that advance justice as fairness
- Perpetuating the spirit of volunteerism as a life-long professional responsibility and commitment to social justice
- Advocating for social justice by serving on a political action group, participating in a petition or letter writing campaign, or engaging in another form of public activism
- Working on a local or national campaign for a candidate or legislation dedicated to advancing social justice in health care

CONCLUSION

The commitment we nurture during medical school to care for the least advantaged must transcend throughout one's career. We must never mistake enlightened self-interest for altruism. Only through an enduring commitment to all members of society, both the advantaged and disadvantaged, can the profession of medicine be true to its responsibilities as an instrument of social justice in a democratic society. Whether through insights into the well-being of each patient, or advocacy in the design of societal institutions and the application of the difference principle on a national policy level, physicians must keep their focus on the health of all citizens. It is a privilege to serve the public, one person at a time. This is the legacy of medicine; it is the profession's responsibility freely taken and pledged at graduation, "on our honor."

Thomas J. Nasca, M.D., MACP
Chief Executive Officer
Accreditation Council for Graduate Medical Education
Professor of Medicine
Formerly the Gertrude M. and Anthony F. DePalma Dean (2001–2007)
Jefferson Medical College

Linda L. Blank
Vice President, The Culliton Group, Washington, DC
Robert G. Petersdorf Scholar (2006–2007),
Association of American Medical Colleges, Washington, DC

REFERENCES

1. Mosca L, Banka CL, Benjamin EJ, et al. Evidence-based guidelines for cardiovascular disease prevention in women: 2007 update. *Circulation.* 2007;**115**(11): 1481–1501.
2. Tobin JN, Wassertheil-Smoller S, Wexler JP, et al. Sex bias in considering coronary bypass surgery. *Ann Intern Med.* 1987;**107**(1):19–25.
3. Anand SS, Xie CC, Mehta S, et al. Differences in the management and prognosis of women and men who suffer from acute coronary syndromes. *J Am Coll Cardiol.* 2005;**46**(10):1845–1851.
4. Daly C, Clemens F, Lopez Sendon JL, et al. Gender differences in the management and clinical outcome of stable angina. *Circulation.* 2006;**113**(4): 490–498.
5. Kennedy JW, Killip T, Fisher LD, Alderman EL, Gillespie MJ, Mock MB. The clinical spectrum of coronary artery disease and its surgical and medical management, 1974–1979. The coronary artery surgery study. *Circulation.* 1982; **66**(5 Pt 2):III 16–23.

6. Douglas PS, Ginsburg GS. The evaluation of chest pain in women. *N Engl J Med.* 1996;**334**(20):1311–1315.

7. Heidenreich PA, Shlipak MG, Geppert J, McClellan M. Racial and sex differences in refusal of coronary angiography. *Am J Med.* 2002;**113**(3):200–207.

8. Saha S, Stettin GD, Redberg RF. Gender and willingness to undergo invasive cardiac procedures. *J Gen Intern Med.* 1999;**14**(2):122–125.

9. Stramba-Badiale M, Fox KM, Priori SG, et al. Cardiovascular diseases in women: A statement from the policy conference of the European Society of Cardiology. *Eur Heart J.* 2006;**27**(8):994–1005.

10. Guru V, Fremes SE, Austin PC, Blackstone EH, Tu JV. Gender differences in outcomes after hospital discharge from coronary artery bypass grafting. *Circulation.* 2006;**113**(4):507–516.

11. Glaser R, Herrmann HC, Murphy SA, et al. Benefit of an early invasive management strategy in women with acute coronary syndromes. *JAMA.* 2002;**288**(24):3124–3129.

12. Lorber J. Doctor knows best: Gender and the medical encounter. In: *Gender and the Social Construction of Illness.* Thousand Oaks: Sage Productions; 1997.

13. Wizemann TM, Pardue M, eds. *Exploring the Biological Contributions to Human Health: Does Sex Matter?* Washington, D.C.: National Academy Press; 2001.

14. Dracup K. The challenge of women and heart disease. *Arch Intern Med.* 2007;**167**(22):2396.

15. Grady D. In heart disease, the focus shifts to women. *The New York Times.* April 18, 2006.

16. Wenger NK. You've come a long way, baby: Cardiovascular health and disease in women: Problems and prospects. *Circulation.* 2004;**109**(5):558–560.

17. Canto JG, Goldberg RJ, Hand MM, et al. Symptom presentation of women with acute coronary syndromes: Myth vs reality. *Arch Intern Med.* 2007;**167**(22):2405–2413.

18. Clinical Researcher. What women want: Taking sex differences seriously in clinical trials. *Understanding the Biology of Sex and Gender Differences.* Vol. 1 No. 8. Washington, D.C.: 2001.

19. Merz C, et al. Insights from the NHLBI-sponsored Women's ischemia syndrome evaluation (WISE) study: Part II, gender differences in presentation, diagnosis, and outcome with regard to gender-based pathophysiology of atherosclerosis and macrovascular and microvascular coronary disease. *Journal of the American College of Cardiology.* 2006;**47**(3 suppl):21s–29s.

20. Anderson FW, Hogan JG, Ansbacher R. Sudden death: Ectopic pregnancy mortality. *Obstet Gynecol.* 2004;**103**(6):1218–1223.

21. Bouyer J, Coste J, Fernandez H, Pouly JL, Job-Spira N. Sites of ectopic pregnancy: A 10 year population-based study of 1800 cases. *Hum Reprod.* 2002;**17**(12):3224–3230.

22. Murray H, Baakdah H, Bardell T, Tulandi T. Diagnosis and treatment of ectopic pregnancy. *CMAJ.* 2005;**173**(8):905–912.

23. Ankum WM, Mol BW, Van der Veen F, Bossuyt PM. Risk factors for ectopic pregnancy: A meta-analysis. *Fertil Steril.* 1996;**65**(6):1093–1099.

24. Ethics Co. Code of professional ethics of the American College of Obstetrics and Gynecology. 2004.

25. Aristotle. *Nichomachean Ethics*, Book V. Translated by Ross, WD. USA: Oxford University Press; 1998.

26. Blanchard J, Lurie N. R-E-S-P-E-C-T: Patient reports of disrespect in the health care setting and its impact on care. *J Fam Pract*. 2004;**53**(9):721–730.

27. Smedley BD, Stith AY, Nelson AR, eds. *Unequal Treatment: Confronting Racial and Ethnic Disparities in Healthcare*. Washington, D.C.: National Academy Press; 2003.

28. Wilson-Stronks A, et al. Hospitals, Languages and Culture Study. http://www.jointcommission.org/PatientSafety/HLC/. Accessed April 7, 2008.

29. The National Committee for Quality Assurance. Recognizing Innovation in Multicultural Health Care. http://www.ncqa.org/tabid/451/Default.aspx. Accessed April 7, 2008.

30. American Medical Association. Cultural Competency in Medicine. http://www.amsa.org/programs/gpit/cultural.cfm. Accessed April 7, 2008.

31. American Association of Medical Colleges. Tools for Assessing Cultural Competence Training and Resource Guide. http://www.aamc.org/meded/tacct/start.htm. Accessed April 7, 2008.

32. US Department of Health and Human Services Office of Minority Health. A Physician's Practical Guide to Culturally Competent Care. https://cccm.think culturalhealth.org/. Accessed April 7, 2008.

33. U.S. Department of Health and Human Services Office of Minority Health. Assuring Cultural Competence in Health Care: Recommendations for National Standards. The Office of Minority Health Web site. http://www.omhrc.gov/templates/browse.aspx?lvl=2&lvlID=15. Accessed April 7, 2008.

34. American Academy of Pediatrics Committee on Environmental Health. Lead exposure in children: Prevention, detection, and management. *Pediatrics*. 2005;**116**(4):1036–1046.

35. Annest JL, Pirkle JL, Makuc D, Neese JW, Bayse DD, Kovar MG. Chronological trend in blood lead levels between 1976 and 1980. *N Engl J Med*. 1983;**308**(23):1373–1377.

36. Centers for Disease Control (CDC). Preventing lead poisoning in young children – United States. *MMWR Morb Mortal Wkly Rep*. 1985;**34**(5):66–8, 73.

37. Wear D. Insurgent multiculturalism: Rethinking how and why we teach culture in medical education. *Acad Med*. 2003;**78**(6):549–554.

38. Novack DH, Epstein RM, Paulsen RH. Toward creating physician-healers: Fostering medical students' self-awareness, personal growth, and well-being. *Acad Med*. 1999;**74**(5):516–520.

39. Smedley BD, Stith AY, Nelson AR, eds. *Unequal Treatment: Confronting Racial and Ethnic Disparities in Health Care*. Washington, D.C.: National Academic Press; 2002.

40. Gabriel B. Confronting "unequal treatment": The institute of medicine weighs in on health care disparities. *AAMC Reporter*. 2002;**11**(9):6–7.

41. Hall MA, Schneider CE. The professional ethics of billing and collections. *JAMA*. 2008;**300**(15):1806–1808.

42. U.S. Census Bureau. Health Insurance Coverage: 2007. http://www.census.gov/hhes/www/hlthins/hlthin07.html. Accessed September 4, 2008.

43. Ethics04. Section 3: The Impact of Managed Behavioral Health Care on Core Ethical Principles. http://www.ceuinstitute.bizhosting.com/ManCareE/Ethics04.htm. Accessed September 4, 2008.

44. Gordon PH, Nivatvongs S. Anorectal abscesses and fistula-in-ano. In: Gordon PH, Nivatvongs S. *Principles and Practice of Surgery for the Colon, Rectum, and Anus*. 3rd ed. Informa Health Care; 2002:191–233.

45. Jobst MA, Thorson AG. Anal sepsis and fistula. In: Yeo CJ, ed. *Shackelford's Surgery of the Alimentary Tract*. 6th ed. Saunders; 2007:2045–2061.

46. Kessler DP, Sage WM, Becker DJ. Impact of malpractice reforms on the supply of physician services. *JAMA*. 2005;**293**(21):2618–2625.

47. Agency for Healthcare Reserach and Quality. The Impact of State Laws Limiting Malpractice Awards on the Geographic Distribution of Physicians.

48. Office of Technology Assessment. Impact of Legal Reforms in Medical Malpractice Costs; 1993.

49. Principles of medical ethics: Adopted by the AMA Houseof Delegates, June 2001.

50. AMA code of medical ethics: E10.018 physician participation in soliciting contributions from patients, October 2006.

51. Council on Ethical and Judicial Affairs. Code of medical ethics of the American Medical Association. 2006;15.

52. Ibid. at 317.

53. Ibid. at 272.

54. Garner BA, ed. *Black's Law Dictionary*. 8th ed. Eagan, MN: Thomson West; 2004.

55. See, e.g., Alaska stat. § 09.17.010 (2006); cal. civ. code § 3333.2(2006).

56. See generally Finley LM, The hidden victims of tort reform: Women, children, and the elderly, *53 Emory L.J.* **1263**(2004).

57. Congressional Budget Office. Limiting Tort Liability for Medical Malpractice 6. http://www.cbo.gov/ftpdocs/49xx/doc4968/01–08-MedicalMalpractice.pdf. Updated 2004. Accessed September 4th, 2008.

58. See generally Vidmar N, et al. "Judicial hellholes": Medical malpractice claims, verdicts and the "Doctor exodus" in Illinois, *59 Vanderbilt L.Rev* **1309**(2006).

59. Lang AE, Lozano AM. Parkinson's disease. first of two parts. *N Engl J Med*. 1998;**339**(15):1044–1053.

60. Poewe W. Drug therapy: Dopamine agonists. In: Schiapira A, Olanow CW, eds. *Principles of Treatment in Parkinson's Disease*. Philadelphia: Butterworth Heinemann Elsevier; 2005:25–47.

61. Holloway RG, Shoulson I, Fahn S, et al. Pramipexole vs levodopa as initial treatment for Parkinson disease: A 4-year randomized controlled trial. *Arch Neurol*. 2004;**61**(7):1044–1053.

62. Trenkwalder C, Paulus W, Walters AS. The restless legs syndrome. *Lancet Neurol*. 2005;**4**(8):465–475.

63. Levine SR. The interplay of age, access to health care, and insurance status: The good, the bad, and the ugly. *Arch Neurol.* 2007;**64**(1):15–16.

64. Freeman VG, Rathore SS, Weinfurt KP, Schulman KA, Sulmasy DP. Lying for patients: Physician deception of third-party payers. *Arch Intern Med.* 1999; **159**(19):2263–2270.

65. Lo B. *Resolving Ethical Dilemmas; A Guideline for Clinicians.* Baltimore: Williams and Wilkins; 1995.

66. Dickman RL. Bending the rules to get a medication. *Am Fam Physician.* 2000;**61**(5):1563–1564.

67. Bloche MG. Fidelity and deceit at the bedside. *JAMA.* 2000;**283**(14):1881–1884.

68. Free Medicine Foundation for All Ages. http://www.freemedicinefoundation. com/our_mission.html. Accessed September 6, 2008.

69. Rawls J. Justice as fairness. *The Journal of Philosophy.* 1957;**54**(22):653–662.

70. Rawls J. *A Theory of Justice.* Cambridge, MA: Harvard Press; 1971.

71. Rawls J. *A Theory of Justice.* 2nd ed. Cambridge, MA: Harvard Press; 1998.

72. Rawls J. *Justice as Fairness, A Restatement.* Cambridge, MA: The Belknap Press of Harvard University Press; 2001.

73. Ibid. chapter 2.3, page 7.

74. Gough JW. *The Social Contract: A Critical Study of Its Development.* Oxford, England: The Clarendon Press; 1957.

75. Steinbrook R. Disparities in health care – from politics to policy. *N Engl J Med.* 2004;**350**(15):1486–1488.

76. Bloche MG. Health care disparities – science, politics, and race. *N Engl J Med.* 2004;**350**(15):1568–1570.

77. Lurie N. Health disparities – less talk, more action. *N Engl J Med.* 2005;**353**(7): 727–729.

78. Institute of Medicine. Unequal treatment: Confronting racial and ethnic disparities in health care. 2003.

79. Liaison Committee on Medical Education Web site. http://www.lcme.org/ standard.htm. Accessed November 3, 2008.

80. Powers M, Faden R. *Social Justice. the Moral Foundations of Public Health and Health Policy. Issues in Biomedical Ethics.* New York, NY: Oxford University Press; 2006.

81. Iglehart JK. Medicare, graduate medical education, and new policy directions. *N Engl J Med.* 2008;**359**(6):643–650.

82. Terry K. How do you compare? *Med Econ.*:30–38.

83. Baker CD, Caplan A, Davis K, et al. Health of the nation – coverage for all Americans. *N Engl J Med.* 2008;**359**(8):777–780.

84. ABIM Foundation. American Board of Internal Medicine, ACP-ASIM Foundation. American College of Physicians-American Society of Internal Medicine, European Federation of Internal Medicine. Medical professionalism in the new millennium: A physician charter. *Ann Intern Med.* 2002;**136**(3):243–246.

85. Pellegrino E, Thomasma D. *The Virtuous Physician.* New York, NY: Oxford University Press; 1993.

86. Nagel T. *The Possibility of Altruism*. Princeton, NJ: Princeton University Press; 1978.

87. Nasca TJ. Graduation address, Jefferson Medical College.

88. O'Neill O. *Autonomy and Trust in Bioethics*. Cambridge, United Kingdom: Cambridge University Press; 2002.

89. Gruen RL, Pearson SD, Brennan TA. Physician-citizens – public roles and professional obligations. *JAMA*. 2004;**291**(1):94–98.

90. Colby A, Ehrliche T, Beaumont E, Stephens J. Educating citizens: Preparing America's undergraduates for lives of moral and civic responsibility. 2003.

Cases and Commentaries

Following an episode of rectal bleeding, a fifty-six-year-old man is diagnosed with metastatic colon cancer. His family physician of the past thirty years reflects on this case. Upon review of the patient's outpatient records, he realizes that fifteen years ago he noted that the patient's father had colon cancer diagnosed in his sixties, and the physician wrote several entries in the chart that the patient was to have a screening colonoscopy at age fifty. The patient has been seen five times in the past six years (for treatment of upper respiratory infections and check-ups) and the physician now realizes that he never recommended a screening colonoscopy to him.

A Perspective from a Primary Care Physician

Clinical Background

For colon cancer screening, many of the national professional organizations, including the American Cancer Society and the U.S. Preventive Services Task Force, recommend the following screening options for average risk individuals starting at fifty years of age: fecal occult blood testing annually, flexible sigmoidoscopy every five years, annual fecal occult blood test plus flexible sigmoidoscopy every five years, double contrast barium enema every five years, or colonoscopy every ten years. Each one of these tests or combination of tests has different sensitivities and specificities.[1] Colonoscopy is the "gold standard" for screening. It is estimated that 10 percent of polyps greater than 1 cm in diameter become malignant within ten years, and about 25 percent become malignant after twenty years. It is possible that this patient may have had a significant polyp at age forty-one, and it could be argued that he should have undergone his first colonoscopy then, not at age fifty. Perhaps the family physician was not aware of this.

It is a reasonable assumption that if one follows the guidelines for colo-rectal cancer screening, most premalignant, adenomatous polyps can be detected and advanced colorectal cancer prevented in the average risk pa-tient. Most recommend that those with higher risk get screening earlier and possibly genetic testing and counseling.[1] The patient's father having colon cancer in his early sixties places him in a higher risk category. The father's medical history of cancer was obtained from the patient when he was forty-one years of age, and at that point the family physician recommended screening colonoscopy at age fifty. Since he wrote it in the chart several times, one assumes he also shared that recommendation with the patient.

Professionalism Considerations

The family physician served as the patient's personal physician for thirty years. This suggests a trusting relationship. It was unclear why there was no follow-up to the written recommendation for screening colonoscopy at age fifty. This could possibly be related to poor charting by the physician and the lack of timely "flagging" of a recommendation. Installing an electronic medical record system (EMR) would make it much easier to follow up on preventive services. The EMR can serve as a reminder for both the patient and physician for time-sensitive recommendations.

It is also unclear why the patient did not follow up on the physician's recommendation, which, if included in the chart, was probably shared with him. It could be argued that the patient had a shared responsibility for follow-up. Perhaps he denied potential colorectal cancer as a risk for himself, or perhaps he was concerned about the cost of colonoscopy, the preparation, and the potential risk associated with such an exam. One might expect he should have recognized how serious cancer of the bowel is, for his father had colon cancer. In a contractual type of doctor–patient relationship there is a shared responsibility for care, whereas in the paternalistic type of relationship the patient expects and accepts the physician's recommenda-tions every step of the way. This can also absolve a patient from his own responsibility.

Unfortunately, failure to follow up on a screening recommendation resulted in the patient's presenting with rectal bleeding and metastatic can-cer at age fifty-six. It is safe to say that undoubtedly the family physician recognized the oversight, and the patient and his family may have as well. The family physician should go back and examine the patient's chart to de-termine what went wrong and how it could have been avoided. It might also be of some value for him to review the literature for the risk of colorectal cancer in first degree relatives and when and what screening/preventive measures should be taken.

Now that the patient has advanced colorectal cancer, a difficult issue for the family physician to consider is whether or not he should sit down with the patient and his family to discuss how the oversight occurred. As with all such discussions, there are potential benefits and harms, and the physician must weigh these in each individual situation, always keeping the patients' best interests as paramount. Oftentimes, this is best accomplished with gentle, probing, open-ended questions, in order to assess what the patient would like to discuss. A hazard associated with this is the possibility that neither the patient nor his family may want to relive or hear this, particularly realizing that the patient also knew about the screening recommendation and did not follow up. At least initially, some patients do not like to look back, but rather are focused on the immediate problem and the future. Raising the issue could just make them feel worse and result in pointing fingers to blame. In other words, the physician could do harm. Therefore, it may be best not to raise the issue unless the patient seems to want to address this and asks specific questions. Then the physician must be completely honest and open. The long relationship and trust between the patient and his family physician depend upon this. Once the patient doubts the physician's veracity, it will be difficult for him to believe anything the physician tells him about his illness. Participating in his chronic care and maintaining hope would be impossible if the patient did not trust the physician. Bok sums this up by pointing out that patients who are lied to are resentful, disappointed, and suspicious. They feel wronged and are wary of new overtures. On the other side of the relationship, Bok points out that physicians who lie find that subsequent lies come more easily, psychological barriers wear down, and the ability to make moral distinctions can coarsen.[2]

Some physicians are hesitant to be open for fear of a malpractice suit. The current tort system built on a personal fault foundation is very threatening to physicians. A no-fault system, where avoidability rather than negligence is considered, could alleviate this and allow one to look at medical errors in an organized, open aggregate manner. This could lead to more constructive recommendations for the overall improvement of care.[3] Openness may not always prevent a malpractice suit, but, should it occur, the physician will have acted in a much more professional manner than if he attempted to conceal the truth.

Opinion

As a family physician I would attempt to provide a supportive role by answering all questions in a direct manner, coordinating the patient's care, supporting the family, and continuously promoting an optimistic and hopeful atmosphere. Rather than sit down with the patient and attempt to cover the entire scenario in one visit, I would rather schedule frequent visits to see how the patient and his family's reaction to this illness would unfold over time. I would attempt to work very hard to do no harm, and would try to maintain a positive balance between risk and benefit. I would be quick to use consultation when needed – both to help me realize what might be best for the patient, and also to reassure the patient and the family that he was getting the very best care.

Paul Brucker, M.D.
President Emeritus, Thomas Jefferson University
Professor of Family and Community Medicine,
Jefferson Medical College

A Perspective from a Bioethicist and Attorney

In reflecting upon this vignette, I wanted to address a couple of initial concerns. A traditional critique of bioethics is that it often reduces ethical issues to "quandary ethics." What should we do in a certain case? What is the best solution? With the growth of professionalism as a movement within medical education, I would like to avoid reducing professionalism to "quandary professionalism." Rather, striving for professionalism means taking seriously the virtues that the Accreditation Council for Graduate Medical Education outlines: "respect, compassion, integrity, responsiveness, commitment, and excellence."[4] The details of this case are too thin to adequately reflect on all of the aspects of these virtues, but we can try to address the following questions:

1. What does respect for the patient mean here?
2. What does integrity demand of the physician?
3. Is the physician compassionate?
4. Has the physician been sufficiently responsive?
5. What kind of commitment does the physician have?
6. How can the physician show excellence?

Respect and integrity go hand in hand. Respect suggests that the physician will not manipulate the patient for his or her own means. Integrity suggests that the physician will not deceive the patient. Compassion means that the physician will want to do what is of benefit for the patient. Responsiveness demands that the physician will not neglect important duties but address them in a timely manner. Commitment calls for a greater obligation of caring that may create some hardship on the physician. Lastly, excellence demands more than what is customary.

In this vignette, we have a physician who has been committed to his patient for three decades. Such a long-standing relationship is increasingly rare in health care, so it's a true testament to both the physician and patient that such a relationship has lasted for so long. Discovering that his patient has metastatic colon cancer requires a great deal of compassion from the physician toward his patient. Such compassion, however, may be mixed with his own feelings of potential inadequacy and guilt. Does he blame himself for the fact that this patient did not receive adequate screenings earlier? Did he not have an effective reminder system? Does he feel that he did not adequately respond to his patient's needs earlier, perhaps averting such a terrible outcome for this patient? Unfortunately, such mistakes are not uncommon in health care. As the Institute of Medicine report *To Err Is Human* noted, tens of thousands of patients lose their lives every year due to medical mistakes.[5]

A great strength of professionalism is that it asks physicians to reflect upon their calling as healers and not just disease managers. A great weakness is that it presumes that the physician is the only person who is responsible for the care of the patient when in fact it's a team of individuals who are caring for the patient. A blame-oriented culture would try to punish this physician – why didn't you do this screening? Alternatively, a culture of professionalism and patient safety would create a system where easy-to-commit human errors are prevented.

Recently, a guest speaker at our medical school, in a discussion of the topic of patient safety, mentioned that physicians still think of health care as a cottage industry when in fact it is a $2 trillion industry. Moreover, he stated "this system for patient safety has total reliance on individual responsibility and individual perfection. The reason it doesn't work is no one is perfect."[6] This comment reflects a challenge for the professionalism movement – just focusing on physicians' behaviors is not enough. Rather, professionalism means everyone involved in the care of the patient has to be on the same page. Even the most vigilant and caring physicians make mistakes. A health care system that is serious about professionalism must ensure that there are fail-safe mechanisms in place. Thus, having an EMR system that regularly reminded the physician about colonoscopy screenings might have prevented this tragic outcome.

Lastly, admitting mistakes and expressing genuine remorse is an ideal that addresses all of the concerns I have outlined. As ethicist John Banja has observed, patients want a heartfelt apology when a medical error has occurred.[7] Such an acknowledgment by a physician to a patient should sustain the trust of the patient. Although there is always the fear of litigation with such an apology, the consensus among physicians and ethicists is that physicians should disclose errors rather than cover them up. Admitting a mistake not only requires humility but some measure of courage. The goal of professionalism and patient safety is to ensure that fewer mistakes are committed and that then when they do occur, physicians and other health care professionals have the ability to express regret in a non-punitive environment. This is what patients want and presumably what the patient in this vignette would want as well.

Kayhan Parsi, J.D., Ph.D.
Associate Professor of Bioethics and Health Policy
Neiswanger Institute for Bioethics and Health Policy
Stritch School of Medicine, Loyola University

HONESTY WITH PATIENTS – PEDIATRICS

A ten-year-old girl is receiving chemotherapy for sarcoma that was diagnosed last year. The family moves to another town and have their first visit with the pediatric oncologist. During a discussion with the family about the care of the patient, it becomes evident that the child does not understand she has cancer. The parents are concerned that if their child learns of the diagnosis, she may become overly anxious, since her grandfather recently died of cancer.

A Perspective from a Pediatric Oncologist

Clinical Background[8]
Ewing sarcoma is the second most common type of malignant bone tumor in childhood. Treatment consists of combination chemotherapy with surgical resection or radiation for control of the primary tumor. The treatment is intensive and extends over a period of almost a year, during which patients spend a great deal of time in the hospital, isolated from their peers. There are also many serious side effects. Short-term effects include profound myelosuppression which can result in life-threatening infection or bleeding, nausea, vomiting, mucositis and alopecia among others. Long-term effects may include cardiomyopathy, infertility, and second malignancies as well as significant orthopedic impairment depending on the location of the primary tumor. Despite all of this, long-term disease-free survival for patients with localized disease approaches 70 percent. Ewing sarcoma can metastasize, most commonly to the lungs but also to other bones. The outlook for patients with metastatic disease is much poorer, with less than 30 percent long-term survival.

Professionalism Considerations[9–11]
It is not uncommon for parents of children newly diagnosed with cancer to try to protect their child from learning their diagnosis. They are experiencing

intolerable anguish as they are bombarded with terrifying information. What parent would wish to expose their child to such pain? However, a doctor's primary responsibility is to the patient. For pediatricians, the unique, symbiotic parent–child bond necessarily blurs that primary relationship, but it remains the physician's duty to respect the child's individual rights at a developmentally appropriate level.

Cancer will dramatically affect virtually every aspect of life for the child and family. The child will realize that something is seriously wrong in the face of such disruption. Even if the child is not directly informed of her diagnosis, she will read its implications on her parents' worried faces. Kept in the dark, the child may believe that her situation is hopeless and that she will certainly die. Why else would the parent avoid telling the truth? If open lines of communication are not established between parent, medical team, and child, the child may be afraid to ask questions or express emotions for fear that the answers will be too scary, or that they will upset the parent. In the case described, although the diagnosis is serious, there is effective treatment and chances are good that the child will recover. It is likely that the child's imaginings would be far worse than the truth.

Children with cancer are treated in specialty centers where they will be surrounded by other children with cancer and their families. In addition to their primary treatment team, there will be many specialists, trainees, technicians, and housekeeping personnel who will enter their room and interact with them. Even if the child does not figure out on her own that she is being treated in a cancer ward and therefore must have cancer, it is virtually inconceivable that someone – another patient, visitor, or staff member – would not let slip to the child that she indeed has cancer. In addition, a ten-year-old would likely have had enough exposure through the media and other interactions to recognize that people who get sick and lose their hair have cancer. The child would then learn her diagnosis without access to accurate, and potentially reassuring, information and emotional support. The news may be more frightening to the child than it was for the parents, who were told in a setting where they could be supported by physicians, nurses, and social workers. Children often have misconceptions about cancer. They often feel guilty, thinking that they somehow brought it on themselves by being "bad." They may believe that their cancer is contagious and thus avoid friends or siblings in fear of making them sick. In the absence of open communication, these misconceptions will not be addressed.

Children learn from infancy to trust their parents, and trust is fundamental in any successful physician–patient relationship. If a child finds that critical information was withheld by their parents and physician, her ability to trust those individuals will be compromised. She may not be able to believe reassuring information, such as news that the treatment is working, or that the pain will be relieved.

Patients are active participants in their own care. They must comply with their medications and treatments, and report symptoms so that side effects can be identified and managed appropriately. An understanding of why a treatment is being carried out and what to expect from it is essential for the patient to be an effective participant.

Understanding what motivates a family's request that information be withheld is essential. In this case, the child recently experienced the death of her grandfather from cancer. The parents worry that if the child learns that she has cancer, she will believe that she too will die. I would argue that it is even more important in this situation that the child be told the truth. It can be explained that "cancer" is not a single disease, but rather a general term for many different disorders that behave very differently, and that whereas the grandfather's disease could not be cured, the child in fact has a very curable illness and should expect to recover. The child can then be offered the opportunity to meet other children who have survived cancer.

Opinion

Certainly children are different, depending on their developmental stage and level of anxiety, in terms of how much information is appropriate. Although I strongly encourage families to be honest and provide accurate information, I rely on the child and family to guide me in terms of how much detail to provide. The ten-year-old with Ewing sarcoma must know the name of her disease and be aware that it is cancer. She must know she did not cause it, could not prevent it, and that it is not contagious. She must understand that her disease is curable, that we expect and hope that she will get well, but her life will be significantly altered for awhile. She should be told in general terms about the treatment and expected side effects. She must be informed of any procedures or surgeries that will be done and what measures will be taken to prevent discomfort. I would tell her family that I would not be able to care for her effectively if she were not given at least this amount of information.

One need not be brutally honest. The child does not need to be present for the lengthy consent discussion with the family where every possible side effect is described in detail. Allowing the parents some opportunity to meet with the oncologist alone gives them the freedom to ask their most difficult questions without concern for scaring the child. However, if a child asks a question, it should be answered with honesty. For instance, I might not choose to tell this newly diagnosed child with Ewing sarcoma that she could die from her disease. If she asked me, I would tell her that although we did not expect her to die and that we expect treatment will prevent death, that indeed some children do die from this disease.

Convincing parents to be honest with their children is often a gradual process requiring many conversations with different members of the health care team. It is important to avoid jeopardizing a relationship with a family early on by becoming too confrontational over this common issue. Often once they themselves reach an understanding of the diagnosis and learn to trust the providers, the parents will accept the child's need to know, and information will begin to flow naturally.

Robin Miller, M.D
Division of Hematology-Oncology
Alfred I. duPont Hospital for Children
Wilmington, DE

A Perspective from Parents of Medically Fragile Children

Our experience as parents of seriously ill children is that, all too often, physicians respond negatively to us when we disagree with or question their recommendations. They often do not adequately try to understand our perspective or patiently try to explain their reasons for recommending a course of action that we are hesitant or unwilling to endorse. We have often been left feeling abandoned or forced to accept a course of action we are neither comfortable with nor fully understand.

These parents may be advocating for a decision that may not appear to be in the best interest of the child. Yet their reasoning needs to be understood as the physician helps the family to make the right decision for their child. In this case, there may be many underlying reasons for the parents' decision not to tell their daughter her diagnosis. One reason may be a version of denial. By not telling her, it is somehow less true or real. They may not be ready to provide the support she would need upon hearing her diagnosis and prognosis until they receive it themselves. Another reason might be that they do not want to tell her such bad news without being able to reassure her that everything will be "OK." Possibly, they do not fully understand her prognosis and their fears may be overblown due to their lack of knowledge. They may need time and assistance to process the fact that they may not, ultimately, be able to reassure her that all will be fine. Finally, for their daughter, whom they know better than the treating clinicians do, it might be a terrible mistake for her to know.

She might become so frightened and hopeless that her course of illness would actually worsen. Until these, and other possibilities, are clarified it would be inappropriate for the physicians to impose their preference on this family.

We feel that the key issue for the treatment team is understanding the myriad of confusing and painful feelings that this family is experiencing. This understanding is the foundation for discussions about whether and how to inform the child about her cancer. The parents are scared and are facing the most painful experience any parent can face, that is, their inability to assure the safety and well-being of their daughter. Their motivation is purely to act in a way to protect their child. They are facing this horrific situation with no preparation and tremendous fears. It is critically important that the treating physicians understand the parents' motivations and establish a relationship with them to help them assist their child in the most appropriate manner.

A critical error would be to allow the situation to proceed in a manner in which the physicians and the parents take opposing positions allowing a power struggle to emerge. The decisions and strategy of the treatment team in addressing this issue will determine whether the family and the medical team are aligned so that together they can develop a plan that offers the best chance for recovery. Tension between the treatment team and family over whether to inform the child of her cancer needs to be avoided because it will detract from the effectiveness of the treatments offered.

What would help this family and child most with this issue is for members of the treatment team to reach out to the family to understand what this medical situation means to them. This illness does not exist in a vacuum but, rather, in a broader familial and societal context. The most effective treatment takes that broader context into account when developing a clinical plan of action. One difficulty may be the treating team's discomfort with addressing issues relating to the emotional functioning of the child and her family. In this case there may still be unresolved issues relating to the grandfather's death that need to be explored.

Overall, as parents, we must stress that the treating team needs to be patient and compassionate and understand these issues in their broadest context. The efficacy of the treatment offered to this child will be the result of the combination of the medical care provided and the support and involvement of the family. The clinical outcome will be optimized by assuring that the child and the family's emotional needs are understood and met and the family is supported in their efforts to care for their daughter.

Michael Golinkoff and Elizabeth Kramer
Bala Cynwyd, PA

HONESTY WITH PATIENTS – PSYCHIATRY

A fifty-four-year-old woman, placed last year on the antipsychotic drug olan-zapine (Zyprexa) for her schizophrenia, develops diabetes. After the diagnosis of diabetes is made, the patient is agitated and at her next visit with her psychiatrist, she questions why this side effect of olanzapine was not men-tioned when the drug was initially prescribed.

A Perspective from a Psychiatrist

Clinical Background

Whenever treatment options are being discussed, the physician is obligated to make full disclosure to the patient.[12–14] The only exceptions to this rule are when (1) the patient is unconscious and harm from failure to treat is immi-nent; or (2) disclosure poses such a serious psychological threat of harm to the patient that disclosure would be medically contra-indicated.[15]

There are many reasons why a physician may not fully disclose informa-tion in any given situation, and disclosure should be tailored to each unique situation. One reason is that physicians may be reluctant to fully disclose side effects out of fear that the patient may refuse the proposed intervention.[12] However, it is not accepted practice to remain silent in order to ensure that the patient will consent to treatment.[15]

When disclosing information to obtain informed consent, three areas are involved: information (from the physician), decisional capacity (on the part of the patient), and voluntarism (on the part of the patient).[16]

Professionalism Considerations

In this particular case, it is presumed that the patient was psychotic in order for an antipsychotic drug to be prescribed. This particular issue complicates this case, as the decisional capacity of the patient may have been compro-mised. In light of the paranoia, it might have been very difficult (if not im-possible) for the patient to trust the physician (or anyone), and this may have affected the physician's decision to withhold information from the patient.

Deciding if a patient has the capacity to make his or her own decisions is often a very difficult task, especially in psychiatric matters, where the treat-ment options are not shared with the family without the patient's consent. This is different from medical illnesses, where a surrogate can make decisions until the patient's physical situation improves to the point where the patient can then take over decision making.

As a result, psychiatric patients often are caught in the gray area of having diminished mental capacity, but needing treatment for that diminished mental capacity and there being no way to gain consent for that treatment without a court order. This is another reason why the physician may have withheld information from the patient at the time of initial treatment.

Opinion

In my opinion, when the psychotic patient is offered treatment, the psychiatrist must make a decision as to how much and what type of information the patient can understand and assimilate.[13,17] If the symptoms are serious enough that the psychiatrist feels that the treatment must be initiated (for example, a paranoid patient pointing a gun at a perceived threatening person), then the psychiatrist may only tell the patient that the medication will help the patient feel better (less anxious, less angry, etc.). Those things are true, but it does not give the whole story.

As soon as the patient had improved to the point where the details of the treatment can be understood and a reasonable decision can be made, then the physician should have discussed with the patient the entire scope of the proposed treatments and possible side effects. If the patient at that time consented to take the medication, the physician could have provided nutritional and lifestyle information to the patient so as to minimize the effects of the drug being prescribed, such as the increased risk of diabetes. After this discussion occurred, the patient and physician are working together, both with the same information.

Josephine Albritton, M.D.
Assistant Professor, Department of Psychiatry and Health Behavior
Medical College of Georgia

A Perspective from a Health Consumer Advocate

Whenever I read that yet another drug that has been on the market for many years is found to have a major adverse effect, I wonder how the prescribing doctors inform their patients. Do they call each one immediately? Or do they wait until the patient comes in for the next follow-up visit? My question became less abstract recently when my husband read about a warfarin vs. aspirin trial, published in the *New England Journal of Medicine* and reported in the local paper. The trial participants with intracranial arterial stenosis had been randomly assigned to take either warfarin or high-dose aspirin for nearly two years. Those, like my husband, who were on warfarin had more than twice the rate of death, major hemorrhage, heart attack and sudden death than those on aspirin. We didn't wait for a call or the next visit. His stroke specialist was contacted immediately and his warfarin was changed to aspirin.

Perhaps the fifty-four-year-old woman in this case study was agitated because she recently learned that the diabetes–Zyprexa link had been known for many years before her own diagnosis. A 2006 news report revealed that the pharmaceutical company Eli Lilly inappropriately promoted Zyprexa to primary care physicians.[18] According to the claim, in late 2000, Eli Lilly's own marketing documents disclosed that the company began a campaign instructing its sales representatives to suggest that doctors prescribe Zyprexa to older patients with symptoms of dementia (an off-label use). Documents also showed that Lilly encouraged primary care doctors to treat the symptoms and behaviors of schizophrenia and bipolar disorder even if the doctors had not actually diagnosed these diseases in their patients.[18] By March 2008, Lilly paid $1.2 billion to settle 30,000 lawsuits from people who claimed they had developed diabetes while taking Zyprexa.[19]

In time, Zyprexa carried a prominent warning from the FDA, saying that the drug should not be prescribed for dementia or dementia-related psychosis because it would increase the risk of death in older people. And by 2007, Zyprexa carried the warning about the risk of diabetes. Still, sales of Zyprexa continued to rise. In 2007 Zyprexa became Lilly's best-selling product with $4.8 billion in sales.[19]

In the story of Zyprexa, I see several depressingly recurrent themes associated with many over-marketed drugs (Vioxx, Neurontin, and Procrit to name a few), years after it goes on the market. Zyprexa appears to have harmed some people (but we don't know how many); FDA warnings didn't make much of a difference; off-label use is common; a head-to-head trial showed it is not much better than older, less expensive competing drugs;[20] the pharmaceutical company initially denied knowing of the potentially serious risks; and a lawsuit uncovered in-house documents showing that the company officials did, in fact, know about the risks.

When we started our Center for Medical Consumers (http://www.medicalconsumers.org/) in 1976, it was a dark era of medical information for the public. With a few notable exceptions such as oral contraceptives, no written information came with prescription drugs. *The Physician's Desk Reference*, now available in most public libraries and bookstores, was only for doctors. One of the first things we did was open a free medical library to the public. A steady stream of people came in for a variety of purposes, but looking up drug side effects was always a major draw. We heard many complaints from people who said their doctors told them virtually nothing about side effects. Over the years, particularly with online resources, it has become easier for people who want information about their drugs.

But serious distortions and gaps in information remain despite today's pro-liferation of consumer drug reference books and Web sites. Pharmaceutical research has become a high-stakes business and positive study results are be-coming more and more suspect now that we know how many drug trials go unpublished.[21] Most post-market drug trials are sponsored by the drug com-panies; most drug company-sponsored trials produce results that are favorable to their products;[22] head-to-head comparison trials, needed to compare the newer, more expensive drug to the older drug are relatively rare; the reporting of effectiveness and harms outcomes from randomized trials is often incom-plete;[23] drug reference books and their Internet equivalents do not include findings from phase 4 trials; and many committees that set treatment guidelines are dominated by physicians with financial conflicts of interest.[24] Even govern-ment researchers are now on the payroll of the pharmaceutical industry.[25]

These are the things that come to mind whenever I'm offered a prescription by my doctor . . . and I wonder how much my physician knows about the safety of the drug and the magnitude of its benefit.

Maryann Napoli
Associate Director, Center for Medical Consumers
New York, NY

HONESTY WITH PATIENTS – SURGERY

A fifty-two-year-old woman is referred by her primary care doctor to a surgeon after breast cancer is diagnosed. Mammography showed a 2 cm suspicious lesion in the upper outer quadrant of the left breast and a core needle biopsy was diagnostic for cancer. Following the evaluation of the patient, the surgeon explains the risks and benefits of a lumpectomy, a sentinel node biopsy, and a possible axillary lymph node dissection. A mastectomy, as an alternative approach, is also discussed. During the entire thirty-minute discussion with the surgeon, the patient appears anxious and depressed and is frequently tear-ful. She explains that she has no close family or friends that can help with this decision. Following the discussion, she elects to have the lumpectomy and signs but does not read the informed consent. After the patient leaves, the surgeon wonders whether the patient has the capacity to make the decision regarding her surgery.

A Perspective from a Surgeon

Clinical Background
This fifty-two-year-old woman has a 2 cm malignancy in the upper outer quadrant of her left breast. The standard of care demands that she be

presented with the basic options of breast cancer treatment, mastectomy vs. breast conservation therapy, and the risks and benefits of each option. Proper explanation of these alternatives requires discussion of at least eight key issues. (1) Breast conservation therapy, which allows a patient to retain her natural breast, requires excision of the breast mass to clear margins. (2) This procedure (also called lumpectomy, or partial mastectomy) should be followed by radiation therapy, otherwise chances for local recurrence are unacceptably high.[26] (3) Lumpectomy should be accompanied by a sentinel node biopsy to assess lymph node status. (4) If lymph nodes are positive, sentinel lymph node biopsy should be followed by axillary lymphadenectomy.[27] (5) Mastectomy will also be accompanied by assessment of nodal status, but is generally not followed by radiation therapy. (6) Mastectomy may be accompanied by immediate or delayed breast reconstruction. (7) Reconstruction may take the form of implants or autologous tissue transplant.

These aforementioned general points relate to the local treatment of the breast and the axilla. Given that my patient is fifty-two years old and the lesion is 2 cm, she will undoubtedly require adjuvant chemotherapy, regardless of whether her nodes are positive or negative.[28] As I like to present the entire treatment package "up front," I explain that (8) adjuvant chemotherapy is an "insurance measure," to be taken once all gross disease has been removed. Explanation of the entire treatment package before therapy commences maximizes chances for a well-informed and satisfied patient, as well as a successful outcome.

I have numbered the basic concepts of the clinical considerations in order to underscore the fact that adequate explanation of these concepts requires time (at least thirty minutes), patience, and compassion. It is important to be prepared to review and repeat this information since one should not expect that the average patient will comprehend and assimilate these issues at the time of the initial consultation.

Professionalism Considerations

For me this scenario raises three issues of professionalism:

1. Can I enable my patient to understand these complex issues and to arrive at a decision with which she is comfortable?
2. Have I identified the support system upon which my patient will rely during this next difficult period of her life?
3. If, as in this case, the patient appears to lack a satisfactory support system, what is my responsibility as the patient's physician (captain of the ship regarding her breast cancer treatment) to help provide a support system for her?

Opinion

From a practical standpoint, I am not particularly concerned about the validity of the consent in this case. My intent is to explain clearly, and I will subsequently determine at my next meeting whether the patient understands. I would neither expect nor encourage the patient to make a final decision about treatment at the time of my initial consultation. I usually indicate that there are additional consultations to be obtained and more time to think about this. Obviously, if there is some real concern that the patient is incapable of understanding the issues, I would involve appropriate consultants (such as a psychiatrist) to determine if the patient is truly competent to make a decision.

In general, my first task is to reassure the patient that though this mass is a cancer, "it's been growing slowly for a while and is not likely to move anywhere in the next days." I try to dispel the notion that treating breast cancer is an emergency and I emphasize to the patient that first I need to help her become educated in the issues of breast cancer treatment. I indicate that she will be seeing a radiation oncologist, a medical oncologist, and perhaps a plastic surgeon before we make a decision regarding definitive treatment. I emphasize that I want her to be as well informed as possible about her options for treatment. It is my intention to empower the patient by assuring her that she herself will ultimately have sufficient information to make the best decision for her own treatment.

Given my patient's lament that "she has no close family or friends that can help with this decision," I recognize that she lacks the support system that she will require to see her through the next weeks/months of surgery, possible radiation, and possible chemotherapy.

How far need I, the physician/surgeon, go to provide the patient with appropriate support? As professionals, it is our responsibility to help our patients construct such a support system. Any technician can perform a breast biopsy. Professionalism requires that we, as physicians, look at the bigger picture of our patients' needs. In endeavoring to link the patient to resources available for support, I would do the following:

- In this instance, I would press to find out if there is a relative, friend, old friend, acquaintance, or neighbor whom my patient might trust as a companion during these times. If identified, I would arrange a repeat consultation together with that individual.
- I would consider having this patient talk to one of my own patients who has been through a similar decision-making process.
- Breast cancer support groups can be identified in most major cities.[29]

- Depending upon my assessment of the patient's psychological status, I would consider referring the patient to an appropriate counselor during this time. Were she truly depressed, I would consider a psychiatric referral.

Being diagnosed with a malignancy makes people highly aware (often for the first time) of their own mortality. This recognition often causes their (neglected) psychological issues to surface. A bad spousal relationship, an estranged child, a previous death in the family with unresolved feelings, may all figure prominently in the patient's conscious or subliminal thought processes. The time of crisis precipitated by a diagnosis of malignancy is often a rich time for patients to deal with such issues.[30] I frequently refer patients to counseling to examine these issues. In order to minimize the stigma (which unfortunately is still attached by many to the counseling process), I emphasize to my patients that they are likely to benefit from counseling because they are human and normal, and I suggest that this process could help them sort out their feelings and make better decisions through the course of treatment.

Barry D. Mann, M.D.
Professor of Surgery, Jefferson Medical College
Program Director, Lankenau Surgical Residency Program,
Wynnewood, PA

A Perspective from a Bioethicist

This case raises two issues: capacity assessment and the adequacy of informed consent. Logically, capacity assessment takes precedence because lacking capacity a patient cannot provide informed consent. However, in most routine consultations, physicians do not treat capacity assessment as a discrete task. Instead they handle it in the course of standard interactions which typically, if incompletely, address some of the areas covered by capacity assessment queries, such as appropriate awareness of time and setting. Research has shown that this strategy works most of the time for two groups of patients: those who clearly are capable of making decisions and those who clearly are not.[31]

In the case of the fifty-two-year-old breast cancer patient, the surgeon seems to be conducting such an assessment: His concerns about the patient's capacity to consent to treatment emerge out of his interactions with her over the course of a half-hour consultation. However the patient's behavior does not clearly identify her as belonging at either of the far ends of the competency spectrum and research has also shown that physicians are far less successful at making these judgments, evaluating the capacity of patients who fall somewhere in the middle.[32] The surgeon could at this point choose to conduct a formal capacity assessment, preferably relying on a standardized assessment tool developed specifically to assess capacity to consent to treatment such as the MacArthur Competence Assessment Tool – Treatment (MacCAT-T),[33] as opposed to one developed for more general mental status assessments, such as Mini Mental Status Examination (MMSE). Or he could refer the patient for a psychiatric consultation. From the latter, he might learn that the patient is indeed depressed, although he also might learn from the psychiatrist that this diagnosis in itself would not mean necessarily that the patient could not provide consent to surgery.[34] Alternatively, were the surgeon to embrace informed consent as a model for shared decision making between physicians and patients or their surrogates,[35] he might save both himself and his patients the extra effort.

Admonitions about the need to obtain authentic informed consent to medical treatment are often accompanied by the axiom that informed consent is a process, not a moment. The phrase is meant to do two things. First it directs attention away from the formal features of informed consent, specifically that it is represented by a document which, when signed, signifies an agreement between signers. This does not mean that the consent form should be ignored. Rather the point is to make sure that one does not mistake its signing for the process of reaching the understanding it represents or to suggest that once signed, the need for dialogue ends. And second, it is to this dialogue that the axiom directs attention. The dialogue is part of a process that takes place between patient and physician[35] that establishes not only that the patient has the capacity to make decisions but that decisions to accept, or refuse, treatment also are informed and voluntary.

The requirement to be informed is particularly important because voluntariness in part hinges on it: without adequate information about the range and implications of various choices, one cannot be said to have chosen freely among them. Thus, in this context, being informed is held to a higher standard than the phrase might otherwise suggest. The objective is not simply to inform in the sense of notify, or even tell. Rather the goal is to explain the treatment and its reasons, risks, benefits, and alternatives in such a way that the patient can grasp what implications the information has for him or her personally. This can be a time-consuming discussion and one that typically requires a certain amount of exchange before both parties can be reasonably certain that they are seeing eye-to-eye, at least about the key issues.

Aware of the full demands of informed consent, the physician might allot more time to appointments where recent or serious diagnoses and associated treatment options are addressed. In the case of a fifty-two-year-old woman with a new breast cancer diagnosis, a first encounter with a surgeon to evaluate the disease and review three different treatment options might have called for more than the allotted thirty minutes. Pressed for time, the surgeon might instead enlist other staff[35] to continue talking with the patient, or have on hand a brochure, videotape, or other decision-making aid to help explain the patient's options and which she can review at her own pace.[36] In any case, for this woman, and likely for all patients facing decisions of similar magnitude, the clinician should encourage the patient to take home the consent form to review and discourage her from signing it without reading it. Responding to the woman's claim that she has no one with whom to discuss her treatment options, the physician might suggest that she contact her primary care doctor who referred her or provide her with the contact information for any of several breast cancer information and support organizations.

Achieving mutual understanding on complex treatment issues can be challenging and the difficulty can vary with many factors including the condition, the treatment, the patient, and the physician. In this case, by packing so many tasks into a first meeting, the surgeon might have contributed to an already difficult interaction. The patient's recent breast cancer diagnosis could reasonably explain some of her despondency and the fact that she is being asked to choose among treatment alternatives she might not understand could account for her sustained anxiety. Or, the patient's tears and anxiety might be signs of possible depression and might indicate she is unable to decide among her treatment options. Without building a more robust relationship with the patient and without providing her with more time and resources on which to base her decisions, the surgeon will be left to wonder which it is.

Pamelar Sankar, Ph.D.
Associate Professor, Department of Medical Ethics
University of Pennsylvania School of Medicine

HONESTY WITH PATIENTS – NEUROLOGY

A patient with myasthenia gravis in crisis was placed on plasmapheresis. During the procedure, the patient developed chest pain and hypotension and the medical team was notified. The patient's blood pressure quickly improved with intravenous fluids and the chest pain resolved within a few minutes. While the patient was being stabilized, it was noted by the plasmapheresis technician and physicians that the machine had been incorrectly programmed by the technician, and a red blood cell removal procedure, rather than plasma removal procedure, was underway. The patient has no permanent residua – the exam, electrocardiogram, and later laboratory evaluation were all unchanged. Later in the day, the patient asks the physician what happened.

A Perspective from an Internist and Authority on Disclosure of Medical Errors

Clinical Background

Myasthenia gravis (MG) is an autoimmune disorder characterized by weakness in ocular, bulbar, limb, and respiratory muscles. This weakness results from an antibody-mediated injury of the neuromuscular junction. The most serious form of MG involves weakness of respiratory muscles, which when severe can be a life-threatening problem called "myasthenic crisis." Patients with mild MG can sometimes have their symptoms controlled with acetylcholinesterase inhibitors alone, but most patients require an immunomodulating treatment during their illness such as corticosteroids and other immunosuppressive drugs or plasma exchange.

Treatment of myasthenic crisis typically involves admission to an intensive care unit and rapid therapy with plasmapheresis or intravenous immune globulin. Plasmapheresis works by removing the acetylcholine receptor antibodies from the circulation. In the case outlined in the vignette, rather than receiving plasmapheresis as ordered, the patient was inadvertently started on a red blood cell removal procedure. Hypotension and chest pain ensued, which resolved with intravenous fluid. While the case history does not allow one to determine with certainty the etiology of the chest pain, myocardial ischemia due either to anemia (related to red blood cell removal) or due to blockages in the patient's coronary arteries is high on the differential diagnosis.

Professionalism Considerations

The cornerstone of medical professionalism is acting in the best interests of the patient. Therefore, it is understandably distressing to health care workers when patients suffer harm from their medical care, generally known as "adverse events." A subset of adverse events are classified as "medical errors," defined as "the failure of a planned action to be completed as intended or the use of a wrong plan to achieve an aim."[37] Considerable progress has been made over the last decade in understanding the relationship between adverse events and medical errors. The vast majority of adverse events are not due to medical errors; that is, they are not preventable. Likewise, most medical errors do not harm patients. Furthermore, much progress has been made in understanding the causes of adverse events and errors. Previously, medical errors were thought to stem mostly from "bad apples," health care workers who were either incompetent or lazy. Experts in health care quality now believe that this "bad apple" model is seriously flawed, and stress instead the importance of system breakdowns in the delivery of health care in causing medical errors. Similarly, considerable emphasis has been placed on moving the culture of health care from one where "blame and shame" predominate following medical errors to a "blame-free" culture that focuses on learning from adverse events and errors.

An important component of reducing adverse events and errors has been promoting greater transparency following these events. Previously when adverse events and errors happened, there was a natural tendency among health care workers to keep information about the event to themselves for fear of punishment. This secrecy led to lost opportunities to learn from adverse events and errors and prevent recurrences. Now, health care workers are encouraged to openly report adverse events and errors to their institutions so proper analysis can be undertaken and the quality of care can be enhanced.

Transparency also involves communicating openly about adverse events and errors with patients. The disclosure of adverse events and errors to patients has long been endorsed by professional organizations and increasingly is required by accreditation standards and some state laws.[38-40] Patients clearly favor disclosure of even minor errors, and want to be told explicitly that an error occurred, why the error happened, how recurrences will be prevented, and to receive an apology.[41] Unfortunately, it is also apparent that open disclosure of adverse events and errors to patients is the exception rather than the norm. Common barriers to open disclosure of these events to patients include health care workers' fear of litigation, embarrassment, or uncertainty about how best to communicate in difficult situations such as the one described here.[42]

Several features of this case make it difficult to decide whether and how to disclose this event to the patient. The patient appears not to have suffered any permanent injury, and health care workers might adopt a "no harm, no foul" mentality. Furthermore, while the patient is aware that an unusual clinical event occurred, he or she may not know that this event was caused by an error. Physicians have been shown to disclose less information when patients might be unaware that an error has occurred.[43] Physicians may hope that a nonspecific explanation that highlights the adverse event but ignores the error will mollify patients and avoid awkward discussions about whether the adverse event was preventable. Lastly, this error occurred in the setting of team-based delivery of health care. In this case, the error may have resulted solely from a technical error on the part of the individual operating the plasmapheresis machine. This fact may cause the physician to feel less personal responsibility for the error, leading the physician to inform the patient that the error was made by the technician and did not involve physician error.

These challenges emphasize the importance of getting help before disclosing an adverse event or error to a patient. Oftentimes, what appears to have been a harmful error turns out not to have been preventable once the event has been subjected to formal analysis. In addition, disclosures are relatively rare events for any one clinician. Therefore, many institutions are using "disclosure coaches" to provide just-in-time disclosure training immediately before these conversations. Such coaching involves careful consideration of what should be disclosed to the patient as well as anticipating likely questions and formulating appropriate responses. Role-plays can also provide an important opportunity to practice the disclosure conversation prior to conducting the actual disclosure. Fortunately, research shows that the vast majority of these disclosure conversations go well. In one study, 85 percent of physicians who had disclosed a serious error were satisfied with how the conversation had gone.[44] In their thoughtful commentary accompanying this case, Drs. Pichert and Hickson delve deeper into the important issue of exactly what information should be disclosed to the patient and why.

Opinion

Professionalism in this case requires a dogged and open-minded commitment to understanding exactly what happened to this patient, communicating the information transparently to the patient, and making ample use of the institutional resources available to assist in this process. An adverse event such as this is often less straightforward than it may appear. Careful consultation with clinical and patient safety experts can help determine whether the inadvertent red cell removal was, in fact, associated with the patient's chest pain, as well as help ascertain the exact etiology of the chest pain itself. Root cause analysis can also help understand exactly why the error happened and formulate plans for preventing recurrences, information that is important to share with the patient to highlight the lessons learned from the event. Careful inspection of the pheresis machine can help determine whether human error was to blame for the event, if device redesign might reduce future error, or whether the device itself malfunctioned. All of this information would be important to report to appropriate regulatory agencies. This high level of transparency is difficult, but will help patients make more informed decisions about their health care and enhance patients' trust in the honesty and integrity of the health care system.

Thomas H. Gallagher, M.D.
Carolyn D. Prouty, D.V.M.
Department of Medical History & Ethics
University of Washington

A Perspective from a Center for Patient and Professional Advocacy

To medical professionals, this case describes an obvious error with obvious (but transient) adverse consequences.[43,45,46] The patient, however, knows only that doctors initiated unexpected treatments for chest pain and wonders if he or she is okay. Consider the pros and cons for four ways physicians might (and do) respond:[47]

1. *No disclosure/safe facts:* "Your myasthenia crisis was severe. Your antibody level – what made you feel bad – was so high that plasmapheresis was required. . . . Sometimes treatments make patients feel worse before getting better. That's what happened, so now we'll focus on getting you well."

2. *Facts, promise more later:* ". . . severe crisis . . . ordered plasmapheresis . . . we need to review the events before and after your chest pain . . . learn why chest pain occurred . . . when review is complete we'll discuss the results."

3. *Disclose error:* ". . . ordered plasmapheresis . . . machine was set incorrectly – an error – initially removed red cells instead of . . . , which may or may not have contributed to your chest pain . . . we're reviewing the events . . . trying to learn any other causes so we can rule out other medical problems . . . we'll discuss . . ."

4. *Disclose error, assign responsibility:* ". . . started plasmapheresis . . . our team [or a technician] erred by using a wrong setting . . . removed red cells . . . anemia caused your chest pain . . . I'm very sorry the error happened; I apologize for all of us. I want to address your questions, share what we're doing . . ."

No matter how you would respond, consider why caring physicians might choose or reject each alternative. List each alternative's pros and cons for patients and providers in this case (e.g., alternative no. 1 might retain patient confidence and no. 2 buys time for review, but both allow inadvertent, premature (before all facts are known), or deliberate disclosure by others, leading to suspicions of cover-ups; no. 3 and no. 4 are honest, but patients might lose confidence in providers). Now list follow-up questions patients might reasonably ask in response to each alternative (e.g., no. 2 may prompt, "Doctor, why do you think I had chest pain?"). This exercise helps you anticipate how patients might "push" you along the continuum and prepares you to answer.

When patient data are fully known, we advocate "full disclosure," but what does that mean? Table 6.1 lists its elements and suggests some words (not scripts) for answering the "what happened" question in this case.

Table 6.1. Table elements and suggested communications

Disclosure element	Suggested communications
1. Apology (be *precise*); nature of error, harm	Mr./Ms. ____, I'm sorry to report that the machine was set incorrectly, red cells were removed, and your chest pain resulted. On behalf of us all, I apologize for the incorrect setting and for being unaware until your chest pain began.
2. When, where error occurred	We thought the machine was giving the right treatment, but we were mistaken. So your initial treatment was wrong.
3. Causes, results of harm; actions taken to reduce gravity of harm; actions to reduce or prevent re-occurrence	We corrected the machine setting, but not in time to prevent your chest pain. Once you got IV fluids and the setting was corrected, you got better. I don't expect any lasting bad effects, but we'll continue monitoring to minimize any further problems. We have a team that reviews errors and recommends how to prevent recurrences. All of us will study their report. If you return don't hesitate to ask us to double check our settings.
4. Who will manage ongoing care	If you allow me to continue, your primary doctor and I will work together on your care.
5. Describe error review process, reports to regulatory agencies; how systems issues are identified	We take mistakes very seriously. Everything will be reviewed by experts. The results will be reported to me [and, if applicable, to the ____ Agency]. If the review reveals ways we can better manage myasthenia crises, we will make those changes.
6. Provide contact info for ongoing communications	I [or Dr. ____] will communicate about your continuing care. When questions arise, please have me paged. Or call my assistant, [name] who can help or find me.
7. Offer counseling, support	People in the hospital's ___ office can talk with you and connect you with support services. Here's their card. May I call them or anyone else for you?
8. Address bills for additional care	The review I requested will fairly address the charges resulting from the error. The focus now is returning you to health . . .

We've summarized full disclosure when an error likely caused transient harm. More common are cases with significant adverse outcomes but with errors uncertain or disputed.[47] At such times consider using the "balance beam approach" (see figure 6.1, page 265) for critically examining the how and when, and the pros and cons, of alternative disclosure strategies. If you do, we're confident you'll get it "right" far more often than not.

James W. Pichert, Ph.D.
Gerald B. Hickson, M.D.
Center for Patient and Professional Advocacy
Vanderbilt University School of Medicine

SUMMARY – COMMITMENT TO HONESTY WITH PATIENTS

Background

Honesty is a cornerstone of the doctor–patient relationship. Honesty allows physicians to act with their patients' best interests in mind, engender trust, engage their patients in shared decision making, and ensure that each patient receives health care that reflects the patient's particular circumstances and values. And yet, while acknowledging that honesty is of paramount importance to our patients and to our profession, we may find ourselves facing dilemmas about how to act, particularly when our commitment to honesty appears to conflict with our pledge to "do no harm." If we look to mentors and role models for help in resolving these conflicts, we may find that even those that we admire the most engage in some forms of deception from time to time. This raises important questions for our practice. Is deception ever justified and, if so, when? What kinds of clinical situations are more likely to lead physicians to engage in deceptive practices? How should we handle those situations? Thinking through these issues ahead of time may help us to make better decisions when confronted with such dilemmas in the course of actual patient care.

Deception and Lying

Lying is the willful communication of information we know to be inaccurate in order to mislead another person. Deception encompasses much more than outright lying and includes concealment, distortion, and deflection also with the intent to mislead.[48] When we conceal or withhold information, we tell the literal truth but avoid telling the whole truth. When we distort, we tell the truth but we may adjust our emphasis, highlighting and downplaying information according to our purpose. When we deflect, we tell the truth but avoid addressing our patient's question directly. In order to deceive, we carefully select the information to convey, the words we use to convey it, and the context we choose to place the information in.

Imagine you've ordered a chest radiograph on a smoker who has developed a new cough and has lost a little weight. It shows a 4 cm lung mass that is almost certainly cancer. When the patient comes in for follow-up, you tell her that her X-ray shows a "nodule" and that in order to get a better look at it she will need a CT scan (concealment – you haven't told her that it is highly suspicious for cancer). She asks what the nodule could be and you tell her that it could be a benign growth but that the worst-case scenario is that it could be cancer (distortion – you've placed greater emphasis on the possibility that it could be benign than you actually believe). She asks if you think it looks like cancer and you tell her that benign and cancerous growths can look very similar on X-ray (deflection – you avoid giving your opinion and provide her with related information instead). While it is literally true that without a biopsy you do not know for sure that the patient has cancer, important information is being withheld from this patient.

Each of these types of deception has the potential to mislead the patient and to compromise her ability to make a fully informed health care decision. For example, believing in the possibility that this is benign, she may delay scheduling her CT scan. If discovered, each type of deception has the potential to erode her trust in you and in the medical profession. And yet each type of deception also has the potential to preserve hope, defuse fear, reduce stress, and improve patient function. Physicians may also employ deception to promote compliance with effective therapies, to respect cultural values and traditions, and to avoid their own discomfort discussing painful topics with patients.

Ethical Perspectives

Ethicists have long debated the merits of honesty and whether deception is ever justified. There are two main schools of thought: consequentialist and deontologic. Consequentialism judges an act according to the result it produces. If the result is on balance good, then the action must have been good. If the result is bad, then the action was bad. The deontologic school judges an act according to how it lines up with accepted moral precepts. If we accept the precept that honesty is good, then, by contrast, all deception is considered bad until proven otherwise.

Sissela Bok, a modern ethicist, argues from the deontologic approach: "Lying requires explanation, whereas truth ordinarily does not."[48] Without honesty, there can be no trust and without trust, society falls apart. Lies also lead to an unequal distribution of power: When you lie to a person, you take away their ability to make an informed decision.

Imagine you have gallstones that are causing frequent abdominal pain. You consult with a surgeon about having a cholecystectomy. Now imagine not being able to trust the surgeon to be honest about his credentials, experience, and complication rate. What if the hospital could not be trusted to have properly sterilized its surgical instruments? If you knew this, you wouldn't go to this surgeon or this hospital. No one else would either. The surgeon and the hospital would likely go out of business. If this were true of all surgeons and hospitals, the medical system would fall apart.

Now imagine that the surgeon and hospital are dishonest but that you are unaware of this fact. You'd likely proceed with the cholecystectomy. In this case, the lack of disclosure impairs your ability to make a good decision for yourself and deprives you of the power to protect yourself from potential harm. In this scenario, the deontologic viewpoint is exemplified: Lying violates our moral expectations for honesty, and widespread adoption of lying clearly leads to bad outcomes.

In contrast to Bok, David Nyberg argues from the consequentialist perspective: Deception in some circumstances is not only allowable but may be desirable, and is necessary for the "smooth running of our social lives."[49] We use it to promote good relationships with our friends, co-workers and relatives.

Imagine that you are seeing a patient whom you have been treating for depression. He has lost his job and suffers from low self-esteem. At a follow-up appointment, he finally appears to be turning the corner. His affect is brighter and in honor of his new positive outlook on life he has bought a suit that he wears to his appointment with you and which he intends to wear to future job interviews. He wants to know if you like it but, in fact, you don't like it. Do you tell him your true thoughts – that it's garish and makes him look silly – or do you tell him that he's looking great, assuring yourself that this is technically true, since his improved affect and energy level do make him look better, while letting him think that you are actually approving his suit? The deception supports his damaged self-esteem and avoids criticism that you fear could thrust him back into depression again.

Nyberg would argue that in a case such as this the ends justify the means and that if this deceptive act supports his ongoing recovery from depression, then it was wisely and beneficently chosen. Bok, however, would have qualms about this and would ask whether you really knew what was best for your patient. Maybe it would have been better for him to hear the truth and to know that you respected him enough to be honest with him. Maybe it would have been more therapeutic for him to know that you had enough faith in the durability of his recovery to say something that might be hard for him to hear. Maybe, by being honest, you could have empowered him to make a change in his attire that would positively affect potential employers' perceptions and increase his chances of getting a new job. Additionally, you might not have identified all the possible consequences of your deception. What if he finds out later that you lied? How would that affect your relationship?

Historical Perspectives

Truly honoring our commitment to always avoid deception and be honest with patients can be extremely challenging. Early practitioners of medicine valued the avoidance of harm over the precept of honesty to the point of actively encouraging deception. The lack of any mention of honesty in the Hippocratic Oath was no oversight; Hippocrates himself said "perform these duties calmly and adroitly, concealing most things from the patient while you are attending to him ... reveal nothing of the patient's future or present condition, for many, on learning what is to come, have taken a turn for the worse."[50] As recently as the 1960s, it was the norm not to tell a patient that he had cancer.[51] Society accepted this because in the paternalistic practice of medicine, it was assumed that the beneficent physician was unbiased and always practiced in accord with his patients' best interests.

Since the 1960s, however, many forces have impacted the practice of medicine and in the latter half of the twentieth century, the values of society and organized medicine began to change. The 1960s saw many Americans losing trust in their government and authority figures in general. People wanted a say in the big decisions that affected their lives. At the same time, doctors began to have more choices to offer people with previously untreatable diseases such as cancer. Chemotherapy now offered the hope of cure for patients with testicular cancer and leukemia, albeit at significant cost and risk. In the 1980s, managed care introduced incentives for physician reimbursement that had the potential to create conflicts of interest. Under some of these schemes, interventions that had the potential to benefit the patient might negatively impact the financial well-being of the physician or the health plan. And finally, fear of medical malpractice suits led to the practice of "defensive medicine," the ordering of tests and procedures that have more potential to protect the physician from liability than to help the patient. Patients thus had more therapeutic options, a greater interest in being involved in the decision-making process, and physicians could no longer be assumed to be acting solely with their patients' best interests in mind.

What ensued from these events was the medical profession making an explicit commitment to honesty and transparency in medicine, as well as recognizing that patients are autonomous and have the right to be involved in medical decision making. In the 1970s, informed consent, which had long been an important element of clinical research, emerged as the means to achieve transparency and shared decision making in clinical practice as well. In 1980 the American Medical Association amended its ethics code to explicitly state (for the first time) that "physicians should deal honestly with patients and colleagues."[52] And in 2002, the American Board of Internal Medicine along with the American College of Physicians and the European Federation of Internal Medicine published a physician charter for the new millennium which identifies commitment to honesty with patients as a key professional responsibility.[53]

Modern Dilemmas

While honesty and transparency are now basic tenets of modern medicine, the clinician still frequently finds himself in situations where it is not necessarily clear that "honesty is the best policy." What patients want and how physicians act in these situations has become a focus of research during the past several decades.

Breaking Bad News. Breaking bad news to patients brings our pledge to avoid harm into potential conflict with our duties to deal honestly with our patients, to engage them in shared decision making regarding their treatment and to provide informed consent. Previously, withholding information about bad news from patients was relatively commonplace in medicine. Yet several research studies demonstrated that this practice was not in keeping with what patients wanted. In eight studies of patient preferences, over 90 percent indicated that they would want their doctor to fully disclose information about their diagnosis.[54–61]

However, while some progress has been made in the last twenty years toward being more open with patients about bad news, important barriers persist. For example, in a study conducted in 2001, only 42 percent of physicians believed that their patients wanted this information.[59] Additionally, a recent study suggests that concealing information regarding the diagnosis and prognosis of cancer may be less stressful for physicians than revealing it.[62] Those physicians who did disclose bad news described using a number of potentially deceptive techniques, including using euphemisms such as "growth" or "swelling" to describe cancer and avoiding an explicit discussion of prognosis.[55,63,64] While tenets of honesty and the overwhelming preference of patients would seem to support disclosure of bad news despite physicians' apparent discomfort with this approach, there remain some gray areas where consensus has not been reached. These include disclosure of bad news to patients whose cultural background and values do not support it and to patients with cognitive impairment related to dementia or psychiatric illness.[65,66]

Disclosing Medical Errors. Ethically, physicians have a duty to disclose errors to patients. Hospital accreditation standards and some state laws require that patients be informed about "unanticipated outcomes" in their care.[40] In multiple studies of patient preferences regarding error disclosure, over 88 percent of patients indicated that they would want to know if an error in their care occurred, especially if it was a serious error.[41,67–75] However, a significant gap exists between these expectations for disclosure and current practice. Several studies suggest that harmful errors are disclosed to patients approximately one-third of the time.[41,67,76,77] In those circumstances where disclosure does occur, physicians report choosing their words carefully and phrasing things in such a way as to avoid using the word "error."[42,43] No consensus currently exists regarding whether patients should be told about errors that do not cause harm, also known as "near misses."[78]

Revealing Level of Training. Training future physicians requires altruism on the part of patients. They must be willing to let students and residents participate meaningfully in their care and they must be comfortable with any additional risk that this entails. Students and their mentors may fear that, if informed, patients would refuse student involvement, thus jeopardizing the training of future physicians. While the temptation to conceal training status exists, ethical guidelines state that "all trainees should inform patients of their training status and role in the medical team."[14] In seven studies addressing patient preferences, most patients (66–100 percent) wanted to be informed and to have an opportunity to either grant or deny permission for a student to participate in their care.[79–85] Despite this, a study of internal medicine residents found that a majority (62 percent) had performed procedures on patients without first revealing their paucity of experience with the procedure.[86] Residents felt the need to develop procedural skills and feared that, if fully informed, patients would refuse to allow the trainee to undertake the procedure.[87]

Other Dilemmas. In the modern practice of medicine there are many other situations related to honesty that can pose dilemmas for the physician. Genetic testing is becoming more common and can yield unexpected results, such as revealing that a child's father could not be his biologic father. Physicians may contract transmittable diseases such as chronic hepatitis and HIV (see Schwartz's and Wainapel's commentaries in Chapter 3) that could pose risks for their patients. More and more physicians are employees rather than independent practitioners. Employers may offer financial incentives to physicians that could impact patient care. Physicians need to think about how to handle disclosure to patients in all these difficult circumstances.

In addition, physicians now deal more frequently with insurers and may find themselves torn between advocating for their patient and dealing honestly with the insurer. Contesting a denied service can be time consuming, and physicians may be tempted to save time by finding an acceptable (if erroneous) justification for the service (see Spandorfer's and Gordin's commentary in Chapter 3).

Even interactions with colleagues can prove difficult. Acknowledging an oversight, a mistake, or a gap in knowledge to a colleague can be embarrassing. However, if we fail to disclose these events and allow a colleague to act on the basis of incomplete, inaccurate, or misleading information, that clinician could initiate care that was unnecessary or even dangerous to the patient.

The available data make it clear that physicians struggle with each of the aforementioned situations. For example, most geneticists don't feel comfortable revealing misattributed paternity;[88,89] physicians seldom initiate discussions about financial conflicts of interest;[90,91] 39–44 percent of physicians acknowledge misleading an insurer in order to access care for their patients;[92,93] and, finally, surveys of residents in training indicate that the stresses of the training environment do lead them to deceive their colleagues from time to time, typically in order to maintain an appearance of competence.[86,87,94] While we may like to think of ourselves as honest people, it is apparent that when under duress we are not always equal to the challenges that a commitment to honesty creates.

Review of the Cases and Commentaries

The cases in this chapter provide an opportunity to explore some questions related to our commitment to truth telling in the course of everyday medical practice.

What Clinical Situations Challenge Our Commitment to Honesty?

Each of the cases illustrating honesty with patients presents the clinician with a scenario in which complete honesty and transparency has the potential to cause harm. A child might be devastated if she was told she had cancer. A psychotic patient might refuse effective therapy and descend deeper into her thought disorder if she was informed upfront of all a proposed medication's potential side effects. Some, including the student commentator (see Lewis' commentary, Chapter 2), have argued that if students were to disclose their training status prior to performing procedures, patients could suffer needless anxiety.[95] If we agree that this constitutes harm, then a student could be seen as beneficently avoiding escalating the parents' anxiety by deciding not to inform them of her inexperience with lumbar punctures. By extension, when faced with a patient who is acutely distressed, such as the patient with breast cancer, we might choose to delay or withhold information in order to avoid increasing her distress at that moment. What about situations where harm has already happened? Is there any benefit to focusing a cancer patient's attention on a lost opportunity for prevention? Might this also constitute harm if it provokes regret, guilt, or anger? And finally, if we assign therapeutic importance to the doctor–patient relationship, then deceptions that help to foster good relations might also be viewed as avoiding harm. "Paternalistic deception," that is, deception with the intent of avoiding harm to the patient and with the overarching goal of acting in the patient's best interests, might also provide a rationale for withholding information regarding medical errors as well.

These cases challenge the clinician to weigh the benefits of honesty and full disclosure against the potential to cause harm. The tension between these two goods is an inescapable part of the environment in which we practice. Because of this, it is important that we develop habits of mind that lead us to examine reflexively all possible outcomes of a deceptive act such as withholding information, and to scrutinize closely our motivations when we are considering honoring our duty to avoid harm over our duty to deal honestly with our patients. Bok warns us that "after the first lies . . . others come more easily. Psychological barriers wear down; lies seem more necessary, less reprehensible; the ability to make moral distinctions can coarsen."[48]

The cases also illustrate settings that may be distressing for the clinician. The first of these is the training environment. Students and residents feel the pressure to gain experience and to appear competent before their peers and preceptors. In the face of these pressures, putting patients' needs before their own can create considerable stress for trainees. The second is the medico–legal environment. Fear of litigation, and the harm to the doctor that may ensue, can also make full disclosure of errors very stressful for the clinician. When under stress, the clinician may be more susceptible to or may over-value arguments favoring nondisclosure.[96]

When Is Nondisclosure Justified?

One recognized exception to the ethical and legal expectation for honesty with patients is known as the therapeutic privilege, that is, nondisclosure in order to avoid direct harm to the patient. Early legal cases that tested the boundaries of the therapeutic privilege involved circumstances where physicians withheld important information about the risks of a procedure out of concern that if these risks were shared with the patient they would refuse a beneficial surgery.[97] Due to the ease with which we can rationalize nondisclosure in any number of clinical situations, the potential for abuse of therapeutic privilege is high. Therefore, use of the therapeutic privilege is severely restricted to cases when there is compelling evidence that disclosure could lead to an immediate and serious harm, such as suicide or homicide.[98] In the case of the psychotic patient who was prescribed olanzapine (see Albritton's and Napoli's commentary in this chapter), therapeutic privilege could only have been invoked if it was clear that disclosure of information about the medication would have resulted in immediate danger to the patient

or to another person. Case law makes it clear that therapeutic privilege cannot be invoked if a physician simply fears that disclosure could lead to discomfort or cause a patient to refuse therapy. Thus, therapeutic privilege
would not justify nondisclosure in any of the scenarios described above.

What Do the Cases Tell Us about How to Fulfill Our Commitment to Honesty, Transparency, and Full Disclosure under Difficult Circumstances?

Trainees and Procedures. The student commentator suggests that our current training climate may value the development of procedural skills over the
development of patient interaction skills (see Lewis' commentary, Chapter 2).
And yet it seems clear that a trusting trainee–patient relationship is a pre-
requisite if patients are to allow trainees to "practice" on them. Once a trainee
is adept at developing patient relationships marked by open communication,
trust, and respect, it becomes possible – and perhaps easier – to ask patients
to allow them to play an increasing role in their care. Wilfond provides
a checklist to help students and their preceptors determine when it would
be reasonable for a trainee to propose attempting a procedure on a patient
(see Wilfond's commentary, Chapter 2):

Readiness: does the student understand how to do the procedure and do
they have the basic skills necessary to be successful?

Necessity: is this a skill that the student needs to develop? Will it be an
integral part of their future practice or will they never do it again?

Risk: what is the magnitude of risk to the patient if there are complications
related to the student's inexperience?

Imagine how the case scenario might change had these three points been
discussed. As it stands, the resident encourages third-year student Rebecca
Green to be assertive and tells her that she should perform the lumbar
puncture. He then introduces her as "student Dr. Green" and later as
"Dr. Green." Utilizing Wilfond's approach, the scenario might start with
the resident and student discussing whether she is ready to do the procedure and whether it will be necessary for her career. They would then
discuss the risks to the patient and, if these were felt to be reasonable, speak
with the parents about her doing the procedure. In the course of the
informed consent discussion, they might describe their deliberations in
order to explain why they believe it would be appropriate for the parents
to consider allowing the student to perform the procedure. Regardless of
whether the student does the procedure or not, this type of transparent
communication is likely to foster parental trust in the care team and may

increase the likelihood that the student will be allowed to attempt sub-sequent procedures.

Informed Consent. Informed consent is what allows patients to make auton-omous decisions about health care and to participate in shared decision mak-ing, and hinges on the patient being told truthful information. While the informed consent process is broadly valued by patients, there are exceptions. Certain cultures prefer not to inform their elders of bad news, such as life threatening illness and, as illustrated in this chapter, parents may not be comfortable revealing all things to young children.[99–101] Most doctors are willing to withhold information when it is culturally appropriate to do so.[63] The pediatric oncologist who comments on the case included in this chapter, however, makes strong arguments for disclosing bad news to children. Both commentators assert that before the child can be informed, however, the oncologist and the parents need to achieve trust, a mutual understanding of all the issues at play, and agreement regarding how to proceed. Skipping this step jeopardizes the therapeutic relationship and has the potential to com-promise care. Thus, while physicians might reflexively respond negatively to a request to withhold a diagnosis from the patient, it is important to step back from that reaction in order to first understand what is truly being asked for. In this case, in asking for the oncologist to keep the diagnosis of cancer from their daughter, the parents may really have been voicing their own needs for information and reassurance. Understanding what is motivating such a re-quest may help the physician enlist the parents in sharing this important information with their child in ways that are most comfortable for all involved.

The process of conveying truthful information during informed consent can be frustrating for physicians. The information regarding the procedure, its risks, benefits, and reasonable alternatives is frequently complex and takes time to discuss with the patient. When the physician feels that she knows what the best choice for the patient is, it can be difficult to present options in an unbiased manner and to wait while the patient develops understanding and deliberates. The case of the woman with breast cancer illustrates this. Both Sankhar and Mann stress the importance of allowing enough time. It is important that neither the doctor nor the patient feel rushed. Giving the patient written material to review and scheduling several appointments may facilitate the patient's understanding. Additionally, the commentators remind us that it is not enough to simply convey the information. One must remember to leave time for the patient to speak in order to demonstrate understanding and to communicate her desires fully. Informed consent is only achieved when this happens. When done correctly, the actual signing of the consent document is a mere formality.

Another challenging aspect of informed consent is illustrated by the case involving a woman with psychosis who wasn't informed of a medication side effect. Assuming for the moment that she was able to participate in informed consent at the time the medication was prescribed, this highlights the difficulty of knowing how much information to share with patients. Medications and procedures have innumerable potential risks and it is impossible to discuss every single one. Thus the clinician must decide what to include and what to leave out. In general, one must disclose severe risks such as death, organ failure, and severe functional impairment even if these are not common. Additionally, one must disclose common risks, even if these are not severe.[98] As Albritton points out, disclosing the risk for diabetes not only informs the patient but enables her to take precautions to protect herself from harm.

Medical Errors. Errors are relatively common in the practice of medicine and they are greatly feared by patients and physicians alike. Making an error that harms a patient is one of the most stressful events in clinical practice.[96] Unfortunately, few if any clinicians will be fortunate enough to go through an entire career without being involved in a serious error. Learning how to respond to errors is thus a critical skill for all physicians to have. When done well, the disclosure of error may actually enhance the doctor–patient relationship and reduce the risk of a lawsuit.[42,102]

When a primary care physician forgets to refer his patient for a screening colonoscopy and the patient is subsequently diagnosed with metastatic disease, we sense that the physician is likely to be wracked with guilt and may need emotional support himself. This highlights the importance of moving away from the "culture of blame" in health care that may encourage concealment, deprive a physician of needed support, and lead to a lost opportunity to develop systems that will prevent similar errors in the future.[103] Physicians can contribute to a "blame-free" culture by adopting a stance of curiosity and inquiry with the goal of learning from mistakes. Brucker suggests that this starts with the physician carefully reviewing the chart to determine the source of the error and addressing any knowledge gaps that might have contributed to the error.

The next task for the doctor will be to decide whether the error needs to be disclosed to the patient. It is quite possible that the omission of prophylactic antibiotics will not ultimately harm the woman who had a hysterectomy and that she would never be aware of any problem. If we've addressed the error at a systems level and implemented processes that will make it unlikely that such an error will happen again, have we done our job? Or do we need to go further and disclose the error to the patient? Just as reciting every potential

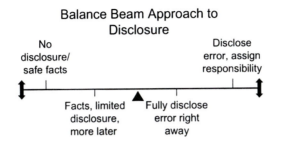

Figure 6.1. Balance Beam Approach to Disclosure

side effect of a medication has the potential to scare patients, some feel that disclosing all errors – including those that are trivial – has the potential to scare patients unnecessarily and is actually counterproductive. In focus groups, patients had mixed feelings about whether they wanted to hear about errors that were caught just in time or ultimately did no harm.[41] Some felt that knowing about them would help them to better protect themselves from future errors, while others felt that hearing about every error would just make them more anxious. Most physicians oppose disclosing trivial and non-harmful errors to the patient while agreeing that it is important to address them from a systems standpoint.[41] Pichert and Hickson propose a "balance beam" approach (figure 6.1) to weighing the risks and benefits of disclosure. This approach highlights the utility of thinking forward to how patients would respond to various degrees of disclosure, and then using this information to guide your decision.

If disclosing trivial and non-harmful errors is a gray area, the ethical and legal imperatives regarding disclosure of harmful errors are clear, as are patients' strong desires for disclosure of such errors.[78,104,105] The key components of error disclosure include:

What: an explicit statement that an error occurred

Why: an explanation of why the error happened

How: how this error will be prevented in the future

Apology: a clear statement indicating your regret that the error occurred

When a single clinician is involved, disclosure is relatively straightforward. When, as in the case of the patient with myasthenia gravis, a team of individuals is involved, the process of disclosure can become more complicated. In this event, the team needs to meet first to review the error and to discuss how to disclose the error to the patient. It is important that the team reaches a mutual understanding of the event and accepts shared responsibility as disclosure discussions that are marked by disagreement and finger-pointing do not inspire patient confidence or enhance the therapeutic relationship.

Finally, the case of the missed antibiotic (see Rabinowitz's and Hoffman's commentary, Chapter 2) raises the question of how to document medical errors. From both a patient safety standpoint and from a legal standpoint, the commentators make it clear that errors should be documented in the medical record. Issues relating to why the error occurred, how systems will be adjusted to prevent it and assignation of blame, however, may more properly be recorded in quality assurance systems.

CONCLUSION

While honesty is one of the most important qualities of a good doctor, situations abound in medicine that can make us contemplate deception, particularly if we can convince ourselves that withholding information will reduce harm for our patient. Professionalism demands that we maintain an awareness of risks associated with being less than truthful with patients, and that we reflect critically on our motivations and justifications for not being truthful because, in most cases, honesty remains the best policy.

Caroline Rhoads, M.D.
Associate Professor of Medicine
Department of Medical History & Ethics, University of Washington

Carolyn Prouty, D.V.M.
Research Coordinator
Department of Medical History & Ethics, University of Washington

Thomas H. Gallagher, M.D.
Associate Professor of Medicine
Department of Medical History and Ethics, University of Washington

REFERENCES

1. Levin B, Lieberman DA, McFarland B, et al. Screening and surveillance for the early detection of colorectal cancer and adenomatous polyps, 2008: A joint guideline from the American Cancer Society, the US Multi-Society Task Force on Colorectal Cancer, and the American College of Radiology. *CA Cancer J Clin.* 2008;**58**(3):130–160.
2. Bok S. *Lying: Moral Choice in Public and Private Life.* New York: Vintage Books; 1999.

3. Studdert DM, Brennan TA. No-fault compensation for medical injuries: The prospect for error prevention. *JAMA*. 2001;**286**(2):217–223.

4. Leach D, Surdyk P. Practicing professionalism. In: Parsi K, Sheehan M, eds. *Healing as Vocation: A Medical Professionalism Primer*. Lanham, MD: Rowman and Littlefield; 2006.

5. Institute of Medicine. To err is human. 1999.

6. Doctor and former astronaut says rocket science not needed to improve patient safety. *Inside the System*. May 2007:4.

7. Banja J. *Medical Errors and Medical Narcissism*. Sudbury, MA: Jones and Bartlett; 2004.

8. Ginsbert J, et al. Ewings sarcoma family of tumors: Ewings sarcoma of bone and soft tissue and the peripheral primitive neurectodermal tumors. In: Pizzo P, Poplack D, eds. *Principles and Practice of Pediatric Oncology*. 4th ed. Philadelphia: Lippincott and Wilkins; 2002:973.

9. Bibace R, Walsh ME. Development of children's concepts of illness. *Pediatrics*. 1980;**66**(6):912–917.

10. Beale EA, Baile WF, Aaron J. Silence is not golden: Communicating with children dying from cancer. *J Clin Oncol*. 2005;**23**(15):3629–3631.

11. Disclosure of illness status to children and adolescents with HIV infection. American Academy of Pediatrics Committee on Pediatric AIDS. *Pediatrics*. 1999;**103**(1):164–166.

12. Kaplan HI, Sadock BJ. *Comprehensive Textbook of Psychiatry VI*.New York: Williams and Wilkins; 1995.

13. Jonsen AR, Siegler M, Winslade WJ. *Clinicial Ethics: A Practical Approach to Ethical Decisions in Clinical Medicine*. 6th ed. New York: McGraw-Hill Medicinal; 2006.

14. Snyder L, Leffler C, Ethics and Human Rights Committee, American College of Physicians. Ethics manual: 5th ed. *Ann Intern Med*. 2005;**142**(7):560–582.

15. American Medical Association. *American Medical Association Code of Medical Ethics: Current Opinions*. 1996–1997 ed. American Medical Association.

16. Roberts LW. Informed consent and the capacity for voluntarism. *Am J Psychiatry*. 2002;**159**(5):705–712.

17. Junkerman C, Shiedermayer D. *Practical Ethics for Students, Interns, and Residents*. Frederick, MD: University Publishing Group; 1994.

18. Berenson A. Drug files show maker promoted unapproved use. *New York Times*. December 18, 2006.

19. Berenson A. Lilly settles Alaska suit over Zyprexa. *New York Times*. March 26, 2008.

20. Carey B. Little difference found in schizophrenia drugs. *New York Times*. September 20, 2005.

21. Lee K, Bacchetti P, Sim I. Publication of clinical trials supporting new drug applications: A literature analysis. *PLos medicine* 2008;**5**(9):E191.

22. Lexchin J, Bero LA, Djulbegovic B, Clark O. Pharmaceutical industry sponsorship and research outcome and quality: Systematic review. *BMJ*. 2003;**326**(7400): 1167–1170.

23. Chan AW, Hrobjartsson A, Haahr MT, Gotzsche PC, Altman DG. Empirical evidence for selective reporting of outcomes in randomized trials: Comparison of protocols to published articles. *JAMA*. 2004;**291**(20):2457–2465.

24. Johnson LJ. Groups blast new cholesterol guidelines. *Associated Press*. July 17, 2004.

25. NewScientist.com News Service. U.S. Reopens Conflicts-of-Interest Drug Research Cases. http://www.newscientist.com/channel/health/mg19425993.600-us-reopens-conflictofinterest-drug-research-cases.html. Accessed August 4, 2008.

26. Fisher B, Bauer M, Margolese R, et al. Five-year results of a randomized clinical trial comparing total mastectomy and segmental mastectomy with or without radiation in the treatment of breast cancer. *N Engl J Med*. 1985;**312**(11): 665–673.

27. Schwartz GF, Guiliano AE, Veronesi U, Consensus Conference Committee. Proceeding of the consensus conference of the role of sentinel lymph node biopsy in carcinoma of the breast April 19–22, 2001, Philadelphia, PA. *Breast J*. 2002; **8**(3):124–138.

28. Pritchard KI, Shepherd LE, O'Malley FP, et al. HER2 and responsiveness of breast cancer to adjuvant chemotherapy. *N Engl J Med*. 2006;**354**(20):2103–2111.

29. How Can I Find Breast Cancer Support in My Area. http://www.breastcancer.org/faq_support.html. Accessed August, 4, 2008.

30. McArdle JM, George WD, McArdle CS, et al. Psychological support for patients undergoing breast cancer surgery: A randomised study. *BMJ*. 1996;**312**(7034): 813–816.

31. Etchells E, Darzins P, Silberfeld M, et al. Assessment of patient capacity to consent to treatment. *J Gen Intern Med*. 1999;**14**(1):27–34.

32. Sturman ED. The capacity to consent to treatment and research: A review of standardized assessment tools. *Clin Psychol Rev*. 2005;**25**(7):954–974.

33. Grisso T, Appelbaum PS, Hill-Fotouhi C. The MacCAT-T: A clinical tool to assess patients' capacities to make treatment decisions. *Psychiatr Serv*. 1997; **48**(11):1415–1419.

34. Desan PH, Powsner S. Assessment and management of patients with psychiatric disorders. *Crit Care Med*. 2004;**32**(4 Suppl):S166–73.

35. Bernat JL, Peterson LM. Patient-centered informed consent in surgical practice. *Arch Surg*. 2006;**141**(1):86–92.

36. Whelan T, Levine M, Willan A, et al. Effect of a decision aid on knowledge and treatment decision making for breast cancer surgery: A randomized trial. *JAMA*. 2004;**292**(4):435–441.

37. Institute of Medicine (U.S.). *To Err is Human: Building a Safer Health System*. Washington, D.C.: National Academy Press; 2000.

38. *American Medical Association Council on Ethical and Judicial Affairs. Code of Medical Ethics, Annotated Current Opinions*. 2004–2005 ed. Chicago, IL: American Medical Association; 2005.

39. Clinton HR, Obama B. Making patient safety the centerpiece of medical liability reform. *N Engl J Med*. 2006;**354**(21):2205–2208.

40. The Joint Commission. *Hospital Accreditation Standards, 2007.* Oakbrook Terrace, IL: Joint Comission Resources; 2007.

41. Gallagher TH, Waterman AD, Ebers AG, Fraser VJ, Levinson W. Patients' and physicians' attitudes regarding the disclosure of medical errors. *JAMA.* 2003; **289**(8):1001–1007.

42. Gallagher TH, Studdert D, Levinson W. Disclosing harmful medical errors to patients. *N Engl J Med.* 2007;**356**(26):2713–2719.

43. Gallagher TH, Garbutt JM, Waterman AD, et al. Choosing your words carefully: How physicians would disclose harmful medical errors to patients. *Arch Intern Med.* 2006;**166**(15):1585–1593.

44. Gallagher TH, Waterman AD, Garbutt JM, et al. US and Canadian physicians' attitudes and experiences regarding disclosing errors to patients. *Arch Intern Med.* 2006;**166**(15):1605–1611.

45. Banja J. Moral courage in medicine – disclosing medical error. *Bioethics Forum.* 2001;**17**(2):7–11.

46. Hickson GB, Clayton EW, Githens PB, Sloan FA. Factors that prompted families to file medical malpractice claims following perinatal injuries. *JAMA.* 1992; **267**(10):1359–1363.

47. Pichert JW, Hickson GB, Vincent C. Communicating about unexpected outcomes and errors. In: Carayon P, ed. *Handbook of Human Factors and Ergonomics in Healthcare and Patient Safety.* Hillsdale, NJ: Erlbaum Associates; 2006.

48. Bok S. *Lying: Moral Choice in Public and Private Life.* New York: Random House; 1978.

49. Nyberg D. *The Vanished Truth: Truth Telling and Deceiving in Ordinary Life.* Chicago: University of Chicago Press; 1993.

50. Hippocrates. *Decorum.* Cambridge, MA: Harvard University Press; 1967.

51. Oken D. What to tell cancer patients. A study of medical attitudes. *JAMA.* 1961;**175**:1120–1128.

52. Sun M. AMA's new ethics code is major break from past. *Science.* 1980; **209**(4458):790–791.

53. ABIM Foundation. American Board of Internal Medicine, ACP-ASIM Foundation. American College of Physicians-American Society of Internal Medicine, European Federation of Internal Medicine. Medical professionalism in the new millennium: A physician charter. *Ann Intern Med.* 2002;**136**(3): 243–246.

54. Curtis JR, Engelberg RA, Nielsen EL, Au DH, Patrick DL. Patient-physician communication about end-of-life care for patients with severe COPD. *Eur Respir J.* 2004;**24**(2):200–205.

55. Fallowfield LJ, Jenkins VA, Beveridge HA. Truth may hurt but deceit hurts more: Communication in palliative care. *Palliat Med.* 2002;**16**(4):297–303.

56. Hagerty RG, Butow PN, Ellis PM, et al. Communicating with realism and hope: Incurable cancer patients' views on the disclosure of prognosis. *J Clin Oncol.* 2005;**23**(6):1278–1288.

57. Marzanski M. Would you like to know what is wrong with you? On telling the truth to patients with dementia. *J Med Ethics.* 2000;**26**(2):108–113.

58. Miyata H, Tachimori H, Takahashi M, Saito T, Kai I. Disclosure of cancer diagnosis and prognosis: A survey of the general public's attitudes toward doctors and family holding discretionary powers. *BMC Med Ethics.* 2004;**5**:E7.

59. Sullivan RJ, Menapace LW, White RM. Truth-telling and patient diagnoses. *J Med Ethics.* 2001;**27**(3):192–197.

60. Wenrich MD, Curtis JR, Ambrozy DA, Carline JD, Shannon SE, Ramsey PG. Dying patients' need for emotional support and personalized care from physicians: Perspectives of patients with terminal illness, families, and health care providers. *J Pain Symptom Manage.* 2003;**25**(3):236–246.

61. Yun YH, Lee CG, Kim SY, et al. The attitudes of cancer patients and their families toward the disclosure of terminal illness. *J Clin Oncol.* 2004;**22**(2):307–314.

62. Panagopoulou E, Mintziori G, Montgomery A, Kapoukranidou D, Benos A. Concealment of information in clinical practice: Is lying less stressful than telling the truth? *J Clin Oncol.* 2008;**26**(7):1175–1177.

63. Anderlik MR, Pentz RD, Hess KR. Revisiting the truth-telling debate: A study of disclosure practices at a major cancer center. *J Clin Ethics.* 2000;**11**(3):251–259.

64. Baile WF, Lenzi R, Parker PA, Buckman R, Cohen L. Oncologists' attitudes toward and practices in giving bad news: An exploratory study. *J Clin Oncol.* 2002;**20**(8):2189–2196.

65. Surbone A. Information, truth, and communication: For an interpretation of truth-telling practices throughout the world. *Ann N Y Acad Sci.*1997;**809**:7–16.

66. Surbone A. Cultural competence: Why? *Ann Oncol.* 2004;**15**(5):697–699.

67. Blendon RJ, DesRoches CM, Brodie M, et al. Views of practicing physicians and the public on medical errors. *N Engl J Med.* 2002;**347**(24):1933–1940.

68. Hingorani M, Wong T, Vafidis G. Patients' and doctors' attitudes to amount of information given after unintended injury during treatment: Cross sectional, questionnaire survey. *BMJ.* 1999;**318**(7184):640–641.

69. Hobgood C, Tamayo-Sarver JH, Elms A, Weiner B. Parental preferences for error disclosure, reporting, and legal action after medical error in the care of their children. *Pediatrics.* 2005;**116**(6):1276–1286.

70. Mazor KM, Simon SR, Yood RA, et al. Health plan members' views about disclosure of medical errors. *Ann Intern Med.* 2004;**140**(6):409–418.

71. Schwappach DL, Koeck CM. What makes an error unacceptable? A factorial survey on the disclosure of medical errors. *Int J Qual Health Care.* 2004;**16**(4):317–326.

72. Shapiro RS, Simpson DE, Lawrence SL, Talsky AM, Sobocinski KA, Schiedermayer DL. A survey of sued and nonsued physicians and suing patients. *Arch Intern Med.* 1989;**149**(10):2190–2196.

73. Sweet MP, Bernat JL. A study of the ethical duty of physicians to disclose errors. *J Clin Ethics.* 1997;**8**(4):341–348.

74. Vincent CA, Pincus T, Scurr JH. Patients' experience of surgical accidents. *Qual Health Care.* 1993;**2**(2):77–82.

75. Witman AB, Park DM, Hardin SB. How do patients want physicians to handle mistakes? A survey of internal medicine patients in an academic setting. *Arch Intern Med.* 1996;**156**(22):2565–2569.

76. Schoen C, Osborn R, Huynh PT, et al. Taking the pulse of health care systems: Experiences of patients with health problems in six countries. *Health Aff (Millwood)*. 2005;Suppl Web Exclusives:W5–509–25.

77. The Kaiser Family Foundation/Agency for Healthcare Research and Quality/ Harvard School of Public Health. National survey on consumers' experiences with patient safety and quality information. November, 2004.

78. The Full Disclosure Working Group. *When Things Go Wrong: Responding to Adverse Events. A Consensus Statement of the Harvard Hospitals*. Boston, MA: Coalition for the Prevention of Medical Errors; 2006.

79. Kim HN, Gates E, Lo B. What hysterectomy patients want to know about the roles of residents and medical students in their care. *Acad Med*. 1998;**73**(3): 339–341.

80. Magrane D, Gannon J, Miller CT. Student doctors and women in labor: Attitudes and expectations. *Obstet Gynecol*. 1996;**88**(2):298–302.

81. Santen SA, Hemphill RR, McDonald MF, Jo CO. Patients' willingness to allow residents to learn to practice medical procedures. *Acad Med*. 2004;**79**(2):144–147.

82. Santen SA, Hemphill RR, Spanier CM, Fletcher ND. "Sorry, it's my first time!" Will patients consent to medical students learning procedures? *Med Educ*. 2005;**39**(4):365–369.

83. Williams CT, Fost N. Ethical considerations surrounding first time procedures: A study and analysis of patient attitudes toward spinal taps by students. *Kennedy Inst Ethics J*. 1992;**2**(3):217–231.

84. Hemphill RR, Santen SA, Rountree CB, Szmit AR. Patients' understanding of the roles of interns, residents, and attending physicians in the emergency department. *Acad Emerg Med*. 1999;**6**(4):339–344.

85. Santen SA, Hemphill RR, Prough EE, Perlowski AA. Do patients understand their physician's level of training? A survey of emergency department patients. *Acad Med*. 2004;**79**(2):139–143.

86. Green MJ, Mitchell G, Stocking CB, Cassel CK, Siegler M. Do actions reported by physicians in training conflict with consensus guidelines on ethics? *Arch Intern Med*. 1996;**156**(3):298–304.

87. Rosenbaum JR, Bradley EH, Holmboe ES, Farrell MH, Krumholz HM. Sources of ethical conflict in medical housestaff training: A qualitative study. *Am J Med*. 2004;**116**(6):402–407.

88. Wertz DC. Ethics and genetics in international perspective: Results of a survey. In: Nippert I, Neitzel H, Wolff G, eds. *The New Genetics: From Research to Health Care*. Heidelberg, Germany: Springer-Verlag; 1999:75–94.

89. Wertz DC, Fletcher JC. Ethics and medical genetics in the United States: A national survey. *Am J Med Genet*. 1988;**29**(4):815–827.

90. Gorawara-Bhat R, Gallagher TH, Levinson W. Patient-provider discussions about conflicts of interest in managed care: Physicians' perceptions. *Am J Manag Care*. 2003;**9**(8):564–571.

91. Pearson SD, Hyams T. Talking about money: How primary care physicians respond to a patient's question about financial incentives. *J Gen Intern Med*. 2002;**17**(1):75–78.

92. Rost K, Smith R, Matthews DB, Guise B. The deliberate misdiagnosis of major depression in primary care. *Arch Fam Med.* 1994;**3**(4):333–337.

93. Wynia MK, Cummins DS, VanGeest JB, Wilson IB. Physician manipulation of reimbursement rules for patients: Between a rock and a hard place. *JAMA.* 2000;**283**(14):1858–1865.

94. Green MJ, Farber NJ, Ubel PA, et al. Lying to each other: When internal medicine residents use deception with their colleagues. *Arch Intern Med.* 2000; **160**(15):2317–2323.

95. Greer DS. To inform or not to inform patients about students. *J Med Educ.* 1987;**62**(10):861–862.

96. Waterman AD, Garbutt J, Hazel E, et al. The emotional impact of medical errors on practicing physicians in the United States and Canada. *Jt Comm J Qual Patient Saf.* 2007;**33**(8):467–476.

97. Lo B. *Resolving Ethical Dilemmas: A Guide for Clinicians.* Philadelphia, PA: Lippincott, Williams, and Wilkins; 2005.

98. Paterick TJ, Carson GV, Allen MC, Paterick TE. Medical informed consent: General considerations for physicians. *Mayo Clin Proc.* 2008;**83**(3):313–319.

99. Pellegrino ED. Is truth telling to the patient a cultural artifact? *JAMA.* 1992;**268**(13):1734–1735.

100. Searight HR, Gafford J. Cultural diversity at the end of life: Issues and guidelines for family physicians. *Am Fam Physician.* 2005;**71**(3):515–522.

101. Surbone A. Persisting differences in truth telling throughout the world. *Support Care Cancer.* 2004;**12**(3):143–146.

102. Kachalia A, Shojania KG, Hofer TP, Piotrowski M, Saint S. Does full disclosure of medical errors affect malpractice liability? The jury is still out. *Jt Comm J Qual Saf.* 2003;**29**(10):503–511.

103. Institute of Medicine (U.S.). *Committee on Quality of Health Care in America. To Err is Human: Building a Safer Health System.* Washington, D.C.: National Academy Press; 2000.

104. Amori G. Pearls on disclosure of adverse events. In: *Risk Management Pearls.* Chicago: American Society for Healthcare Risk Management; 2006.

105. Gallagher TH, Denham C, Leape L, Amori G, Levinson W. Disclosing unanticipated outcomes to patients: The art and the practice. *Journal of Patient Safety.* 2007;**3**:158–165.

Commitment to Patient Confidentiality

Cases and Commentaries

PATIENT CONFIDENTIALITY – INFECTIOUS DISEASE

A physician in a small community practice realizes that his hepatitis C-positive patient is dating one of his other patients who is hepatitis C negative. Upon questioning by the physician, the hepatitis C-positive patient reports that he has not told his girlfriend of this infection.

A Perspective from a General Internist

Clinical Background

Hepatitis C virus (HCV) infection is the most common chronic bloodborne infection in the United States with approximately 1.8 percent of the population infected. HCV is transmitted parenterally by transfusion, intravenous drug use, and accidental needle stick.[1] Sexual transmission can occur, although the risk appears to be very low (less than 3 percent in monogamous partners).[2]

Routine testing for HCV is recommended for high-risk individuals such as persons with history of injected drug use or unexplained abnormal ALT levels, for recipients of blood products or organs before 1992, and persons on chronic hemodialysis. It is unclear if long-term monogamous sex partners of HCV-positive persons will benefit from testing.[3] Testing should be preceded by appropriate counseling. All HCV-positive individuals should be counseled to change behaviors that increase the risk of HCV transmission.[1,4]

Professionalism Considerations

The physician in this case faces a dilemma as his HCV-positive patient has not told his girlfriend about his infection. The girlfriend is also his patient and is HCV negative.

The physician has to respect the *privacy rule* which sets limits on the use of individually identifiable health information by providers. The *Code of Medical Ethics* of the American Medical Association (AMA) states that "the information disclosed to a physician during the course of the patient-physician relationship is confidential to the utmost degree. The physician generally should not reveal confidential communications or information without the patient's expressed consent unless required to disclose the information by law."

The physician should counsel the patient regarding prevention of spreading HCV to others, including sexual transmission. If the patient has only recently been diagnosed with HCV, then he should be counseled regarding further evaluation for chronic liver disease, treatment of hepatitis, and HIV testing. The physician should listen carefully to the patient's perspective and try to understand why the patient is reluctant to disclose his HCV seropositivity to his girlfriend. Dissecting the problem and exploring each of its aspects together with the patient may be helpful.

The physician should discuss with his HCV-positive patient the small but present risk of sexual transmission of this disease and advise the patient to use condoms. He should also ask the patient about any illicit intravenous drug use and alcohol consumption. The patient needs to be advised not to share any personal care items that might have blood on them and to cover cuts or sores on his skin.[1] In addition, the physician should stress the importance of full disclosure and counsel abstinence or the use of condoms until his girlfriend becomes aware of the risks. These steps may prevent transmission of the disease.

Often, patients decide not to disclose their positive hepatitis or HIV status because they are afraid of being discriminated against or stigmatized in their community. This becomes even more problematic in small communities. Educating the community will help prevent transmission and nurture compassion and respect for these sick individuals. Workshops, community panel discussions, distribution of factsheets and development of peer education programs are some of the modalities that help raise awareness. These efforts can be further expanded with collaboration at a state and national level.

The fact that the girlfriend is also one of the physician's patients further complicates this case. The principles of beneficence and nonmaleficence require that health care providers do what is considered in the best interest of the person for whom they are providing care. The physician knows that informing the girlfriend about her boyfriend's hepatitis status will benefit her as she might take precautions that will prevent transmission. However, the physician is not allowed to disclose this information as this will violate his HCV-positive patient's autonomy.

The physician may schedule an appointment with the patient's girlfriend for counseling about the risks of sexually transmitted diseases (STD) in general and the negative consequences of unsafe sex. The physician should emphasize the importance of full disclosure and trust in establishing the foundation of a trustworthy relationship. The couple should engage in an honest discussion and share health information, in particular carrier status for any potential STD.

The physician's *primary commitment must always be to the patient's welfare and best interests*, whether the physician is preventing or treating illness or helping patient to cope with illness, disability, and death. Medical care in the United States has rapidly shifted from a paternalistic approach to patients to an emphasis on patient autonomy. According to the "independent choice model" of decision making, the physician objectively presents the patient with options and odds but withholds his own experience and recommendations to avoid overly influencing the patient. Intense collaboration between patient and physician can help the patient to autonomously make choices that are informed by both medical facts and the physician's experience.[5,6]

Opinion

This case underlines the ethical dilemmas that physicians often face in everyday practice. The role of the physician as the patient's advocate can often lead to a crossroads where his effort to protect his patient from physical or psychological harm may be challenged by the societal laws of protecting privacy. The physician might have to balance the needs for privacy against the obligation of protecting the individual.

Whenever conflicts arise, counseling and open discussion with the patient might be the best approach. Building a patient–physician relationship on trust, mutual understanding, and respect can effectively help the patient who faces such a predicament to make a well-informed decision. The risk of sexual transmission of the disease remains controversial and probably very small. However, this low but present risk for the patient's girlfriend of contracting a disease should be explained clearly to the patient. The physician should protect the patient's privacy and autonomy and at the same time he should strongly encourage the patient to discuss his diagnosis with his girlfriend. The final choice belongs to the patient, who hopefully can make the right decision with the physician's guidance.

Irene Alexandraki, M.D.
Assistant Professor of Medicine, Department of Medicine
University of Florida College of Medicine-Jacksonville

A Perspective from a Bioethicist

Doctor–patient confidentiality is a basic tenet of modern medical care, and a core value of professional medical ethics. The primary justification for that tenet is the expectation that a person seeking medical help and advice should not be hindered by a fear that the physician or other clinicians (and, by extension, associated personnel) will disclose any aspect of the patient's concerns or condition to those outside the recognized medical setting (which may include third parties, such as insurance companies). Confidentiality standards include unauthorized disclosure to family members or spouses, except in cases where an individual has legal health care authority over the patient (as in pediatrics, or guardianships, though some degree of confidentiality is appropriate there as well).

Doctor–patient confidentiality is an ethical concept, going back to the Hippocratic Oath. The associated legal concept is "doctor–patient privilege." The law acknowledges a "special relationship" between doctors and patients (as it does, for example, between attorneys and clients, clergy and parishioners). The scope of that relationship, and thus legal protection of doctor-patient communication, varies from state to state. No federal law governs or defines the relationship.

Balancing the physician's obligation to maintain patient confidentiality is the medical obligation to public health. The obligation may be to specific other individuals (e.g., the girlfriend in our scenario) or to the general public welfare, as in the case of a carrier of an epidemic (e.g., Mary Mallon, "Typhoid Mary"). State requirements mandate reporting certain kinds of illnesses (AIDS and Class IV HIV, hepatitis A and B, measles, rabies, tetanus, and tuberculosis), and some injuries as well (gunshot wounds or suspected child abuse), even if disclosure violates patient confidentiality. Of course, legal obligations and ethical obligations are not the same thing, and may even conflict.

The legal obligation to individuals was articulated in the famous Tarasoff case, where the family of a murdered woman sued a therapist for not informing the intended victim that his patient threatened to kill her (the therapist did inform the police). The California Supreme Court ruled, in a much quoted phrase, "The protective privilege ends where the public peril begins." The case has become the touchstone for trying to understand the balance between patient confidentiality and public protection.

In the case in question, the doctor seems to hold two incompatible obligations to two patients – the obligation of privacy and confidentiality to the patient, and the obligation to protect the health and well-being of his girlfriend, also a patient. Let us call the patient John and his girlfriend Jane. The first course, all would agree, is to use all the power of persuasion at the doctor's disposal, based on the (hopefully developed) relationship he has with John, to convince John to inform Jane himself or to allow the doctor to notify her. Failing that, the doctor seems left with a choice of either (a) deciding to inform Jane against John's wishes and so having to explain to John why the doctor must break his confidence, or (b) deciding not to inform Jane, and explaining to a potentially Hepatitis C-positive Jane in a year or two why the doctor knew John was Hepatitis C positive and did not warn her.

Some argue that, as painful as it may seem, the obligation to patient confidentiality is absolute. It also protects public health, as patients who know their confidentiality may be compromised will not come forward in the first place.[7] Others point out that true privacy is abrogated as soon as a patient seeks help from the medical system in any case.[8]

In the case of John and Jane, the obligation of the physician is to do everything reasonable to try to convince John to inform Jane, and, failing that, to inform Jane personally (with full disclosure to John that the physician intends to do so). Too often cases like this are seen as exceptions to a general principle of confidentiality, or a "breach" of confidentiality,[9] rather than a qualifying aspect of that principle. Patient confidentiality as a value exists in a web of competing values that sometimes trump it, as it did in the Tarasoff case or the case of an abused child. John is also a moral agent, and has now enlisted the doctor as a player in this moral drama, and so the relative weights of the competing moral interests must be evaluated.

The bar to violating confidentiality must be set very high. The doctor would not have an ethical obligation to warn if Jane was not his patient. The threat to Jane must be high, as it is in this case where she faces contracting an incurable disease. John must know and understand that he has the disease, and that it is transmitted to Jane sexually or through other transfers of bodily fluids (e.g., intravenous drug use). Ultimately, however, the threat to Jane is a compelling reason to breach John's confidentiality and inform her.

An additional point must be made. Informed consent requires physicians to reveal the circumstances under which they will disclose patient information at the outset of the doctor–patient relationship. If John had been informed by his doctor about the kinds of circumstances that may arise that would require disclosure, including significant health threats to another patient, he would have no standing to oppose the physician's action. Given an informed patient, the ethical issue disappears.

Paul Wolpe, Ph.D.
Asa Griggs Candler Professor of Bioethics at Emory University
Director of the Emory University Center for Bioethics

PATIENT CONFIDENTIALITY – OBSTETRICS-GYNECOLOGY

One evening, a 28-year-old woman, G2, para 2–0–0–2, mentions to her husband that she had an appointment with her gynecologist that morning. The gynecologist prescribed metronidazole for treatment of "vaginitis." The next morning, the husband telephones the gynecologist and asks the physician whether his wife's infection could possibly be related to infidelity.

A Perspective from an Obstetrician-Gynecologist

Clinical Background

Vaginal infections may be classified into three types.[10–12] The most common form is bacterial vaginosis (BV). This infection results from an alteration in the normal vaginal flora and is caused by a combination of several organisms, including anaerobes, *Mobiluncus species*, *Gardnerella vaginalis*, and genital mycoplasms. Risk factors for BV include multiple sexual partners, recent change in sexual partner(s), douching, and changes in the hormonal milieu of the vagina (e.g., transition to menopause). Bacterial vaginosis is not usually considered to be a sexually transmitted disease. Although several treatment options are available, the most cost-effective treatment for bacterial vaginosis in both gynecologic and obstetric patients is oral metronidazole, 500 mg, twice daily, for seven days. Treatment of the patient's sexual partner is not routinely indicated.[13]

The second most common cause of vaginitis is moniliasis, or yeast infection. This infection, like bacterial vaginosis, results from alteration in the normal vaginal flora. Risk factors for moniliasis include young age, nulliparity, being in the luteal phase of the menstrual cycle, use of spermicides, recent broad-spectrum antibiotic therapy, pregnancy, diabetes, and an immunosuppressive disorder. The most common organism is *Candida albicans*; the other two important pathogens are *Candida tropicalis* and *Candida glabrata*. The latter two organisms assume increasing importance in women who have chronic yeast infections.[11] Moniliasis can usually be treated successfully with either topical antifungal medications such as clotrimazole, miconazole, or terconazole, or by an oral medication such as fluconazole. Dosing regimens for the topical medications vary from a one-time application to seven days. Fluconazole is usually administered as a single oral dose, 150 mg. Treatment of the sexual partner is not routinely indicated.

The third cause of vaginitis is trichomonas infection. Unlike bacterial vaginosis and candidiasis, trichomonas is a sexually transmitted disease that is caused by the protozoan, *Trichomonas vaginalis*. The infection is highly contagious, and >50 percent of patients will be infected after a single unprotected exposure to an infected host.[10] The most effective treatment for trichomoniasis is a single 2 g dose of oral metronidazole.[10-13] The sexual partner should be treated with a similar dose of medication in order to prevent reinfection. The sexual partner is most likely to accept treatment if the woman's physician provides a prescription for him. However, many gynecologists are understandably reluctant to write a prescription for an individual who is not actually their patient. Because trichomoniasis is a sexually transmitted disease, affected patients should be tested for all other sexually transmitted infections such as gonorrhea, chlamydia, hepatitis B, syphilis, and HIV infection.

Professionalism Considerations

This case deals squarely with the issue of patient confidentiality. The gynecologist has no legal or ethical obligation to divulge confidential information to the patient's husband. This principle is particularly relevant if the woman simply has bacterial vaginosis or candidiasis because neither of these is a sexually transmitted disease, and neither poses any significant risk to the husband. Under no circumstances should the gynecologist divulge information to the husband without the expressed permission of the patient.

The situation becomes slightly more problematic if the patient is being treated for trichomoniasis. This infection is a sexually transmitted disease, and treatment of the woman's sexual partner is indicated. Most gynecologists would explain this necessity to the patient, request that she inform her sexual partner of the infection, and ask that he seek treatment from his physician.

As noted, anyone with trichomonas infection also should be tested for other sexually transmitted diseases. If diseases such as gonorrhea, chlamydia, syphilis, or HIV infection are identified, the physician has a legal obligation to report these infections to the local public health agency. In addition, although trichomonas does not usually cause a serious illness in the male partner, gonorrhea, chlamydia, syphilis, and HIV infection can cause serious morbidity and, in the case of HIV infection, even mortality. Therefore, if any of these infections are documented, the physician should strongly encourage the patient to explicitly inform her sexual partner(s) of the need to seek treatment. If the woman refuses to do so, the physician faces a major ethical dilemma. His or her principal obligation is to respect the confidentiality of the patient. However, the physician also has an obligation to be fair and just to all parties concerned. Clearly, the sexual partner will benefit from treatment.

The sense of urgency in notifying the sexual partner becomes particularly pronounced if HIV infection is present. In the state of Florida, the physician does not have an obligation to inform the sexual partner if the patient refuses to do so. However, neither is the physician vulnerable to legal action if he/she decides to inform the partner without the patient's consent. In the present case, should a sexually transmitted disease be documented, the ethical principles of justice and beneficence justify firm efforts on the part of the physician to have the woman disclose the nature of her illness to her husband.

Opinion

This physician's first priority is to protect the confidentiality of his/her patient. Therefore, without the expressed consent of the patient, the gynecologist should not discuss her clinical care with her husband. I believe that this principle should be inviolate if the woman simply has an infection such as bacterial vaginosis or candidiasis. If trichomoniasis is present, but no other sexually transmitted diseases are identified, I do not believe that the physician would be justified in violating the confidentiality of the patient. If concurrent STDs are documented, the physician has an obligation to report these infections to the local public health authority. Investigators from the public health unit, in turn, will contact the patient and make an effort to notify her sexual contacts. If HIV infection is documented, I personally believe that the physician is obligated to inform the patient's sexual partner(s) of this infection if the woman refuses to do so. In this situation, there is a compelling sense of urgency about having the sexual partner(s) tested for HIV infection and treated, if infection is identified.

Patrick Duff, M.D.
Department of Obstetrics and Gynecology
Associate Dean for Student Affairs
University of Florida College of Medicine

A Perspective from a Physician and Expert on Patient Confidentiality

The starting point in this case is patient confidentiality. Without assurance of confidentiality, patients might not reveal embarrassing or even illegal actions important for physicians to know in providing optimal care.[14] This ethical principle is complemented by the federal Health Insurance Portability and Accountability Act (HIPAA) of 1996. HIPAA prevents physicians from revealing patients' personal information to third parties, even spouses, without patients' consent except when such disclosures are likely to provide significant benefit and are unlikely to cause harm to the patients.[15] Nonetheless, this particular vignette raises a series of medical, legal, and ethical questions that invite different recommendations concerning the gynecologist's communications with the patient's husband.

Why did the gynecologist prescribe metronidizole? This antimicrobial is used for two types of vaginal infections: bacterial vaginosis and trichomoniasis. Bacterial vaginosis, an overgrowth of bacteria not normally present in the vagina, is not a sexually transmitted disease (STD) and, therefore, the issue becomes relatively simple. The gynecologist will benefit both wife and husband by removing any doubt, anxiety, or suspicion raised by an incomplete understanding of the illness being treated. Providing this information will involve minimal, if any, breaking of confidentiality because the wife has already revealed she is being treated for vaginitis.

If, however, the metronidizole was prescribed for trichomoniasis, the issue becomes complicated. The protozoa *Trichomonas vaginalis* is sexually transmitted and highly contagious. The physician has an ethical responsibility to prevent the further spread of this infection by instructing the patient to tell all her sexual partners that they are likely to be infected and need to seek medical care. Fulfilling this responsibility involves discussing with the patient both *from whom* she might have contracted the protozoa and *to whom* she might have transmitted it.

Does the gynecologist have a legal or ethical responsibility to do more than advise the patient? First, physicians are mandated to report other STDs, namely chlamydia, gonorrhea, syphilis, chancroid, and HIV infections, to their local department of health, which takes responsibility for finding and treating potentially infected contacts. Trichomonas is not, however, a reportable disease. Second, if a physician thinks a patient is likely to kill or cause serious harm to any other person, the physician has, according to the American Medical Association's *Code of Ethics*[15] and the laws of most U.S. states, the duty to try to prevent this by contacting law enforcement agents or even by warning potential victims.[16] This duty might apply to HIV, but surely not to trichomonas since trichomoniasis is not life threatening, causes little suffering in males, and is curable. It seems unlikely, therefore, that the gynecologist would be found liable if the wife did not inform her sexual contacts or if these contacts did not take the necessary measures to protect themselves and others.

To complicate matters further, it is not clear from the vignette whether the husband is calling because he suspects his wife of infidelity, because his wife suspects him of infidelity, or because he has in fact been unfaithful. The gynecologist may already have some knowledge about this from what the wife reported, but does not know, of course, if the wife was reporting the truth. This question is further complicated by the possibility that any particular infidelity might not have been the source of the infection. In men, trichomonas infection is often asymptomatic and carriage is "self-limited and transient." In women, however, asymptomatic carriage can "occur for prolonged periods of time" (with only one-third becoming symptomatic within six months) so that "it is not necessarily possible to ascertain when and from whom the infection was acquired."[17]

In light of these uncertainties, the gynecologist should, in the case of trichomoniasis, explain politely that physicians are not permitted, by medical ethics and federal law, to discuss patients' medical care with anyone but the patients, not even with spouses. If, however, the husband reports specifically that his wife revealed (in accordance with the gynecologist's instructions) that she has an STD or, more particularly, trichomoniasis, the gynecologist would be permitted, in my view, to explain the medical facts. The husband should be told that the protozoa is highly contagious, that infection can be asymptomatic, and that he needs to be evaluated for treatment so that he will not reinfect his wife or anyone else. The gynecologist must remember throughout that her or his primary duty is to the wife, not to the husband, and must refrain from giving advice that might be construed as establishing a patient–physician relationship with the husband.

Finally, the gynecologist's duty to the wife implies an ethical and, possibly, legal responsibility to tell her about the conversation and to offer to help her deal with any marriage problems.

Paul Sorum, M.D.
Professor of Internal Medicine and Pediatrics
Albany Medical College

PATIENT CONFIDENTIALITY – PEDIATRICS

A grandmother brings her thirteen-year-old granddaughter to see her pediatrician for evaluation of poorly controlled type 1 diabetes. The grandparent is concerned that the child's parents are not appropriately caring for her and requests specific information about the diabetes medications and recent lab work.

A Perspective from a Pediatrician

Clinical Background

Causes of poor diabetic control in a thirteen-year-old are numerous and include acute infection, omission of insulin doses, suboptimal dosing, changes in exercise or dietary habits, depression or other mental health issues, barriers to access to care, and unmet needs for family support. The transition from childhood to adolescence is marked by developmental processes, such as changes in the individual's level of independence and self-determination that may impact on diabetes management.

Professionalism Considerations

In the ideal situation, this adolescent and her parents would have already discussed the change in the relationship between the physician and adolescent which should occur at the transition from childhood to adolescence.[18] That conversation would include the agreement between all three parties that the content of adolescent's visits with the physician are confidential from the parent unless the physician has a compelling reason to break confidentiality. Such judgments may include that the patient is not competent to provide informed consent or that the adolescent is a danger to self or others (for instance, if he or she is suicidal, or involved in serious drug use), or if the physician is compelled by law to do so (as in the requirement to report physical or sexual abuse, for instance). Physicians also provide guidance and support to the adolescent for effective communication between the adolescent and the parents, and encourage parental involvement as appropriate, but should not mandate it.

The goal of optimal independence and normalization of everyday life for an adolescent with diabetes must be balanced with the need to prevent life-threatening outcomes of suboptimal management. Diabetes education programs which employ a family-focused approach in which adolescents and parents use a shared management approach results in fewer conflicts and better glycemic control. Such programs can be delivered in the family's home.[19–21]

Regarding the role of the grandparent, the physician would need to better understand her concern and would need to clarify her role in the care of this patient. Grandparents sometime assume a prominent role in the care of their grandchildren. Has the grandparent been specifically granted permission (by the parents and adolescent) to have access to this information and to be involved in the patient's care? If not, the physician is not permitted to give the grandmother access to the information she is requesting.

In this instance, the primary relationship and guarantee of confidentiality (with the stated exceptions) is between the adolescent and her physician. The main portion of the visit would be between the patient and her physician during which the physician would take a detailed history, including what the patient believes causes her diabetes to be poorly controlled; her dietary and exercise habits; her recent insulin regimen in response to blood glucose measurements; how she and her parents share responsibility for management of her diabetes; and discussion of personal-social issues such as school performance, possible depression, or other mental health issues, and substance use. Review of the record of blood glucose measurements and insulin dosing would be reviewed. Adjustments might be made in rules for insulin dosing. If a need for further or repeated diabetes education is identified, that might be carried out by another member of the physician's team.

The adolescent's parents are the only other party with the right to be involved in discussions of the patient's care. If the parents and the patient had given permission for her grandmother to be involved in her care, a signed record of it would be present in the patient's chart.

If the grandparent has written permission to be involved in her granddaughter's care, the visit would involve the grandmother in (1) the initial three-party portion of the visit, during which the patient and the grandmother would state their reasons for the visit and their concerns, and (2) at the conclusion of the visit to wrap up and share with the grandmother any content of the confidential portion of the visit that could be shared (i.e., if the adolescent had agreed to share it).

Concerning the allegation of neglect: Is the grandparent alleging that parental neglect of her granddaughter's care is leading to poor control of her diabetes? If yes, does the alleged neglect reach the level that requires reporting to child protection authorities? The pediatrician should listen to the grandparent's concerns but should not reveal protected information without the parents' consent. The pediatrician would likely want to cross-check reports of parental involvement with the adolescent patient. Ultimately, the physician would weigh all of the information to determine if the allegation of neglect causes a level of suspicion which would require reporting to child protective authorities. If the physician judges that a report is warranted, it would necessitate an exception to the confidentiality agreement with the patient and family, since a report is then mandated by law.

Opinion

This is a complicated situation in which the physician needs to weigh the guarantee of confidentiality in the relationship with this adolescent; evidence (of medical neglect) warranting breaching the confidentiality; and the "official" status of the grandparent with regard to her granddaughter's medical care. While the physician's initial impulse may be to involve an obviously concerned and perhaps well-intentioned grandparent, careful discussion and clinical judgment will lead to the best decision.

Karen Edwards, M.D.
Associate Dean for Primary Care
New York Medical College

A Perspective from a Medical Education Scholar and Grandparent

The complexity of family life in the United States suggests that this hypothetical case might not be too uncommon. In many families both parents work. A growing number of children are raised in single-parent households. Furthermore, it has been estimated that between 11 and 17.5 million children are raised by a parent whose judgment is impaired by alcohol or drugs.[22] It seems reasonable to guess that this grandmother might be doing this because the girl's parents are distracted by other responsibilities, living apart, divorced, or impaired by drugs or alcohol.

I was asked to comment on this case from the perspective of a grandparent, and someone who has been involved in evaluating the knowledge, skills, and attitudes of young physicians in medical school and residency. In particular, a few years ago my wife took our four-year-old grandson to see a physician because his mother, our daughter, had been hospitalized and we needed a physical examination form completed by a physician so that we could make arrangements for child care. We were surprised to learn that many physicians refuse to talk to a grandparent about a pediatric patient because U.S. common law requires parental consent for a physician to care for minor children.[23] Nevertheless, I would expect a physician who is a true professional, when faced with this grandmother and the 13-year-old, to be thinking about the following two issues before turning them away: What are the circumstances surrounding the grandmother's request? What are the benefits and risks of giving her the information she is seeking?

First, I would expect the physician to clarify the grandmother's role in the girl's care and try to infer parental consent. Does she care for the child routinely? For example, the grandmother's role might be clear if she lived in the same home or in the same neighborhood. The granddaughter's demeanor and communication with her grandmother would provide clues about the legitimacy of the grandmother's role. On the other hand, if the grandmother were visiting temporarily from out-of-town or if the granddaughter's behavior did not seem to reinforce her grandmother's role in her care, I would understand if a physician questioned the reasonableness of the grandmother's request and turned her away.

It is obvious that there are emergency exceptions to the need for parental consent. Although the present case is not an emergency, I would expect the professional physician to evaluate the urgency of the request and the potential risk to the granddaughter's health if nothing were done.

In this situation, a family member is eager to be supportive. I would expect the professional physician to give her the information if the granddaughter's condition was not under control and the grandmother might be able to help in correcting this. The benefits of responding seem to outweigh the risks if the grandmother plays a role in the care of the granddaughter. The only risk would be that the parents might challenge the appropriateness of the medical encounter with the child and the small breach of confidentiality.

In summary, from the perspective of a grandparent, I would expect the professional physician to welcome the opportunity to strengthen a relationship with this patient and to establish a new bond with a family member who might be able to make a positive contribution to the patient's health. Cited recently by the Committee on Pediatric Emergency Medicine[19] and originally published in the context of emergency care settings, the following advice might present a useful guideline that a professional could use in situations where there is a need to provide essential care for an adolescent patient without explicit parental consent:

Act like the patient is someone you care about. Act like you have the courage and intelligence to tell the difference between necessary and unnecessary care and testing, and that you have done for the patient what you would have done for your own family member.[24]

Thinking back to our own experience, this is exactly what happened. The physician whom my wife and grandson saw performed exactly as we expected by assessing the credibility of her situation and choosing to complete the physical examination form as requested.

Jon Veloski, M.S.
Center for Research in Medical Education and Health Care
Jefferson Medical College

PATIENT CONFIDENTIALITY – PSYCHIATRY

A thirty-five-year-old man is seeing his psychiatrist for depression. At the end of a visit, he asks the psychiatrist to code the diagnosis as insomnia and not depression because of his concern about the confidentiality of records and discrimination based on diagnosis of depression.

A Perspective from a Psychiatrist

Clinical Background
Insomnia can be either a disorder or a symptom. It can occur as a condition in and of itself, in which case it is referred to as primary insomnia, or can occur in the context of another medical or psychiatric condition, in which case it is referred to as co-morbid insomnia. The term "co-morbid" was

utilized in preference to the term "secondary" in a 2005 NIH State of the Science Conference[25] in recognition of the fact that in such mixed states, the direction of causality between insomnia and coexisting disorders is difficult to establish. It is rarely clear as to whether the insomnia is a result of the co-morbid entity, whether the co-morbid entity is a result of the insomnia, or whether the two conditions coexist independently of one another. This ambiguity is evident in the case of depression, the subject of this clinical scenario; longitudinal studies have revealed that the relationship between insomnia and major depression is bidirectional. Insomnia commonly coexists with major depression, is fomented by major depression, and is associated with an increased risk of developing future depressive disorders in individuals who are currently free of such disorders.[26] From a clinical standpoint, therefore, it is conceivable for insomnia to be the patient's primary diagnosis in this scenario, as long as it does, in fact, coexist with the depression. The patient's request, however, goes beyond this, as he also wishes the diagnosis of depression to be excluded.

Professionalism Considerations

The reasons for the patient's request are not clear. He may be concerned about the stigma of mental illness. Insomnia can be viewed as a "medical" disorder as opposed to a "psychiatric" disorder, a view which is supported by medical coding nosologies such as the ICD-9, which lists insomnia under both the psychiatric (307.41, 307.42) and medical (780.52) sections.[27] In a study of 1,187 depressed patients from 46 U.S. primary care clinics, 67 percent expected depression-related stigma to have a negative effect on employment, 59 percent on health insurance, and 24 percent on friendships.[28] Alternatively, the patient's request may be motivated by financial concerns; a medical disorder may be reimbursable by his insurance carrier, whereas a psychiatric disorder may not be. Also, he may be in denial of the psychiatric nature of his condition. For these and other reasons, miscoding of depression is a common practice in medicine; in one study, 50.3 percent of primary care providers deliberately substituted another diagnostic code for major depression within a two-week period.[29]

The patient's request presents the physician with a difficult conflict. If the psychiatrist were to deny this request, he or she would appear to be violating the principle of primacy of patient welfare, possibly placing the patient at greater risk for stigmatization and discrimination or granting him a greater financial burden. On the other hand, if the psychiatrist were to honor the patient's request, he or she would clearly be violating the principle of social justice, would be compromising medical ethical standards, and might even be placing him/herself at risk from a legal perspective. This apparent conflict can be resolved when it is approached from a psychiatric perspective.

One of the important goals of psychotherapy is to make the patient consciously aware of unconscious thoughts, feelings, and conflicts. This is a critical step in implementing a resolution of symptoms. To this end, the psychiatrist must always be mindful of the potential for intrapsychic meaning in whatever the patient expresses, verbally and nonverbally, in the psychotherapeutic session. Communications that offer opportunities for a high "yield" in intrapsychic material are those which directly involve the psychiatrist or the psychiatrist-patient relationship. Transference is one such phenomenon. It involves feelings, thoughts, and attitudes that the patient has about the psychiatrist, and which have, as their bases, earlier, important, relationships in the patient's life, such as those that exist between individuals and their parents or siblings. These feelings and thoughts are typically unconscious, at least in part. For example, an angry patient may direct his/her anger at the psychiatrist, yet not recognize that the anger is based in infantile relationships. Alternatively, the patient may not feel consciously angry at all, but act, within the psychotherapeutic sessions, in ways that appear to express internal, unconscious, angry feelings. Such may be the case with the patient of this scenario. Rather than expressing anger overtly to the psychiatrist (e.g., "I feel angry with you today,"), he may be expressing anger in disguised form. The patient's request in this scenario may be an example of a transferencial communication, whereby he may be placing the psychiatrist in a difficult position as a way of punishing the physician as an expression of his own underlying anger. A host of other psychodynamic formulations can explain the patient's request and, ultimately, the psychiatrist's deepening knowledge of the patient over time will guide him in arriving at the correct formulation. The main point to be made here is that such interactions must always be viewed in the context of the psychotherapeutic relationship, and the patient's psyche.

Opinion

What, then, might an appropriate response be on the part of the psychiatrist to such a request? Clearly, acting upon the apparent conflict without considering the psychological meanings involved would be an incorrect response. The psychiatrist cannot "take sides" between the two choices the patient presents him, which represent the principles of primacy of patient welfare and of social justice, respectively, as these choices are only disguised expressions of elements of the underlying, more clinically pertinent, psychological conflict. Rather, the psychiatrist must resort to further exploration by asking the patient to explain the reasons for his request. Accordingly, one possible response is "you place me in a difficult position, where whatever I do seems wrong. Please tell me what was going on in your mind when you made the request." Or, "let's discuss the consequences of honoring your request, and of not honoring your request." Other possibilities exist, and the one selected would be determined by the psychiatrist's knowledge of the patient and his psychodynamics.

Both honoring the patient's request for a change in diagnostic coding and refusing to do so, represent direct responses by the psychiatrist upon the manifest request without recognition of the true, underlying, unconscious meanings of this request. Both actions risk the loss of important opportunities for transforming a wealth of unconscious material into the realm of the conscious, a therapeutic faux pas. They also risk the possibility that the underlying primary conflict will find other ways of disguised expression in the future, leading to continued symptomatic difficulties in the patient's life and in the therapeutic sessions.

The psychiatrist's decision to undertake a path of further psychological exploration places the physician and the patient in agreement with both principles of professionalism. Whereas the patient may perceive that his best interests are served by the psychiatrist's changing of his diagnosis, it is actually clinically in his best interest to not "jump into action," but to explore his own request further. It is also in the best interest of society as a whole, and of the psychiatrist's professional integrity, to keep the patient's clinical improvement as his top priority. Ultimately, such a course of action represents good patient care.

Karl Doghramji, M.D.
Professor of Psychiatry and Human Behavior
Jefferson Medical College

A Perspective from a Scholar on Patient Privacy

Under the therapeutic principle of "do no harm" and the Hippocratic Oath a physician may not reveal confidences without patient consent.[30] Since "the quality of the therapeutic alliance is the best predictor of treatment outcome,"[31] breaching confidentiality through disseminating a detrimental diagnosis can hurt the therapy. Medical records deserve confidentiality, particularly about such a potentially stigmatizing condition as depression, because patients may otherwise experience employment or health insurance discrimination.

Yet, embedded in this vignette are questions, dilemmas, practicalities, and alternatives. First, it needs to be clear whether and what kind of depression brought the patient in, how recent and reliable the diagnosis is, and if the patient presented with insomnia initially. Second, discussion of confidentiality needs to occur at the start of therapy before a diagnosis may be clear. Third, such a request may become an opportunity to bring the content and motivation into the therapy while working on the meaning and feelings there.

A series of questions need to be considered. What does the diagnosis mean to the patient? Is this a symbolic or practical concern? Is fear about the diagnosis well founded or consequential in itself? Does the patient accept that he is depressed, not just sleeping poorly, and is his insomnia a symptom of a deeper malaise?

Moreover, there are practical questions that might ease or increase the dilemma, such as if the diagnostic code is used for internal clinic purposes, for example, within an HMO (health maintenance organization) or self-pay, rather than for external insurance reimbursement? Does the patient (or therapist) know if a diagnosis may extend therapy benefits beyond what insomnia might provide, and thus lead to improvement? Or does lack of insurance parity (difference in coverage from physical disorders) mean a psychological diagnosis might end treatment sooner? Does he have a secure job and health coverage, and the means to pay out of pocket expenses? Is either the doctor or the patient aware of cases of discrimination or coverage loss from the diagnosis?

It is important that the psychiatrist maintain an honest and candid relationship with the patient. Does either consider this request a distortion of the relationship? Is insomnia so much a part of the symptomology that it is a valid diagnosis? If not, is there another? Could the doctor be wrong in the diagnosis, particularly early in therapy? Can diagnosis and claims be waited on until this issue is resolved? Can the therapist help the patient through the anxiety and any detrimental consequences?

Though a psychiatrist may not reveal information or diagnosis without patient consent, there needs to be a record of the evidence for the diagnosis. Including the symptoms and perhaps a tentative diagnosis of depression in separately stored process notes would be protected by HIPAA and *Jaffe* v. *Redmond*. Medical records need to be clear and complete for future treatment; yet when whole records can be sent ubiquitously and instantaneously with negative consequences, many are edited or incomplete, for exactly those reasons.

While there is little written on this dilemma, and no surveys of psychiatrists who treat adults, some ethics literature and studies of primary care physicians (PCP) and pediatricians, including child psychiatrists, provide comparisons. Fully half of PCPs have modified depression diagnoses[29] for uncertainty on their validity or concern for the negative consequences for patients, though only one-in-nine patients so requested modification. More than two-thirds of pediatricians coded alternatively, though just over half of child psychiatrists,[32] who were sometimes more (others less) likely to substitute a diagnosis because of concerns for confidentiality, stigma, or insurance.

Moreover, in considering a similar dilemma, Lo describes a nurse in excellent health who has a routine checkup at the hospital where he works. The nurse asks his physician not to write in the medical record that he had been severely depressed several years ago. He knows that many people in the hospital might see his record, and he does not want colleagues to know his psychiatric history. He also fears that he will have difficulty changing jobs if his history is known. From Lo's perspective, psychiatrists ought to keep psychotherapy notes separately.[33] Furthermore, the World Medical Association maintains that "physicians should view with a critical eye any legal requirement to breach confidentiality and assure themselves that it is justified before adhering to it."[34]

Explorations of this dilemma with two groups of colleagues reveal differing approaches. During questions at a medical school psychiatry department grand rounds, colleagues expressed concern about the consequences of a depression diagnosis. One had a client denied health insurance when his insurance ended. Some suggested the alternative diagnosis was appropriate for confidentiality and alliance reasons. Another colleague suggested that coding insomnia and depression sequentially would appear as insomnia, the first diagnosis.

Discussion with forensic psychiatrists focused more on airing the issues within the therapy and dealing with the consequences of the diagnosis, both in and outside the relationship. They advised using and recording the depression diagnosis to avoid insurance deception; one held if the patient disagreed, terminating the therapy or referring, while another suggested paying cash. Perhaps their orientation to the intersection of medicine and law contributed to their perspectives. But what if the patient cannot afford a lengthy therapy, might not get insurance with depression recorded, or the therapist cannot offer a sliding scale?

This dilemma also reinforces the need for stronger confidentiality and anti-discrimination laws, mental health parity, and universal health coverage. As with other complex situations, there are many principles involved and it is unclear what every conscientious physician might do. Discussion within the context of the therapy is likely to lead to better solutions than any hard and fast ethical or practical prescriptions.

Richard Sobel, Ph.D.
Program in Psychiatry and the Law at Harvard Medical School

PATIENT CONFIDENTIALITY – NEUROLOGY

While at a wedding reception, a nurse overhears a neurologist, whom she knows from working at the same hospital, telling others at his table a story involving a hospitalized patient with delirium. While hospitalized, the patient had episodes of bizarre behavior and was ultimately diagnosed with neuro-syphilis. During the story-telling, the neurologist included identifying infor-mation about the patient, who is a prominent local businessman.

A Perspective from a Neurologist

Clinical Background

In this breach of confidentiality the neurologist has revealed information about a patient, information that would be embarrassing and damaging to the man's reputation, in a community where he is well known. He has been entertaining guests with an interesting clinical story by imparting medical information about a patient to a group of people who have no business knowing such information. He would regard the situation as intriguing as neurosyphilis is now rare with the advent of antibiotics and safer sex practi-ces. *Treponema pallidum*, if untreated as a primary infection, may develop into a secondary and then tertiary stage, often decades later, with meningo-vascular syphilis, general paresis or tabes dorsalis. As in this case, those with general paresis will show mental changes, usually dementia and sometimes with agitation and delirium.

Professionalism Considerations

Trust is the cornerstone of the patient–physician relationship, and a compo-nent of this trust is based in confidentiality about matters told to and learned by the physician.[35,36] The principle of trust is a core tenet of medicine and has been central in the code of ethics for medicine as far back as Hippocrates.

All health care professionals have an obligation to keep information about patients confidential. Even if the man in this case was not a prominent busi-nessman who was well known in the community, a serious violation has occurred.

Confidentiality is not an absolute and although there are legal supports for patient confidentiality there are also situations stipulated in law where harm-ful effects to others may require disclosure of specified types of information, such as reportable diseases.

While there can be debatable issues around some specific aspects of confi-dentiality, there is no debate here. The neurologist, and those listening to him (if they thought about it), would know that this was an improper breach of confidentiality. He would know that he should not reveal medical information about a patient even if he thought it was disguised (it wasn't). In addition, most of the public know they should not be hearing about a person's illness from a physician without explicit permission from the person. This is not an arguable situation – the neurologist has committed a serious error, as the patient and his family (and the ethics committee) would undoubtedly tell him if they knew.

The story calls for discussion on at least three points. First, confidentiality is a part of the sacred trust we have with patients and we must always be on guard to assure that their information and their secrets are protected. In telling an interesting medical story at a social event, the neurologist has broken this central tenet of medicine.

Second, it raises the question of what the nurse who overheard the story should do when observing a violation of confidentiality. It is difficult to confront, even gently, the neurologist in this situation, but it would stop further re-telling of the story, and undoubtedly would stop that neurologist from so easily breaking faith with patients in the future. The health care professions have been accused of not effectively policing themselves, which has resulted in increasing external surveillance of our actions. If we take seriously the responsibility of the profession to police itself, we should act appropriately when there are violations. The neurologist is wrong, but is the nurse also wrong if she just listens and does nothing further?

Third, this vignette is representative of a very common ethical breach, one the health professions must address further. Physicians and other health care professionals are intensely involved with their work and find great interest in the patients and the fascinating situations they encounter. It is tempting for them to share the interest with others. But care must be taken as many do not have a right to hear. The legal complexities of confidentiality are not so common but violations occur daily. Doctors talking about patients continue the conversation when they step into a crowded elevator. Nurses talk about patients in the cafeteria. Medical students tell their classmates about the interesting cases with revealing personal details. House staff put up lab tests and magnetic resonance images at rounds, rounds that may be transmitted to other sites around the area, with the name of the patient clearly displayed. Clinic and office staff may leave charts lying around. Sheets containing patient identifiers and medical information are improperly disposed of. The list goes on, and each person has a responsibility not only to avoid breaches of confidentiality, but to take steps to minimize the possibility, and to take corrective steps when it happens.

Opinion

Keeping medical information confidential is a cornerstone of professional practice, and we must not only be personally vigilant, but take steps when we see an infraction. The nurse who overheard should quietly speak to the neurologist. If she were reluctant, but she mentioned it to me, I would speak to the neurologist. Only by addressing these serious infractions are we going to stop a common pattern of professional misconduct.

Jock Murray, M.D., FRCP(C), MACP
Professor Emeritus
Dalhousie University, Halifax, Nova Scotia

A Perspective from a Nurse

The physician's actions in this vignette are immoral, unethical, and illegal. Respect for human dignity and confidentiality are basic ethical principles mandated in the Hippocratic Oath,[37] the *Principles of Medical Ethics*,[38] the *International Code of Medical Ethics*,[39] and the Declaration of Geneva.[40] Divulging this private information is also a violation of the privacy rule of the Health Insurance Portability and Accountability Act of 1996,[41] and could result in monetary damages at civil trial. The physician's behavior is egregiously wrong and the nurse must make a decision. This commentary focuses on the nurse's role, professional mandates, salient features, compelling forces, and the ideal response.

The nurse faces a serious problem and must decide how to respond. Ethical decision making, after all, is the responsibility of every professional. A professional code of ethics offers guidance, but the nurse may feel constrained by a social system that engenders real or perceived inequality. Nevertheless, the nurse's decision is important because of harm to the patient.

The physician's act causes present and potential future harm and offers no benefit. The physician immediately harms the patient by violating his dignity. The potential harm to this patient includes disruption of personal and business relationships and loss of income. Additionally, the physician potentially harms the health care system as a whole, since those who hear the story will distrust physicians to guard their privacy when they become patients. Finally, if no one challenges the physician, he will likely repeat this behavior in the future and thus harm other patients.

The *Code of Ethics for Nurses* (Code of Ethics) guides nurses by directing them to embrace the ideals and moral norms of the profession.[42] The Code of Ethics is based upon ethical principles, including beneficence and the idea of obligatory duties. The ethical principle of beneficence requires the nurse to act in such a way as to benefit patients and prevent harm. The Code of Ethics establishes several points related to beneficence and duty that are specifically applicable to this case. The nurse (1) has a primary duty to the patient;

(2) maintains respect for the inherent dignity of every individual; (3) is a vigilant advocate for dignified and humane care; and (4) protects the rights of the patient. Further, the Code of Ethics instructs the nurse to take specific actions to prevent or stop any unethical or illegal action by any person that jeopardizes the rights or the best interest of the patient.

Imagine the same scenario occurring in the hospital hallway within earshot of the patient's nurse. A nurse in that setting would certainly speak to the physician and likely report the case to a supervisor or administrator. Unfortunately, the Code of Ethics fails to specify in what setting the rules apply. Since this case occurs at a wedding party, many questions are unanswered by the Code of Ethics. Do ethical codes apply outside of the professional setting and role? Does the nurse have a duty to all patients or only those who are direct recipients of care? Since the infraction occurred outside of the facility, what is the appropriate chain of command? Contemporary codes of ethics answer none of these questions.

The ideal nurse would manifest character traits and virtues consistent with the values of the profession and would always act courageously and according to principle. The nurse should seek a solution that honors the patient, the physician, and the nurse. Since the physician is a moral being worthy of respect, the nurse should confidently, yet discreetly, approach the physician and broach the subject. If the physician's behavior continues despite the nurse's intervention, the nurse should later notify authorities at the physician's licensing board.

One would like to think that nurses always demonstrate moral virtue and integrity, but doing what is morally right is seldom easy. In a real-life situation most nurses would struggle with this decision. Because physicians are sometimes perceived to be more powerful than nurses, the nurse might be frightened to challenge the physician, especially in public. By approaching the physician, the nurse may worry about serious risks. The nurse may hesitate to make waves or may be concerned about loss of employment since physicians generate revenues for hospitals. The nurse may realize that some medical licensing boards reveal the names of those who file complaints. Given an atmosphere that has evolved from an historical tradition of power imbalance and gender stereotyping, it is not surprising that moral convictions might take a backseat to fear and intimidation. The nurse's eventual action will depend upon the balance between these factors and the nurse's courage, moral integrity, and awareness of professional ethics.

Compelling questions arise from the particulars of this situation: the diagnosis, the setting, and the relative social positions of nurses and physicians. But each case challenges professionals to critically examine their own moral values and search professional ethics for the best solution. Each person should courageously act in a manner that is consistent with professional and personal moral values. Like physicians, nurses must make critical judgments and take actions to protect patients, uphold professional ethics, and maintain moral integrity.

Alvita Nathaniel, Ph.D., FNP-BC, FAANP
Associate Professor
Coordinator, Nurse Practitioner Track
West Virginia University School of Nursing

SUMMARY – COMMITMENT TO PATIENT CONFIDENTIALITY

Background

Confidentiality within the physician–patient relationship has been a core ethical precept since antiquity. The Hippocratic Oath specifically discusses confidentiality as an ethical imperative:

> What I may see or hear in the course of the treatment or even outside of the treatment in regard to the life of men, which on no account one must spread abroad, I will keep to myself, holding such things shameful to be spoken about.

Much later, in the late eighteenth century, the Scottish physician John Gregory wrote his influential *Lectures upon the Duties and Qualifications of a Physician* (1772). Gregory continued to exhort physicians to protect patient confidentiality in these lectures. In 1847, the American Medical Association (AMA) established its first code of ethics. One of the core requirements was patient confidentiality. The Code stated:

> Secrecy and delicacy, when required by peculiar circumstances, should be strictly observed; and the familiar and confidential intercourse to which physicians are admitted in their professional visits, should be used with discretion, and with the most scrupulous, regard to fidelity and honor ... none of the privacies of personal and domestic life, no infirmity of disposition or flaw of character observed during professional attendance, should ever be divulged by him except when he is imperatively required to do so.[43]

The 2002 Physician Charter on Medical Professionalism, a collaborative work by several medical organizations describing the core components of medical professionalism, included the following about medical confidentiality:

> Earning the trust and confidence of patients requires that appropriate confidentiality safeguards be applied to disclosure of patient information. This commitment extends to discussions with persons acting on a patient's behalf when

obtaining the patient's own consent is not feasible. Fulfilling the commitment to confidentiality is more pressing now than ever before, given the widespread use of electronic information systems for compiling patient data and an increasing availability of genetic information.[44]

The law has looked to these ethical guidelines as a basis for imposing legal obligations of confidentiality. Common law initially established legal precedents of confidentiality. These rights were further strengthened through subsequent state and federal legislation. In addition to establishing confidentiality as a legal right, legislation has determined situations where a physician has an obligation to override confidentiality. These exceptions, as described below, generally involve instances where the public interest is better served by breaching confidentiality.

The Need for Confidentiality

Physicians and patients both depend on the need for physician–patient confidentiality. For physicians, effective treatment requires accurate information. Full, frank, and candid disclosure by the patient facilitates an accurate diagnosis and appropriate medical treatment. For patients, confidentiality is paramount. Having a trusting relationship with a physician allows the patient to feel comfortable revealing sensitive information. If confidentiality is not maintained, then patients may either withhold information or give inaccurate information, to their own detriment. Breaches in confidentiality may lead to stigmatization and even the denial of health care, housing, insurance, and employment.

Despite the clear obligation for providers to maintain patient confidentiality, a significant proportion of patients have misunderstandings about many issues surrounding the confidentiality of their medical information.[45] Further, many patients are unaware of the ethical and legal obligations of physicians to ensure confidentiality. This is particularly true of adolescents, as several studies have shown that they are generally unaware of routine confidentiality protections. This lack of awareness, in turn, leads many to either delay or avoid medical care or to change the details of their illness.[45] Of 1,295 high school students surveyed by Cheng, 68 percent had concerns about the privacy of a school health center, and 25 percent reported that they would avoid care altogether rather than risk information disclosure to parents.[46] Other studies have shown that battered women,[47] patients undergoing genetic testing,[48] and patients with HIV or who are at risk for HIV,[49,50] may decide either to not receive medical care or to alter their complaints to the physician out of concern for medical confidentiality. This is also true in patients with mental health illnesses.[51,52] In a study of seventy-six adult psychiatry patients, slightly more than half were unable to explain what medical confidentiality meant.[52] It is possible that uncertainty over confidentiality led the patient in the case and commentary discussed by Sobel and Doghramji to ask his physician to change the diagnostic coding for depression.

Protected Health Information and Breaches in Confidentiality

Protected Health Information (PHI) is the term for any identifiable health information that could be reasonably used to identify an individual. Examples of PHI may include a patient's physical examination or a past or present medical history. It may also include research records, a unique patient identification number, or records describing payment for a health care service. A breach in confidentiality is the transmission of PHI to a third party who is not directly involved in the patient's medical care or is not authorized by the patient to receive his or her health information.

Confidentiality covers not only what patients say to physicians, but also what physicians may discover independently during examination of the patient or from test results. The duty to maintain confidentiality even continues after the patient is no longer under the care of the physician. Further, the duty to maintain confidentiality continues after the patient is deceased.[53] If confidentiality were not maintained, even for the deceased, then there might be a reluctance on the part of the patient to share medical information prior to death.

Challenges to Maintaining Confidentiality and HIPAA

Even Hippocrates could not have foreseen the many challenges to maintaining confidentiality in today's medical environment. The challenges arise from not only the number of personnel accessing records, but also the methods through which records are accessed and shared. Multiple personnel with various responsibilities in the patient's care increasingly have access to medical records. In addition to treating physicians, others with access to the patients' records may include medical students, house staff, nurses, medical assistants, pharmacists, case managers, social workers, administrators, insurers, secretaries, and transcriptionists. The increasing reliance on electronic health records also adds to this challenge, as many of these providers may readily access the patient's medical history through computers at the hospital, in the outpatient setting, or at home. The temptation exists to view patient's medical charts in the electronic chart for non-medical need purposes. As Sylvester states in his commentary, a medical student may be curious about a former patient's progress and may want to follow up on a patient no longer under his or her direct care. Although such an initial impulse has merit, Sylvester and Goodman argue that phoning the family or, better yet, simply obtaining permission directly from the patient is ideal. Lastly, the improper sharing of faxes, e-mails, and shared databases may lead to further challenges in avoiding breaches of confidentiality. The challenge is that in today's online environment, it only takes a few clicks to copy and paste vast amounts of private health information into a non-secure e-mail environment.

Mindful of the ethical and legal imperatives of maintaining confidentiality, privacy experts and policy-makers voiced concern that confidentiality was not being adequately protected.[54] The increased number of providers that have access to records and the growing implementation of electronic communication and electronic records led to multiple opportunities for confidential information to be disclosed to third parties. With these concerns as a backdrop, in 2003 the U.S. government implemented federal health privacy regulations, referred to as the Health Insurance Portability and Accountability Act (HIPAA). This regulation ushered in a new era of patient privacy.[55] Under HIPAA, patients have multiple areas of privacy protection. One area of protection is to help patients better understand their medical privacy rights. All patients are given a "notice of privacy practices" by their health providers, which gives patients the right to know who will be able to see and use their records. Another area of protection is the provision which allows patients the right to choose who may view their records. Also, patients are, with rare exception, given the right to access their records, although some psychotherapy notes may be exempt, as could notes that endanger the safety of another individual.

In enacting HIPAA, Congress mandated establishing federal standards for privacy of PHI. Prior to HIPAA, medical confidentiality regulation relied on a "patchwork of Federal and State law."[56] Also, prior to HIPAA, PHI could be distributed without consent, for reasons other than health care treatment. For example, pharmacy benefits management companies could disseminate health information to marketers without the permission of patients.[57] Patients who had smoked and used nicotine replacement treatments were contacted by marketers of a newer smoking cessation drug. If companies sold this information to marketers, information on other illnesses, such as mental health illnesses and HIV were also marketable prior to the passage of HIPAA regulations.

Many have felt that HIPAA has been more a bureaucratic impediment to patient care than a true advancement in patient confidentiality.[15] This criticism of HIPAA may result from misconceptions about its specific regulations. For instance, some clinicians believed that their offices required soundproofing, many were uncertain about how to speak with patients in semiprivate hospital rooms, some believed that all PHI needed to be removed from e-mails and faxes, and others believed that obtaining records, even in emergencies, required patient authorization.[15]

The U.S. Department of Health and Human Services replies to several areas of concerns on the frequently asked questions section of their web site.[58] Fortunately, HIPAA regulations allow physicians to use their judgment regarding the patient's wishes or best interests. If, in the course of giving appropriate and reasonable care, incidental disclosure of medical information is given out, the provider is not held responsible for violating HIPAA regulations. Keeping one's voice down should suffice; rarely is there a need to avoid speaking in an area altogether or to avoid speaking to patients in semiprivate rooms. Soundproofing or other expensive modifications should not be required. A physician may consult with another physician by e-mail about a patient's condition and faxes containing PHI can be sent as long as reasonable safeguards are met. Importantly, authorization of release of medical records must not impede the release of information that is essential for medical care. Lo and others suggest that incidental disclosures are permissible in ethical medical practice if the following criteria are met: The communication should be necessary and effective for good patient care; the risks of breaching confidentiality are proportional to the likely benefits; alternatives for communication are impractical, and the communication practice is known to patients.[33] Health care providers should be aware that there are two distinct goals of HIPAA: to protect privacy and confidentiality but also to allow the flow of medical information that is essential for medical care.

Review of the Cases and Commentaries

The seven cases that illustrate patient confidentiality and their accompanying commentaries reflect different perspectives of students, physicians, and educators and help to elucidate the challenges that medical students and professionals confront in maintaining a balance between patient welfare and confidentiality. These cases describe a range of challenging situations: medical students disclosing PHI from a medical lecture to a non-medical student; a student accessing the EMR to follow up on the health status of a former patient; a family member requesting PHI about a patient from the physician without obtaining consent; a husband requesting PHI concerning his spouse for information that bears consequences on his own health but may also disclose information regarding infidelity; a request to code a different diagnosis so the patient may avoid potential stigmatization if the PHI is revealed to a third party; a patient who tells his physician that he will not disclose his blood-borne disease to his girlfriend; and finally a physician discussing PHI at a wedding reception concerning a patient with a serious neurological condition occurring as a result of a stigmatizing disease. The cases and their commentaries reflect the variety of ethical challenges in confidentiality that can arise.

Specific Medical Student Issues

Medical students have the same obligation to maintain patient confidentiality as physicians. With their first patient – the cadaver – students are taught by anatomy professors to be respectful, maintain privacy, and respect confidentiality.[59,60] No PHI should be shared with those outside class. For example, an anatomy professor described a case where a student in a local post office talked on his cell phone loudly and in detail about the recent experience of the dissection of a cadaver.[61] This was overheard by a woman whose mother had recently died and had donated her body to the anatomy lab. The woman, overhearing the conversation in a public space, was horrified. Although the woman's mother was not identified, she believed that the student should have shown more discretion in describing his experience in the cadaver lab. Whether speaking in a public space, such as the wedding reception commented on by Murray and Nathaniel in this chapter, or in a hospital hallway, students and all health care providers need to be mindful that everything reasonable is done to protect patient privacy.

Another pre-clinical encounter that gives rise to confidentiality issues occurs in lectures when PHI is discussed, or when patients themselves are invited into class. To students, it may seem innocuous to discuss a case with non-medical student friends and family. However, as Lerman and Spike write in Chapter 2, this information may be sensitive and confidential. Even when such patients are de-identified in these discussions, one must be sensitive as to what purpose it serves to share this information. Is it for educational purposes or is it simply to share an interesting clinical anecdote? As the New Jersey State Supreme Court wrote, "What policy would be served by according the physician the right to gossip about a patient's health?"[62]

As students begin their clinical work, further confidentiality issues arise and unexpected challenges may develop. First, patients may be more concerned about their confidentiality being breached by a student than by the attending physician. Such a concern may limit the information given to the student. In one British study, 40 percent of 335 surgical patients felt that students should not see their records, and 17 percent were worried that the student would discuss their case outside of surgery.[63] Another study reported patients' concern about whether the students would inappropriately share their medical history. These patients felt that this was a potential barrier when deciding whether to take part in student education.[64] Patients, however, should be reassured that students are held to the same standards as physicians to maintain confidentiality. HIPAA regulations have addressed medical student use of patient record and "permit medical trainees access to patients' medical information, including entire medical records."[58]

A second challenge students may have in the clinical setting is feeling unprepared to take appropriate action when they overhear others breaching patient confidentiality. For example, in a study examining students' attitudes towards confidentiality of computerized medical records, students were able to recognize that they had a responsibility to report a breach in confidentiality; however, many were not knowledgeable about the best course of action to take when confidentiality had been breached.[65]

A third challenge students may face in the clinical setting occurs as students try to balance their educational needs and curiosity with respect for patient confidentiality. Sylvester and Goodman (see Chapter 2) argue a view consistent with the AMA code of ethics and by HIPAA regulations – the curious student should seek the permission of the patient or patient's parent when accessing information months after being involved in the patient's care.

Exceptions to Confidentiality

Despite the expectation of confidentiality in the physician–patient relationship, confidentiality is not absolute. Physicians may have competing ethical obligations, such as a duty to warn or report. There are situations where maintaining confidentiality may lead to harm. Legally, to protect a third party, it is permissible to breach confidentiality if certain conditions apply.

Codes, professional guidelines, and the courts have recognized that there are instances when society's welfare, as well as the need to protect a third party, may require exceptions to physician–patient confidentiality.[33,44] As stated by the California Supreme Court following the Tarasoff case, "the protected privilege ends where the public peril begins."[66] In breaching confidentiality, Lo states that five elements must be in place:[33]

1. Potential harm to third parties is serious
2. Likelihood of harm is high
3. No alternative for warning or protecting those at risk
4. Breaking confidentiality will prevent harm
5. Harms to the patient are minimized and acceptable

A common clinical encounter in which breaching confidentiality may be appropriate involves the decision whether to notify the partner of a patient with an STD. As discussed earlier in the chapter in the commentaries written about the woman with vaginitis and the man with hepatitis C, the physician should make great effort to encourage the patient to disclose the infection to his or her partner. Failing that, physicians should consider whether the decision to breach confidentiality meets the five elements listed. For instance, it seems clear that in the case commentary involving the woman who had vaginosis (a form of vaginitis), it would be inappropriate to breach the patient's confidentiality and inform her spouse. However, if there was evidence of other STDs associated with "serious harm," such as HIV or hepatitis C, the physician would have an obligation to report this to her partner. The decision to breach confidentiality may seem clearer when the partner is also the physician's patient, as described in the commentaries by Alexandraki and Wolpe.

In cases where it is discovered that the patient may be experiencing elder abuse, child abuse, or domestic violence, confidentiality may be breached for the sake of the patient. States typically have a sliding scale of duty to report instances of abuse; for example, as discussed by DeJong (in Chapter 3), child abuse is a legally mandated reporting obligation, whereas elder abuse and domestic abuse are not.[67,68]

Certain medical situations could result in harm to society at large if not reported to public officials. For example, physicians must report gunshot wounds in order to serve the public interest.[69] Medical conditions that affect the ability to drive – such as seizure disorders – need to be reported to the driver's licensing authorities. A suspected occupational disease in an individual worker should be reported to local health authorities and/or a regulatory agency, such as Occupational Safety and Health Administration or the Environmental Protection Agency. In some states, laboratories are required to report abnormal findings of public health significance (for example, elevated levels of heavy metals). This reporting may be critical in protecting others in the same community, work, or home environments.[70]

Adolescent Issues

Adolescents present particular challenges with regard to confidentiality. As discussed by Veloski and Edwards, in most cases the legal right to consent to treatment resides with the adolescent's parent or legal guardian. However, in the case of an emancipated minor (one freed from control by a parent or legal guardian) or a "mature" minor, the adolescent has the right to maintain confidentiality from his/her parent or legal guardian. Most adolescents are not aware of these protections and, in turn, may avoid necessary medical care or give incomplete information.[45] Additionally, physicians need to be aware of the specific laws in their jurisdiction related to adolescent confidentiality protection.[71]

Conclusion

These cases in patient confidentiality illustrate the sometimes competing values of public health, patient autonomy, protection of third parties and confidentiality. As evidenced in the commentaries, these values may look different to the medical student, to the patient, and to the physician. In this increasingly complex world of electronic communication and record keeping, maintaining confidentiality is difficult. When confidentiality conflicts with other core values, the solutions may be challenging. Hopefully, by consulting authoritative ethics documents (e.g., codes and professional guidelines), examining the relevant literature, and seeking the input of professional colleagues, we can all better address the many ethical challenges in the area of confidentiality.

David Axelrod, M.D., J.D.
Assistant Professor of Medicine
Jefferson Medical College

Kayhan Parsi, J.D., Ph.D.
Associate Professor of Bioethics and Health Policy
Neiswanger Institute for Bioethics and Health Policy
Loyola University Chicago Stritch School of Medicine

John Spandorfer, M.D.
Associate Professor of Medicine
Jefferson Medical College

REFERENCES

1. CDC National Center for HIV, STD, and TB Prevention. National hepatitis C prevention strategy. 2006.
2. Osmond DH, Padian NS, Sheppard HW, Glass S, Shiboski SC, Reingold A. Risk factors for hepatitis C virus seropositivity in heterosexual couples. *JAMA.* 1993;**269**(3):361–365.
3. Chou R, Clark EC, Helfand M, U.S. Preventive Services Task Force. Screening for hepatitis C virus infection: A review of the evidence for the U.S. preventive services task force. *Ann Intern Med.* 2004;**140**(6):465–479.
4. De Rosa CJ, Marks G. Preventive counseling of HIV-positive men and self-disclosure of serostatus to sex partners: New opportunities for prevention. *Health Psychol.*1998;**17**(3):224–231.
5. Quill TE, Brody H. Physician recommendations and patient autonomy: Finding a balance between physician power and patient choice. *Ann Intern Med.*1996; **125**(9):763–769.

6. Snyder L, Leffler C, Ethics and Human Rights Committee, American College of Physicians.Ethics manual: 5th ed. *Ann Intern Med.* 2005;**142**(7):560–582.

7. Kipnis K. A defense of unqualified medical confidentiality. *Am J Bioeth.*2006;**6**(2): 7–18.

8. Hodge JG. The legal and ethical fiction of "pure" confidentiality. *Am J Bioeth.* 2006;**6**(2):21–2;discussion W32–4.

9. Gibson E. Medical confidentiality and protection of third party interests. *Am J Bioeth.* 2006;**6**(2):23–5; discussion W32–4.

10. Eckert LO. Clinical practice. acute vulvovaginitis. *N Engl J Med.* 2006;**355**(12): 1244–1252.

11. Sobel JD. Vaginitis. *N Engl J Med.* 1997;**337**(26):1896–1903.

12. ACOG technical bulletin. Vaginitis. no. 226, July 1996 (replaces no. 221, March 1996). Committee on Technical Bulletins of the American College of Obstetricians and Gynecologists. *Int J Gynaecol Obstet.* 1996;**54**(3):293–302.

13. Centers for Disease Control and Prevention, Workowski KA, Berman SM. *Sexually transmitted diseases treatment guidelines*, 2006. MMWR Recomm Rep. 2006;**55** (RR-11): 1–94.

14. AMA (Ethics) AMA Code of Medical Ethics. http://www.ama-assn.org/ama/pub/category/2498.html. Accessed July 11, 2008.

15. Lo B, Dornbrand L, Dubler NN. HIPAA and patient care: The role for professional judgment. *JAMA.*2005;**293**(14):1766–1771.

16. Guedj M, Sastre MT, Mullet E, Sorum PC. Do French lay people and health professionals find it acceptable to breach confidentiality to protect a patient's wife from a sexually transmitted disease? *J Med Ethics.* 2006;**32**(7):414–419.

17. Sobel JB. Trichomonas vaginitis. *UpToDate.* 2007.

18. Ford C, English A, Sigman G. Confidential health care for adolescents: Position paper for the society for adolescent medicine. *J Adolesc Health.* 2004;**35**(2):160–167.

19. Golden MP. Incorporation of quality-of-life considerations into intensive diabetes management protocols in adolescents. *Diabetes Care.* 1998;**21**(6):885–886.

20. Task Force on Community Preventive Services. Recommendations for health-care system and self-management education interventions to reduce morbidity and mortality from diabetes. *Am J Prev Med.* 2002;**22**(4 Suppl):10–14.

21. Silverstein J, Klingensmith G, Copeland K, et al. Care of children and adolescents with type 1 diabetes: A statement of the American Diabetes Association. *Diabetes Care.* 2005;**28**(1):186–212.

22. Fraser JJ, Jr , McAbee GN, American Academy of Pediatrics Committee on Medical Libility. Dealing with the parent whose judgment is impaired by alcohol or drugs: Legal and ethical considerations. *Pediatrics.* 2004;**114**(3):869–873.

23. Committee on Pediatric Emergency Medicine. Consent for emergency medical services for children and adolescents. *Pediatrics.*2003;**111**(3):703–706.

24. Henry GL. Common sense. *Ann Emerg Med.* 1991;**20**(3):319–320.

25. National Institutes of Health. National Institutes of Health state of the science conference statement on manifestations and management of chronic insomnia in adults, June 13–15, 2005. *Sleep.* 2005;**28**(9):1049–1057.

26. Ford DE, Kamerow DB. Epidemiologic study of sleep disturbances and psychiatric disorders: An opportunity for prevention? *JAMA.* 1989;**262**(11):1479–1484.

27. World Health Organization. *ICD-9: International Classification of Diseases.* Vol. 9.

28. Roeloffs C, Sherbourne C, Unutzer J, Fink A, Tang L, Wells KB. Stigma and depression among primary care patients. *Gen Hosp Psychiatry.* 2003;**25**(5): 311–315.

29. Rost K, Smith R, Matthews DB, Guise B. The deliberate misdiagnosis of major depression in primary care. *Arch Fam Med.* 1994;**3**(4):333–337.

30. Program in psychology and the law (PIPATL), amiscus brief to the U.S. Supreme Court. *Citizens for Health v. Leavitt.*

31. Schacht TE. Making psychotherapy work in primary care medicine. *Am Fam Physician.* 2006;**73**(1):34, 37.

32. Rushton JL , Felt BT, Roberts MW. Coding of pediatric behavioral and mental disorders. *Pediatrics.* 2002;**110**(1 Pt 1):e8.

33. Lo B. *Resolving Ethical Dilemmas: A Guide for Clinicians.* Philadelphia, PA: Lippincott, Williams, and Wilkins; 2005.

34. World Medical Association. *Medical Ethics Manual.* World Medical Association ; 2005.

35. Winslade WJ. Confidentiality. In: Reich WT, ed. *Encyclopedia of Bioethics.* Vol. 1. revised edition ed. New York: Simon and Schuster Macmillan; 1995:451–459.

36. American Psychiatric Association Committee on Confidentiality. Guidelines on confidentiality. *Am J Psychiatry.* 1987;**144**(11):1522–1526.

37. NOVA Online: Survivor M.D. The Hippocratic Oath–Classical Version. http://www.pbs.org/wgbh/nova/doctors/oath_classical.html. Accessed July 11, 2008.

38. AMA (Ethics) Principles of medical ethics. http://www.ama-assn.org/ama/pub/category/2512.html. Accessed July 11, 2008.

39. WMA– Policy: International Code of Medical Ethics. http://www.wma.net/e/policy/c8.htm. Accessed July 11, 2008.

40. Declaration of Geneva: Physician's Oath. http://www.cirp.org/library/ethics/geneva/. Accessed July 11, 2008.

41. HHS–Office for Civil Rights–HIPAA. http://www.hhs.gov/ocr/hipaa/. Accessed July 11, 2008.

42. Code of Ethics for Nurses. American Nurses Association Web site. http://www.nursingworld.org/ethics/code/protected_nwcoe303.htm. Updated 2001. Accessed March 11, 2007.

43. American Medical Association. Code of Medical Ethics of the American Medical Association. http://www.ama-assn.org/ama/upload/mm/369/1847code.pdf. Accessed December 20, 2008.

44. ABIM Foundation. American Board of Internal Medicine, ACP-ASIM Foundation. American College of Physicians-American Society of Internal Medicine, European Federation of Internal Medicine. Medical professionalism in the new millennium: A physician charter. *Ann Intern Med.* 2002;**136**(3):243–246.

45. Sankar P, Mora S, Merz JF, Jones NL. Patient perspectives of medical confidentiality: A review of the literature. *J Gen Intern Med.* 2003;**18**(8):659–669.

46. Cheng TL, Savageau JA, Sattler AL, DeWitt TG. Confidentiality in health care: A survey of knowledge, perceptions, and attitudes among high school students. *JAMA*. 1993;**269**(11):1404–1407.

47. Rodriguez MA, Craig AM, Mooney DR, Bauer HM. Patient attitudes about mandatory reporting of domestic violence. Implications for health care professionals. *West J Med*. 1998;**169**(6):337–341.

48. Lerman C, Narod S, Schulman K, et al. BRCA1 testing in families with hereditary breast-ovarian cancer: A prospective study of patient decision making and outcomes. *JAMA*. 1996;**275**(24):1885–1892.

49. McDonald R,Free D, Ross F, Mitchell P. Client preferences for HIV inpatient care delivery. *AIDS Care*. 1998;**10** Suppl. 2:S123–35.

50. Erwin J, Peters B. Treatment issues for HIV+ Africans in London. *Soc Sci Med*. 1999;**49**(11):1519–1528.

51. Weiner MF , Shuman DW. What patients don't tell their therapists. *Integr Psych*. 1984:28–32.

52. McGuire JM, Toal P, Blau B. The adult client's conception of confidentiality in the therapeutic relationship. *Prof Psych Res Pr*. 1985;**16**:375–384.

53. Robinson DJ, O'Neill D. Access to health care records after death: Balancing confidentiality with appropriate disclosure. *JAMA*. 2007;**297**(6):634–636.

54. Welch HG. Informed choice in cancer screening. *JAMA*. 2001;**285**(21):2776–2778.

55. Annas GJ. HIPAA regulations–a new era of medical-record privacy? *N Engl J Med*. 2003;**348**(15):1486–1490.

56. Office for Civil Rights–HIPPA. United States Department of Health and Human Services Web site. http://www.hhs.gov/ocr/hipaa/. Accessed August 9, 2008.

57. Lo B, Alpers A. Uses and abuses of prescription drug information in pharmacy benefits management programs. *JAMA*. 2000;**283**(6):801–806.

58. U.S. Department of Health and Human Services Web site. http://www.hhs.gov/hipaafaq/index.html. Accessed December 20, 2008.

59. Graham HJ. Patient confidentiality: Implications for teaching in undergraduate medical education. *Clin Anat*. 2006;**19**(5):448–455.

60. Escobar-Poni B, Poni ES. The role of gross anatomy in promoting professionalism: A neglected opportunity! *Clin Anat*. 2006;**19**(5):461–467.

61. Carmichael SW, Pawlina W. Loose lips sink ships. *Acad Med*. 2004;**79**(10):1002.

62. Shannon TA, Manfra JA. *Law and Bioethics: Texts with Commentary on Major U.S. Court Decisions*. New York: Paulist Press; 1982.

63. O'Flynn N, Spencer J, Jones R. Consent and confidentiality in teaching in general practice: Survey of patients' views on presence of students. *BMJ*. 1997;**315**(7116):1142.

64. Howe A, Anderson J. Involving patients in medical education. *BMJ*. 2003;**327**(7410):326–328.

65. Davis L, Domm JA, Konikoff MR, Miller RA. Attitudes of first-year medical students toward the confidentiality of computerized patient records. *J Am Med Inform Assoc*. 1999;**6**(1):53–60.

66. Tarasoff v. Regents of the University of California, *551 P2d 334 (Cal.* 1974).

67. Krueger P, Patterson C. Detecting and managing elder abuse: Challenges in primary care. the research subcommittee of the elder abuse and self-neglect task force of Hamilton-Wentworth. *CMAJ*. 1997;**157**(8):1095–1100.

68. Eisenstat SA, Bancroft L. Domestic violence. *N Engl J Med*. 1999;**341**(12):886–892.

69. Frampton A. Reporting of gunshot wounds by doctors in emergency departments: A duty or a right? some legal and ethical issues surrounding breaking patient confidentiality. *Emerg Med J*. 2005; **22**(2):84–86.

70. Barker LR, Burton JR, Zieve PD, eds. *Principles of Ambulatory Medicine*. 6th ed. Baltimore, MD: Lippincott, Williams, and Wilkins; 2003.

71. Diaz A, Neal WP, Nucci AT, Ludmer P, Bitterman J, Edwards S. Legal and ethical issues facing adolescent health care professionals. *Mt Sinai J Med*. 2004;**71**(3): 181–185.

8 Commitment to Improving Quality of Care

Cases and Commentaries

IMPROVING QUALITY OF CARE – ADULT PRIMARY CARE

A primary care physician who directs a large primary care clinic is notified of an insurance company audit that for the second consecutive year reports that a higher than predicted fraction of patients in that practice has cholesterol levels that are not at goal (Adult Treatment Panel III (ATP-III)). Following the audit last year, the physician notified his colleagues of these findings and spoke at a business meeting of the need to adhere to lipid-lowering recommendations. Despite the reminder given by the clinic director, the overall lipid results are slightly worse this year than last year.

A Perspective from an Internist and Quality of Care Scholar

Clinical Background

A strong body of evidence documents that elevated LDL cholesterol is a major risk factor for cardiovascular disease and that LDL-lowering interventions reduce the risk for cardiovascular disease events in both primary and secondary prevention settings. The effectiveness of cholesterol management in the prevention of cardiovascular morbidity and mortality has prompted many quality improvement efforts such as the Ambulatory Quality Alliance to develop quality measures related to cholesterol management.[1]

The ATP-III recommends measurement of fasting lipoprotein levels (total cholesterol, low density lipoprotein (LDL) cholesterol, high density lipoprotein (HDL) cholesterol, and triglycerides) every five years, beginning at age twenty years.[2] The ATP III identifies optimal lipoprotein levels as total cholesterol < 200 mg/d, LDL cholesterol < 100 mg/dL, and HDL cholesterol > 60 mg/dL. ATP-III recognizes different targets for patients with different cardiovascular risk profiles. The LDL goal is <100mg/dL for patients with existing coronary heart disease or its risk equivalent. Risk equivalent is defined as the presence of diabetes, peripheral arterial disease, abdominal aortic aneurysm, symptomatic carotid artery disease, or a Framingham risk score that indicates a ten-year risk for coronary heart disease >20 percent. The Coordinating Committee of the National Cholesterol Education Program has recommended such patients have an LDL less than 70 mg/dL.[3] For patients with two or more cardiac risk factors who do not have existing coronary heart disease or its risk equivalent, ATP III guidelines recommend target LDL levels are <130mg/dL. LDL <160 mg/dL is the recommended goal for patients with 0–1 risk factor. ATP guidelines will be updated in late 2009.

Diet, exercise, and pharmacologic therapy are the major modalities for optimization of lipoprotein levels. Clinical trials demonstrate the effectiveness of LDL-lowering interventions in reducing cardiovascular morbidity and mortality among persons with and without existing cardiovascular disease. Because clinician and patient adherence to ATP-III recommendations is necessary to approximate the benefits demonstrated in clinical trials, the ATP-III advocates the use of multidisciplinary strategies to achieve the full benefit of the recommendations at the population level.

Professionalism Concerns

Several forces compel physicians to follow authoritative clinical guidelines such as the ATP-III recommendations. Among these forces are the desirability of achieving optimal patient outcomes, the recognition that performance will increasingly determine compensation as the pay-for-performance movement gains hold, and the pride that comes from having one's clinical practice rated highly. Maintenance of high levels of quality of care is also a matter central to medical professionalism.

Recognition that quality improvement is a matter of professionalism is likely to be a particularly powerful force in motivating physicians to integrate quality improvement into their daily work. Physicians who view quality improvement as something foisted on them by external parties will no doubt be less enthusiastic participants in quality improvement efforts than those who view quality improvement as a professional duty. In 2002, the American College of Physicians-American Society of Internal Medicine, the European Federation of Internal Medicine, and the American Board of Internal Medicine developed a physicians' charter that outlines a set of principles to which medical professionals should aspire. Other codes of professional ethics such as the American Medical Association *Code of Ethics* echo many of the same elements of professionalism as the charter.[4] Consideration of these principles should guide the physician director's behavior in this scenario described.

The primacy of patient welfare is a fundamental principle of professionalism. This principle mandates that physicians dedicate themselves to serving the best interest of the patient despite market forces, societal pressures, and administrative exigencies that may try to erode this dedication. It is clearly in the best interest of patients cared for in the practice described in the vignette to have cholesterol levels consistent with ATP-III targets. Thus, physicians who behave in accordance with principle of the primacy of patient welfare are obligated to work towards achievement of ATP-III goals since doing so will optimize patient outcomes.

Among the professional responsibilities outlined in the charter on professionalism are commitments to professional competence, to scientific knowledge, to professional responsibilities, and to improving quality of care. These commitments should guide the behavior of the physician director and his colleagues in responding to their practice audits. Maintenance of professional competence and scientific knowledge involves keeping abreast of current evidence and authoritative guidelines relevant to the types of patients that a physician cares for. Consequently, the physician director and his colleagues should be knowledgeable about the ATP-III recommendations. They must also understand that a professional commitment to improving quality of care extends beyond that of maintaining personal competence. The charter on professionalism calls for physicians to take an active role in the development and implementation of quality of care measures, participate in processes for routine assessment of performance, and states that physicians are responsible for developing and implementing strategies to continuously improve the quality of care delivered by them and the organization that they work within. The vignette does not contain sufficient information to judge whether the physician director and his colleagues failed to maintain competency and currency of knowledge, but it does document a lack of commitment to the professional responsibility to improve quality of care.

A physician's primary commitment is to the welfare of his or her patients. In recent years, there is increasing recognition both within and outside of the United States that this commitment extends beyond a physician's relationships with individual patients and also encompasses active engagement of physicians in modern, systematic approaches to the assessment and improvement of health care quality.[4,5]

Opinion

The physician director's passive response to the initial audit did not honor the fundamental principles and professional responsibilities. Professionalism mandates that he take a more active response to the current audit findings. In his supervisory role, the physician director in the vignette has a professional responsibility to motivate himself and his colleagues to do the right thing for their patients. Further, his director role confers an additional responsibility of determining whether the audit accurately reflects his practice's true performance.

To behave in a professional manner worthy of the trust the public places in physicians, the director must motivate his colleagues to learn why their practice failed to meet ATP-III targets. Once they have confirmed and identified potential explanations for suboptimal performance, the physicians need to develop quality improvement interventions to address the identified reasons and implement these interventions. Among the interventions they should consider are those that the ATP-III advocates: physician and patient education, reminder systems for clinicians and patients, patient advocates, patient education about preventive care, development of standardized treatment plans, and use of feedback from past performance to foster change in future care. Implementation of such strategies would be a professional response to sequential reports of suboptimal lipid control among patients in the practice. Inertia is an unacceptable and highly unprofessional response to data that suggests suboptimal care.

Christine Laine, M.D., M.P.H.
Editor, Annals of Internal Medicine

A Perspective from a Health Services Researcher

The quality of care delivered in physicians' offices is suboptimal,[6] and the care of patients with abnormal lipid profiles is no exception.[7,8] Data from a 2005 assessment of care delivered to more than 70 million people enrolled in health plans across the United States showed that fewer than half of those patients at high risk for myocardial infarction have adequately controlled lipids.[9] This "care gap" – the underuse of statin medications – and efforts to improve the use of these medications in the treatment of lipid disorders, can illustrate the general challenge of quality improvement. The case scenario prompts several questions that this commentary will address:

- Why do care gaps exist?
- How do organizations – health plans, integrated delivery systems, practice groups, governments – try to change physicians' practice to reduce care gaps?
- Which strategies are effective at changing physicians' behavior?
- Does audit and group-level feedback, as described in the case scenario, change behavior and improve the quality of health care?

Care Gaps

The care gaps in the management of lipids arise from numerous barriers to optimal practice at the level of the system, the patient, and the physician. At the system level, poor access to care (e.g., inadequate physician supply) and lack of insurance coverage keep many patients from receiving adequate treatment. Patient-level barriers include the patients' general predisposition toward treating symptoms over preventing disease. It is much easier for a patient to accept a short-term course of antibiotics to treat a painful sore throat than to commit to a lifelong regimen of lipid-lowering therapy to lower the chances of having a heart attack or stroke that may be years or even decades in the future. Barriers that prevent physicians from adhering to guidelines for best practice include lack of time in routine office visits, lack of information or knowledge (i.e., many physicians are not aware of current recommended guidelines), forgetfulness, and a phenomenon called clinical inertia (i.e., the perceived high "activation energy" required to make a change from the status quo).

Changing Physician Behavior

For more than three decades, researchers and health care administrators have implemented and evaluated the effectiveness of a variety of interventions to improve how clinicians prescribe medications. While passive interventions, such as lectures and mailed information describing clinical guidelines, do not generally improve practice, there are other interventions that have strong evidence for being able to improve how physicians prescribe medications. These effective interventions include audit and feedback with comparison to local peers, real-time clinical reminders, educational outreach (also called academic detailing), local opinion leaders, and computerized physician order entry.[10] Brief descriptions of each of these approaches may be useful for identifying common characteristics that lead to successful changes in physician behavior.

Audit and feedback involves the assessment of how physicians have been practicing (the audit) and then the presentation of that information to the physicians (the feedback).[11] Audit and feedback seems most effective when it is personalized and presented in the context of peer performance; that is, when an individual physician can benchmark his or her performance against peers and gauge the degree of change necessary to reach identified goals. In the case scenario provided, the audit appeared to be performed at the practice level, and there was no indication that each of the physicians in the practice could see how their panel of patients fared in comparison to his peers' panels. This type of high-level audit without peer-comparison feedback is not likely to change behavior.

One of most consistently successful interventions for improving physicians' prescribing practice involves educational outreach, popularly called "academic detailing."[12] This strategy uses many of the same techniques and strategies that are employed by "detail" representatives from the pharmaceutical industry in their efforts to influence how clinicians prescribe their medications. Drawing on adult learning theory and social marketing principles, academic detailing consists of delivering a concise, evidence-based message to physicians with professionally illustrated and simple educational materials from a credible organization, through a face-to-face visit, typically one-on-one but sometimes in small groups. Several states in the United States and provinces in Canada have adopted academic detailing programs, as have a variety of countries, such as Australia. In the case scenario, the business meeting seemed to provide an opportunity for dialogue between the physician-practice director and his colleagues, but this type of interaction lacks the depth of exchange to explore barriers to and facilitators of behavior change that would characterize academic detailing.

Many studies have demonstrated that opinion leaders can change physician practice.[13] Opinion leaders are educationally influential local experts whose practice is emulated by their peers. Physicians in practice seem to rely on peer opinion leaders to guide policy and practice decisions. Not all organizational leaders are recognized by physicians as opinion leaders. In the case scenario, it is uncertain whether the physicians in the practice perceive their director-colleague as an opinion leader and whether they will emulate his practice and respond to his encouragement.

Health information technology (HIT) interventions,[14] such as computerized order entry with clinical decision support, can change the way physicians order medications, but this type of intervention is not a panacea. While clearly effective in reducing the use of medications that may be inappropriate or risky, alerts and reminders in the electronic health record and computerized order entry systems have been less impressive at improving the use of medications in chronic disease management and in increasing the use of preventive services for healthy populations. As HIT interventions continue to improve and expand to wider segments of physician practices, further study will be needed to assess their effectiveness. Some of these technologies might be useful for the practice described in the scenario, but the adoption and expansion of HIT is an expensive and long-term proposition.

Summary

When multiple stakeholders – patients, physicians, and insurance companies – share the common goal of improving quality of care, a variety of opportunities exist to address the barriers to overcoming care gaps. Addressing barriers at the level of the system, the patient, and the physician can have incremental and synergistic effects. Physicians need to recognize the potential for audit and feedback to improve their practice and should feel empowered to participate in efforts to improve the care of their patients.

Steven R. Simon, M.D., M.P.H.
Associate Professor, Department of Ambulatory Care and Prevention
Harvard Medical School and Harvard Pilgrim Health Care

IMPROVING QUALITY OF CARE – GASTROENTEROLOGY

A gastroenterologist has had three patients in the past year who have had colonic perforations following colonoscopy, a complication rate higher than expected. The chairman of medicine is notified of this after the third perforation.

A Perspective from a Chairman of Medicine

Clinical Background

All medical procedures are associated with risk. However, studies over the past decade have led to an understanding of mechanisms that can be utilized to mitigate the risk of many procedures. This new information has often – but not universally – been utilized by professional societies and hospitals to decrease procedural risks. For example, studies have clearly documented that the risk of any procedure is reduced when the operator has the appropriate level of training, performs at least the minimum number of recommended procedures each year, obtains advanced training before performing new procedures and receives follow-up training and maintenance of certification during his or her career. Indeed, these criteria have been used for both credentialing and re-credentialing at many – though not all – hospitals and practices. The availability of appropriate levels of support from both staff and professional colleagues also increases patient safety. In addition, regularly scheduled morbidity and mortality conferences to adjudicate issues involved in adverse events as well as ongoing review of each operator's individual adverse event profile provides important documentation that can be utilized to assess the "quality" of any given interventional program.

Professionalism Considerations

Despite numerous safeguards that are put into place, procedural complications still occur. Deciding whether these complications are consistent with the risk of the procedure or are related to an individual physician's skill level becomes one of the most difficult management issues for medical leaders and often challenges the tenets of medical professionalism.

The difficulty in adjudicating a series of adverse events involving any single physician or group of physicians is that these events can be caused by a system error, a group of patients with severe disease and high risk for an adverse event who just happened to be grouped together temporally, or by poor technical performance on the part of the physician. Technical issues arise in all of the procedural arenas – but most commonly in gastroenterology and cardiology. Any report of adverse events should result in a thorough review of each case and root cause analysis should be performed in order to ascertain whether a system error could have been responsible for the unexpected numbers of adverse events. For example, some years ago we recognized in our monthly morbidity and mortality conference that the number of retroperitoneal bleeds after femoral artery puncture during cardiac catheterization had increased at an alarming rate. On careful review, we found that the increase in adverse events was not due to any single physician but rather to a change in the procedure by which the nursing staff transferred the patient from the catheterization table to the gurney prior to transport back to the room. When we reinstituted "passive" transport rather than "active" transport, the number of bleeds returned to better than expected levels.

In addition, a group of adverse events should be reviewed in the context of the operator's overall experience. For example, three colonic perforations over a period of one year might be significant if the operator performed 100 procedures – but might not be significant if that same operator performed 3,000 procedures. Finally, if it is determined that the adverse events were not "system" problems and were not a statistical aberrancy, the physician should be proctored by one or more colleagues who have the level of experience to assess his or her quality of performance before making any decisions. These proctors should provide a written assessment of the physician's skill level and make recommendations regarding potential mechanisms to remediate any skill-set deficiencies that are identified by the proctors. In many if not most cases, these measures allow the physician to return to all professional activities consistent with his or her training.

Unfortunately, it is sometimes recognized that an individual physician cannot be successfully retrained, that the physician lacks the requisite skills, or is "impaired," thus requiring discontinuation of select privileges, for example, performance of a colonoscopy. It is this situation that is one of the largest professional challenges that confronts a chair or a division chief. While virtually all medical schools have some form of a "grievance" committee that ensures that quality of care assessments are fair and equitable and provides the individual physician with due process, in many cases the physician does not utilize this pathway but rather seeks legal help resulting in a lawsuit against the university, the hospital and the chair for breach of contract or restraint of trade. It is when quality issues are adjudicated in legal offices or in the courtroom that the system of medical professionalism breaks down. For example, it becomes difficult in a court of law to explain to a jury why an individual gastroenterologist who has passed his or her boards doesn't have the requisite skills to perform a colonoscopy. In addition, the plaintiff's attorneys often point to the fact that a group of physicians may be anxious to "unload" one of their physicians if their volumes or reimbursements have decreased and therefore they would like to have fewer mouths to feed. These issues can become even more politically charged and confrontational if the aggrieved physician is a member of the voluntary staff of the hospital and not a member of the full-time academic faculty. Here again the argument is often made that the chair has focused on a physician who is a "competitor." Quality reviews also become more complex if errors are found to be the result of the participation of physicians from other departments (eg., perhaps the anesthesiologist did not adequately sedate the patient) as horizontal accountability across the various departmental silos is often lacking in academic medical centers. Thus, to avoid lengthy legal due diligence and the unpredictability of juries in some locales, universities and hospitals often agree to confidential legal and financial settlements, with the physician's resignation from the institution. However, substantive ethical issues arise when the litigation also provides for a "neutral" letter of recommendation. This allows the physician to practice the same interventional procedures elsewhere.

Opinion

In the face of the challenge of dealing with the possibility that a physician is doing harm as a result of a skill level that is less than optimum, the chair or division chief must keep in mind the tenets of medical professionalism. To this end, the chair should obtain the best possible due diligence and wherever possible this adjudication should come through the auspices of structured morbidity-mortality conferences. In cases in which adverse events are due to possible professional issues involving physicians of another department, the chair should expeditiously inform the appropriate individuals to ensure that peer review occurs in an interdisciplinary fashion. Because it is difficult (if not impossible) to adjudicate adverse events in a procedural area, the chair should take every opportunity to utilize "proctors." Indeed, all new faculty members should be proctored before performing procedures independently to ensure that their skill level is appropriate. When a clear determination is made that a given individual does not have the skill level required to perform a specific procedure, the department and the institution should have no reservations in limiting or removing that individual's responsibilities. Finally, the ability of chairs to ensure the safety of patients will require changes in plaintiff's laws including the creation of physician oversight boards that can ensure that the pragmatism of the legal environment does not obviate the ability to deal appropriately with quality of care issues.

Arthur Feldman, M.D.
Magee Professor and Chairman Department of Medicine
Jefferson Medical College

A Perspective from a Lawyer

Lawyers play two roles. One is as a counselor to the client. The second role is as an advocate for the client. As a counselor, the lawyer gives private, personal, disinterested advice to the client. As an advocate, the lawyer vigorously represents the client's best interest in dealing with others. In order to play either role the lawyer needs to be familiar with all the facts that can be acquired and to know how the client views those facts and how others view those facts.

Each of the five possible lawyers (one for each of the three patients with a colonic puncture, one for the chair of medicine and one for the gastroenterologist) will be told and will read slightly different facts and will come to the client with a different background of experience. Each, as counselor, will give his or her client similar, but far from identical, advice. Each, as counselor, will give the client balanced advice on the strengths and risks of the client's situation. Each, as advocate, will unambiguously assert the certain correctness of the client's position.

How can a lawyer simultaneously view the facts as forming two differing pictures? Perhaps Picasso can explain: In two months in 1967 Picasso painted forty-four different "copies" of Velazquez' painting *Las Meninas*. The forty-five paintings (Picasso's forty-four, and the one by Velazquez) are all of the same room containing the same people and objects (in other words, they are paintings of the same facts) but each picture is different. What changes is the aesthetic representation. Picasso once referred to it as "the dramatic effort from one vision to another," and said "If I search for truth in my canvas, I can make a hundred canvases with this truth."[15]

Similarly each of the five lawyers, as his or her client's counselor, will give the client a disinterested presentation, alerting the client to the risks while advocating the client's best position so that the client understands the dangers but believes that the advocate can forcefully argue his or her case. As an advocate to the other parties, the lawyer can take "the truth" (the facts) and paint a verbal picture which most effectively asserts the client's best interest.

The lawyer for the chair of medicine may have the most complex task. These include the following decisions: (1) What position will the chair take about the quality of care provided by the gastroenterologist? (2) Should disciplinary action be taken, and if so what is the proper procedure? (3) What is the likelihood of a suit by the gastroenterologist against the chair and the institution if disciplinary action is taken? (4) What reports must be filed with governmental agencies and insurers? and (5) What position should be taken before the medical licensure board? As counselor, the chair's lawyer will also point out that any injured patient's lawyer who sues will look for as many defendants as possible and advise the chair how to prepare for this. As advocate, the chair's lawyer must assert each position of the chair vigorously and effectively, first in negotiations and later, possibly, at trial.

The lawyer for the gastroenterologist may advocate to the lawyer for an injured patient that the patient has no claim because there clearly was no negligence while, as counselor, privately warn the client gastroenterologist that the evidence is not as clear as the lawyer wished. As counselor, he will prepare the gastroenterologist for a settlement. As advocate, the gastroenterologist's attorney will negotiate for the physician's economic and reputational interest if there is an effort to limit the physician's privileges.

The lawyer for an injured patient has an unambiguous job – to obtain damages for the injured client. But each lawyer will paint at least two pictures, one as a counselor for his or her client and at least one as an advocate to assert his or her client's interest. These different pictures will resolve into a single final "official" picture at the conclusion of negotiations or litigation. Almost certainly, this final "official" picture will be, like the work of a committee, unsatisfactory to everyone.

One may wonder whether we must have such an expensive, time-consuming process for compensating some patients for injuries incurred in delivering health care, while leaving others with similar injuries uncompensated. The answer is no. Compensation could be provided through something like the workers' compensation system. Through this arrangement an injured worker gets a fixed amount based on the injury ($X for a lost thumb, $Y for a blind eye) without regard to fault. But our medical malpractice system, which provides compensation only if the delivery of health care was found to have been negligent, is too entrenched by, among other things, history, the constitutional right to trial by jury, and the financial interest of plaintiff and defense lawyers. The believers in our present system argue that only with the threat of substantial damage awards for negligence can the pressure on physicians be kept up to cause them to maintain and improve the quality of care.

Peter Mattoon, Esq.
Ballard, Spahr Andrews & Ingersoll, LLP, Philadelphia, PA

IMPROVING QUALITY OF CARE – ENDOCRINOLOGY

An endocrinologist completed his internal medicine residency training thir-
teen years ago and endocrinology fellowship training eleven years ago. Follow-
ing the completion of each of these training periods, he passed the specialty
board examinations. He now has a busy community endocrine practice and
has not taken examinations to maintain his board certification. Three years
ago, he received notification from the American Board of Internal Medicine
(ABIM) that his board certification expired and that he is no longer "board
certified" in internal medicine. Last year, he received notice from the ABIM that
he is no longer "board certified" in endocrinology. Since he is busy and can
practice endocrinology without maintaining his certification, he currently has
no plans to take the examination in either of these specialties.

A Perspective from the President of the American Board of Internal Medicine

Background

This case highlights the new reality of the profession raising standards for
board certification to include the periodic maintenance of certification. In
2002, all twenty-four recognized allopathic specialty boards of the American
Board of Medical Specialties (ABMS) agreed to time-limited certification,
thus requiring those specialists who represent 87 percent of physicians in
the United States to recertify on a regular basis. The osteopathic boards are
headed in the same direction. The concept is called "Maintenance of Certification" rather than "recertification" because it is intended that this become
not an iterative process – focusing solely on an exam of knowledge every
seven to ten years – but instead an ongoing process of self-assessment of
knowledge as well as of performance in practice punctuated by periodic
exams to ensure an up-to-date knowledge base.

In the environment of growing expectations for accountability to consumers and patients, as well as payers and purchasers of health care, it became
clear that lifetime certification was not a meaningful credential. If specialty
certifying boards had not taken this important step, it is quite likely that other
regulatory entities would have evolved to take their place. It is important for
the profession that these regulations be professionally based and generated
by peers with a similar specialty practice. The context for these changes has
been made clear over the last decade by the tremendous impact of the Institute of Medicine reports, most notably *Crossing the Quality Chasm*[16] and
the more than a dozen subsequent reports in that series which focused on the

tremendous gaps in quality of care in the United States and the need to apply efforts from multiple stakeholders to improve that care.

From the perspective of the physician, there are now ample data that a physician's knowledge and performance – in both diagnostic and treatment capacities – declines over the course of a career.[17] While this is obviously not true for every physician, it is overwhelmingly true in a meta-analysis of all systematically reviewed literature. Medical science is advancing rapidly, and research has shown that even when evidence-based clinical guidelines are endorsed by specialty societies there can be a gap of fifteen to twenty years before they are widely adopted.[18] It is safe to say that that is simply too long to wait for evidence-based practice, especially in a world where rising health care costs are creating increasing demands for efficiency, thus also demands to limit unnecessary utilization and to focus on the most effective and evidence-based approaches.

Professionalism Considerations

The Physician Charter on Medical Professionalism states ten important commitments for the profession.[19] One central commitment is quality of care. In order to meet this expectation, physicians have two kinds of responsibilities. One is to ensure their own quality of care, and modern quality science shows us that this includes not only studying and staying up to date, but also measuring the quality of care one provides. An adage of quality science is that you can't improve what you don't measure. Indeed, ABIM's experience has been that in the first five years of required Maintenance of Certification, thousands of physicians who have completed practice improvement modules or other clinical assessment of their practice have discovered areas of improvement that they would not have known about had they not done these Internet-based practice evaluations. Measurement does lead to improvement,[20] so the board requires that diplomates consider and submit plans for improvement as part of Maintenance of Certification. The second major responsibility in professionalism is transparency and to make clear to the public meaningful information about quality of care. While there are many ways in which individual disease-specific data can be misinterpreted, the comprehensive assessment that board certification represents is probably the best and clearest public evidence of a physician's commitment to quality.

This physician has decided that he can practice endocrinology without maintaining his certification because he is too busy to do so. He may find that there is a growing expectation that physicians, particularly specialists, be board certified. Health plans and hospitals are increasing their scrutiny of physician credentials and looking for evidence that physicians are practicing according to high standards. Specialty board certification is the most widely accepted credential, and the only one that indicates a comprehensive approach to that accountability expectation. So, while he may not find a problem in his current practice environment, over time this may become a problem for him. He may also miss opportunities to improve. Most recently, Medicare legislation establishing a new and innovative approach to generalist practice, the Patient-Centered Medical Home, has stipulated that physicians must be board certified. Even someone who is initially certified and lets their certification lapse can no longer claim to be a board-certified physician, and publicly available information on the American Board of Internal Medicine (ABIM) and ABMS web sites makes clear to the public that the physician is no longer board certified.

It is unfortunate that this physician feels he doesn't have time to prepare for Maintenance of Certification. The ABIM has invested significant resources in developing tools that allow physicians to receive continuing medical education credits for CME work they do in conjunction with their societies, and to use quality of care data that they may get from their group practice or health plan in order to get credit for the practice assessment component of Maintenance of Certification. Furthermore, while initial pass rates on specialty exams are in the 80 percent range, physicians who are not successful the first time in taking the exam have a very good chance at success if they invest in a modest course of study and retake the exam. The ultimate pass rate is 95 percent. Physicians are voting with their feet in favor of the Maintenance of Certification process. Between 85 and 87 percent of physicians in all of the subspecialties of internal medicine recertify in their subspecialties. Especially remarkable from the perspective of professionalism, 60 percent recertify in general internal medicine, the underlying certificate, even though they are not required by the ABIM to do so. This suggests that those physicians who know that they see a broad range of patients in their practice want to also keep up to date with general internal medicine as well as with their subspecialty area.

The Joint Commission now requires hospitals to demonstrate that physicians who have privileges on their medical staffs are competent in the six core competencies stipulated by the Accreditation Council for Graduate Medical Education (ACGME) and on which Maintenance of ABMS Board Certification is based. These competencies include patient care, medical knowledge, professionalism, communication and interpersonal skills, systems-based practice, and practice-based learning and improvement. Most hospitals are not equipped to truly evaluate all of these competencies, and yet those are the competencies that form the framework for Maintenance of Certification. Thus, the Joint Commission standards will likely lead more and more hospitals to scrutinize physicians' board certification status.

Opinion

In addition to being the right thing to do, Maintenance of Certification – as a way of maintaining one's professional standing – is an efficient and effective way of assuring oneself as well as one's peers and patients of quality of care. It is also efficient because it is widely recognized and because the certifying boards share the goal of reducing the burden of redundant measures and have made possible links with multiple other stakeholder interests seeking quality measures from physicians. Evidence of the meaningfulness of Maintenance of Certification can be gained by testimonials from individuals who are not required to recertify by virtue of having certified before time-limited certification went into place (1989 for geriatric medicine and critical care medicine and 1990 for all other certificates). Richard Baron, a practicing general internist in Philadelphia, and Troy Brennan, at the time an academic physician at the Brigham and Women's Hospital and currently the chief medical officer at Aetna, wrote compellingly of their experience as physicians who were not required to recertify but did so voluntarily.[21,22] Both found it challenging but meaningful, clinically relevant and useful in their practice.

Christine K. Cassel, M.D.
President and CEO
American Board of Internal Medicine and ABIM Foundation

A Perspective from an Internist and Medical Historian

Many factors have contributed to the rise and growth of medical specialization, but at the core of the specialization phenomenon is the relentless growth of medical knowledge and technology. Medical knowledge has simply grown too vast for any one individual to know it all. To achieve a sense of mastery, physicians have long been forced to focus on smaller and smaller areas of practice.[23,24]

Medical specialization first appeared in the United States and other Western countries in the mid-nineteenth century. Ophthalmology was the first field to be recognized as a specialty. By the end of the century, surgery, internal medicine, obstetrics and gynecology, pediatrics, neurology and psychiatry, otolaryngology, pathology, and other fields had also become recognized as specialties. In the United States, specialty boards in fourteen fields were established in the 1930s. After World War II, as the relentless expansion of knowledge and technology continued, additional specialty fields were created, and numerous "subspecialties" became recognized as well.

How should a specialist be trained? In the early twentieth century, a multiplicity of paths to specialty practice could be found. The most common route was through courses at one of the thirty or so unsupervised graduate medical schools, where educational standards were low and a commercial spirit prevailed. After a few weeks of study, graduates of such programs would proclaim themselves "specialists," even though they had barely scratched the surface of their subject.

Fortunately, in the late nineteenth century another model for specialty training appeared: the residency. The residency was introduced into American medicine at Johns Hopkins in 1889. After World War I, residency programs spread to other teaching hospitals, much as the Hopkins system of undergraduate medical education had spread to other schools the generation before. The residency was defined as "a progressive and graduated educational experience designed to enable a physician to make himself proficient in a special field of practice and to give him the educational background for continued development in this field."[25] By World War II, residency training, followed by specialty certification, had become the sole route to specialization in the United States. After World War II, the principles of residency were extended to fellowship training in the many subspecialties as well. The emergence of this system reflected the belief of medical educators that the public needed to be protected from superficial training and commercialism in specialty education, just as earlier medical educators felt that the public required similar protection in undergraduate medical education.

All doctors, whether specialists or not, have the professional obligation to stay up-to-date throughout their careers in practice. To help physicians do so, medical education has always attempted to produce doctors who are critical thinkers and problem-solvers, equipped with the discipline and mental tools to study, reflect, and remain current as long as they are practicing.[26] In this traditional system, responsibility for remaining up to date resides with the individual physician, who acts on the honor system.

This model began to weaken in the 1980s. The continued explosion of medical knowledge made it more difficult for physicians to stay current. Continuing medical education courses were not seen as particularly effective educational aids, especially as pharmaceutical companies began to take more and more responsibility for their content.[27,28] The discovery of large geographical variations in the incidence of certain medical practices without any discernible difference in outcomes did much to challenge the authority of physicians. So did a growing consumer movement in American society and calls for greater transparency in medical practice. In 1988, the editor of the *New England Journal of Medicine* proclaimed that a new era of assessment and accountability had arrived in medicine.[29] Time-limited specialty certification is one outgrowth of these events.

What is new in today's system of specialty recertification is the greater public transparency that is provided. The underlying objective of remaining up to date is itself hardly new. In this context, recertification can be seen as a continuation of medical education's traditional goals: elevating the level of practice of all certified specialists, lessening the gap between what is scientifically known and what is done in day-to-day practice, and promoting public confidence in the abilities of all certified specialists.

The case study provides no information on whether the physician has remained up to date, only that he has failed to take the recertification examination. It is possible that through reading, conferences, meetings, rounds, and other devices the doctor has stayed on top of his field, even without recertification. The problem this physician faces is that with society now demanding greater transparency and accountability, the public is less inclined than in earlier eras to take his word that he has kept up at face value.

Kenneth M. Ludmerer, M.D.
Professor of Medicine
Washington University in St. Louis School of Medicine

IMPROVING QUALITY OF CARE – HOSPITAL MEDICINE

A fifty-six-year-old man, following an elective cerebral aneurysmal clipping, developed several hospital complications. These complications included a refractory seizure disorder, nosocomial pneumonia, drug-induced hepatotoxicity, and deep venous thrombosis. During the nine week hospitalization, the patient and family became frustrated with the fragmented care in the hospital. Specifically, they complained of a lack of communication among the physicians as one hospitalist covered for another, and a lack of communication among the hospital doctors and the patient's outpatient doctors. They felt this lack of communication led to lapses in the quality of care.

A Perspective from an Internist and Hospitalist

Professionalism Considerations[30–32]

The complexity of caring for inpatients, even those outside the intensive care units, has risen steadily over the past ten to fifteen years. In addition to the higher "average acuity of illness," physicians must also deal with an increased need for subspecialty consultation, rapidly changing technology and an ever-changing armamentarium of medical treatments. Decrements in the average length of stay mean that more tests are being performed, and more consultants are being called in an ever-shorter period of time. Finally, the arrival of hospitalists has brought about the departure of primary care physicians from the hospital. Thus, upon admission, a "familiar face" – like this patient's outpatient physician has, for many patients, been replaced with that of a complete stranger.

In light of these developments, it is no surprise that patients in the hospital lack confidence in their physicians and the health care team because they feel that their care is fragmented, incomplete, or illogical. In many cases the patient's perception is, at least to some extent, accurate. However, even in those cases where the "behind the scenes" work is coordinated, well reasoned and based on good communication among physicians, the patient may experience substantial anxiety unless he or she is kept informed and given the chance to ask questions and have them answered.

Before outlining ideas about how to minimize the likelihood of miscommunication (or perceived lack of care coordination), it is worth acknowledging the magnitude of the tasks facing doctors who serve as the "physician of record" for inpatients. Whether she or he is a hospitalist, intensivist, or a neurosurgeon, the physician of record in the hospital is expected to be the "quarterback" or "field commander" in what is often a highly complicated situation. In a given day, this doctor will likely receive information from as many as four to six different sources, few of which have any direct contact with one another. For example, on a typical day, the care of a single patient, such as the one in this vignette, might require that the primary physician consult a subspecialist, review the report of an EEG, ask a radiologist for the interpretation of an X-ray, discuss medication selection and dosing with a pharmacist, speak to a physical therapist, and touch base with a discharge planning social worker. With that background, I will discuss two possible scenarios: perceived lack of care coordination and true lack of care coordination. It is not uncommon for these to coexist.

Perceived Lack of Care Coordination

As an example of perceived lack of care coordination, consider a case of a patient with atrial fibrillation whose warfarin is held postoperatively by a surgeon. The surgeon elects to delay the resumption of anticoagulation therapy postoperatively after a discussion with the cardiologist reveals that the immediate risk of thromboembolism is substantially lower than the risk of serious postoperative bleeding. Unfortunately, neither the surgeon nor the cardiologist explains this decision to the patient. Thus the patient is left wondering whether his warfarin dose (which he's been repeatedly counseled not to forget by his outpatient physician) has been omitted inadvertently. Relaying this information to the patient and his family is a critical task for the primary physician or team in charge of this patient's care. A similar perceived lack of care coordination may have occurred with the patient in the vignette; the seizure disorder, pneumonia, drug-related hepatoxicity and deep venous thrombosis may have been treated appropriately, but the communication between the providers and family was suboptimal, and the perception was that the care was lacking.

Actual Lack of Care Coordination

Another anticoagulation case to consider might be a true breakdown of inter-physician communication. A patient is admitted with acute myocardial infarction and upper gastrointestinal (GI) hemorrhage (evidenced by coffee-ground emesis). The patient is seen by both gastroenterology and cardiology consultants. Each subspecialist documents in the chart that the procedures or treatments (endoscopy, heparin, beta blockade) they would normally recommend are contraindicated. Indeed, the conscious sedation needed to perform esophagogastroduodenoscopy (EGD) is associated with some increased risk among patients who have recently suffered a heart attack. Similarly, clinicians would like to avoid administering heparin or beta-blockers to a patient who may be at risk for ongoing GI bleeding.

On the other hand, there are certainly risks associated with withholding an EGD and pharmacologic treatments such as heparin. Unless the subspecialists communicate with one another, the individual risks and benefits of each of these interventions cannot be weighed against one another. Ensuring that this communication takes place, and that the strategy with the most favorable risk–benefit ratio is chosen, is the job of the primary physician or team assigned to care for this patient.

During the past ten years, we have seen a significant increase in the number of "hand-offs" associated with inpatient care. Within academic medical centers, house staff work hours have been limited, and residents/interns are "cross-covering" for one another more than ever. Within the private hospitals, it is not uncommon for three or four different hospitalists to take over and relinquish the care of a single inpatient during a five- or six-day hospitalization. Each time a patient's care is transferred from one provider to another, the potential for medical error increases and the perception by the patient and family that the care is disjointed intensifies. The Society of Hospital Medicine has produced guidelines which emphasize the importance of a dialogue between providers when a patient's care is transferred.[33]

Finally, patients and their families may experience significant distress when different clinicians impart contradictory information to them. For example, a nephrologist might advise a patient with advanced liver disease and worsening renal function to consider hemodialysis, whereas the gastroenterologist and primary team have proposed that the patient pursue hospice care. It is likely that the patient and family in this vignette, at some point in his prolonged hospitalization, received contradictory recommendations, which led to further frustration about the care. The importance of delivering a consistent and accurate message (that reflects input from all clinicians involved in the patient's care) cannot be overstated.

Opinion

If providers take the time to communicate with one another and ensure that their consensus decisions are relayed, in a timely fashion, to patients and their families, then the perception of fragmented care (and perceived fragmented care) will be greatly reduced.

David Garcia, M.D.
Associate Professor of Medicine
University of New Mexico School of Medicine

A Perspective from a Spouse

The series of cascading complications following this elective surgery was devastating for the family and, most likely in a different way, for the medical team itself. As the patient's wife, I often felt that the physicians were as confused and disappointed in the sequelae to the surgery as we were. Since my husband was not able to communicate with the medical team, it became my responsibility to fill this gap. It seemed that this series of not-quite-explained events led the medical team to avoid contact and dialogue with me. This was the one crucial response that might have made everything else more bearable.

My husband was transferred from one service to another and then from an attending we knew to one that we had never met. We did not know that this was a routine process in inpatient care as patient needs change. There was no communication from the staff about the "transfer" – a crucial step missed since my husband could not communicate with us in any way. In our eyes, his care became fragmented.

Some of the lapses in communication may have been the result of personal style. For example, when I asked to meet the physician who had taken over my husband's care, he expressed some surprise that I actually wanted a face-to-face meeting with him. Other lapses were much more than style. I initially refused to consent to a shunt because the intern assigned to get consent could not tell me why it was to be done. This did not inspire confidence. It was only after a plea to the nurses that a more senior resident came to speak to me about the indications for this invasive procedure.

Fragmentation of communication escalated to chaos as discharge planning began. New medical professionals who seemed to know little about my husband and his hospital course were brought in. When the social worker arrived to do discharge planning, he was acutely psychotic. The fact that this was an acute change in his status was not apparent. Rather than evaluate the cause of this acute change, the new psychiatry resident ordered a guard and restraints. Based on this evaluation, the discharge plan was that my husband needed to be transferred to a nursing home and that he would need round-the-clock care. After I demanded a full psychiatric assessment, it was determined that his mental status was caused by medication side effects. The psychosis resolved and he was discharged directly to a rehabilitation facility.

When it became obvious that there were serious issues with communication as well as further medical complications, my husband's cardiologist stepped in and became the go-between for the patient and the medical team. He also spoke to the medical team on our behalf, and took responsibility for communicating with us on a regular basis.

This case was extremely complicated and most of the severe and life-threatening complications were unexpected and often unexplained. This caused major stress for everyone, the medical team as well as the family members. How could a family without financial, social, and intellectual resources cope with these circumstances? A medical team leader, one individual who is responsible for coordinating decisions and communicating information, was absent in this case. This resulted in unnecessary angst, delays in diagnosis and treatment, and inefficient care.

It may have seemed more expeditious to proceed without taking time to meet with family members. In the long run, with a critically ill patient with altered mental status, this was not the case. A brief update each day when our concerns could be heard and our questions answered would have not only been greatly appreciated, it would have benefited my husband's care and expedited the work of the medical team. Family members need to identify the spokesperson for the family and the physicians must also identify the spokesperson for the medical team. Many of the medical problems of very sick patients in the hospital are unavoidable. Problems such as poor communication and fragmented care can and should be solved.

Karen M. Glaser, Ph.D.
Associate Dean for Academic Affairs
Jefferson Medical College

IMPROVING QUALITY OF CARE – OBSTETRICS-GYNECOLOGY

A fifty-nine-year-old woman has had uterine bleeding over the past three months, nine years after menopause. A pelvic ultrasound shows a thickened uterine wall. Her gynecologist thereafter recommended an endometrial biopsy and performed the procedure using Pipelle sampling in the office. The gynecologist then asked the patient to return in one week for a review of the biopsy result. Because the physician's schedule was busy, the patient was unable to schedule the visit sooner than eighteen days after the biopsy. Ten days after the biopsy, the patient called the office to obtain the result. Although the receptionist gave the message to the physician, the patient did not receive a return phone call and has to wait for the scheduled follow-up visit to receive her results.

A Perspective from an Obstetrician-Gynecologist

Clinical Background

Postmenopausal bleeding is a common gynecologic issue, occurring in an estimated 10 percent of women.[34] The most serious etiology is endometrial cancer, although in approximately 95 percent of cases postmenopausal bleeding is benign.[35] In the majority of women, bleeding is caused by atrophy of the vaginal mucosa or endometrium; other common causes are endometrial hyperplasia, polyps, and leiomyomata.

The evaluation of a woman with postmenopausal bleeding begins with taking a relevant history and performing a thorough pelvic examination including cervical cytology. Transvaginal ultrasound is often used as a noninvasive means to evaluate the endometrial thickness and identify which patients require further evaluation, including endometrial sampling for tissue diagnosis.[36] Endometrial biopsy is a standard technique for endometrial evaluation. It is highly accurate and can be performed as an office procedure, and is almost always tolerated without local or regional anesthesia.

Perhaps more challenging for clinicians than the initial diagnostic evaluation is interpretation of biopsy results and clear communication of ensuing options for evaluation and treatment. The absence of pathology on biopsy may not be indicative of a benign diagnosis. A significant proportion of endometrial biopsy samples are non-diagnostic, and require further assessment with such techniques as saline infusion sonography or hysteroscopy with endometrial sampling.[37] Further, when the cause of bleeding is determined by the biopsy, a variety of options for clinical management often exist. For instance, choices about further evaluation and treatment for endometrial hyperplasia (including options of medication, IUD placement, and surgery) depend on the histologic findings, a patient's age, her health history, and her values, including views on risk and future childbearing. Thus, the disclosure of endometrial biopsy results usually requires a clear and detailed discussion between a patient and her physician.

Professionalism Considerations

This particular clinical case highlights the tension between the professional's obligation to disclose results in a timely manner and their obligation to disclose results in a clinical setting that facilitates adequate patient understanding and the sensitive disclosure of what may be complicated or difficult news.

Clearly physicians have a professional obligation to make significant efforts to make room in their schedules for timely follow-up whenever a procedure is done. Indeed, timely follow-up ranks in importance with a detailed workup, informed consent, and technical competence as core professional obligations whenever a procedure is performed.

Yet the definition of "timely" may vary depending on how fast a pathologic diagnosis can be expected in a particular institution, anticipated urgency for subsequent intervention, a patient's level of concern or discomfort, and other relevant factors. It may be difficult or impossible to eliminate the stress that many patients experience when waiting for results, particularly when a serious diagnosis such as cancer is considered possible. Further, economic pressures resulting from managed care, increasing liability costs, decreasing reimbursement for services, and the like have generated significant pressure to see more patients in less time, and practitioners' schedules often have little room to "squeeze in" another visit. Nevertheless, physicians should take the patient's experience and their professional obligations into account when they structure their clinical time and undertake procedures necessitating timely follow-up.

While it is unfortunate that this physician's clinic schedule did not accommodate what most would agree would qualify as timely follow-up, the decision not to initiate a phone dialogue may actually be defensible in the context of the doctor's professional obligations to provide information with adequate clarity and support. While some physicians feel comfortable communicating complex information by telephone, a phone follow-up may be neither professionally obligatory nor optimal in this situation.

Since the patient's actual biopsy result is not specified in the case, we can only speculate about the rationale (and thus the justification) for delaying the conversation until the office visit, but there are a number of reasonable possibilities. One justified rationale may be that bad news is best communicated in person. If the biopsy showed cancer, the physician may believe that it would be in the patient's best interest to wait until the scheduled appointment. A significant body of literature indicates that insensitive disclosure of bad news may increase the distress of recipients, have a lasting impact on their ability to adapt and adjust, and can lead to anger toward the physician or staff.[38] Guidelines and recommendations describe how doctors should prepare to disclose bad news, what constitutes an optimum supportive environment, and ways to best provide information, and recommend against disclosure of results by telephone. Still, in the setting of a serious diagnosis, these guidelines also highlight the importance of picking a time and place that is convenient for the patient and her family.[39]

Another justified rationale may be that a small amount of information, especially if misunderstood, can do more harm than good. Suppose the biopsy indicated simple hyperplasia. Though the finding rarely can progress to cancer (<1–3 percent of cases), it is usually reversible with oral progesterone. Yet the distinction between simple hyperplasia and the more worrisome histologic types may only be effectively communicated in the office setting; thus a phone conversation could unduly heighten a patient's anxiety about her diagnosis during the time remaining before her scheduled visit. Finally, misinformation could have the opposite effect. If a biopsy result did not show cancer, and yet further studies were required to rule out the diagnosis, a physician may feel that the importance of continued follow-up would most effectively be communicated during an office visit.

In the end, communication of results in a timely, accurate, and sensitive manner is an important professional obligation. While the balance of timeliness and effective communication may be difficult to achieve in the context of increasing physician workload, those who choose to perform procedures should aspire to structure their practices so that both can be predictably achieved.

Opinion

Because we don't know all the facts of this case, it is not clear whether the delayed disclosure is a breach of professionalism or the result of efforts to provide the best care possible in the context of a strained system. Either way, timely disclosure of results should be a priority – along with informed consent, safety, and the like – whenever diagnostic procedures are done. Physicians who perform such procedures have a professional responsibility to structure their practices so that when face-to-face follow-up is indicated, it will be carried out in a timely manner.

Anne Drapkin Lyerly, M.D., M.A.
Associate Professor, Obstetrics and Gynecology
Core Faculty, Trent Center for Bioethics, Humanities, and
History of Medicine
Duke University School of Medicine

A Perspective from Patient Advocacy Experts

The Patient: "He didn't call me back. It must be bad news. Maybe he was afraid I'd get hysterical or scream or cry – or faint, on the phone. But this is worse – it's like he's abandoned me. I'm surprised after all these years. If I call him again – will he get mad at me? And what if it is cancer?"

Her Husband: "You've got me worried now. I'll just call him and ask him to talk to you. Okay?"

What was the Physician thinking?

Dr. A: "The schedule has just been so packed I haven't had time to call her back! Anyway, once I tell her, it will open a Pandora's box of questions and reactions that will take a lot of time to manage. Besides, I never tell patients bad news over the phone. It's too hard to control the situation. Her appointment is only a week away now. It will be better to wait and talk in person."

Or

Dr. B: "I'm uncertain if I should call and tell her the results over the phone or just wait. She'll be worried, but if I tell her over the phone tonight she may not understand the implications and options, and she may get really upset. I'd much rather tell her to come in, but I have a big OR case tomorrow. It will probably be better to wait until her appointment and tell her in person so I can be sure she understands everything."

Or

Dr. C: "I have worried her! I'll ask my receptionist to contact her and find a good time to talk on the phone tonight. I will apologize for the delay, ask if she wants her husband on the phone as well and share some of the information she needs to know and answer her questions. I'd rather speak with her in person, but I have a big case tomorrow, so I'll check with her to see how she's feeling, and if she isn't comfortable waiting until her appointment, I will see her tomorrow right after I get out of the OR. I'm going to have to work with my staff to block more biopsy follow-up appointments. I'll let her know I'm working on making sure this doesn't happen again."

Medical professionalism requires both technical excellence, which is a given, and an "aspiration to and wise application of the principles of professionalism."[40] Fundamental to the physician–patient relationship is the promise to always put the interests of the patient first, to be accountable, and to advocate for the well-being of the patient as "perceived by the patient."[41] The lack of information and uncertainty about the results of the biopsy have left this patient feeling frightened and vulnerable. This is a normal, predictable reaction. Waiting for test results is difficult. Delays are common. To address these feelings, the patient is actively seeking information from her physician. The physician's failure to call her back has added to her anxiety and left her feeling abandoned. This sequence of events may well lead the patient or her family to question the physician's professionalism and expertise, significantly impairing the doctor's ability to be therapeutically effective as a result of the poor rapport and the distrust and fear of marginalization it has engendered. On the other hand, it could be an opportunity for a busy, compassionate physician to demonstrate his/her professionalism, strengthen the relationship and maximize therapeutic effectiveness.

A physician's response to Mrs. Patient's situation will vary depending on his or her orientation to the physician–patient relationship. Physicians who embrace a relationship-centered orientation, which the IOM suggests belongs at the very center of care, work with patients and their families to co-construct effective partnerships.[42] A patient-centered care orientation entails five essential commitments: understand patients' unique psychosocial context; help patients navigate the health care system; use effective interpersonal and communication skills; practice self-awareness; and integrate biomedical expertise with the human and relational dimensions of care.[43]

Dr. A sees only his/her own perspective, feels burdened, and does not act to relieve the patient's suffering. Although both Drs. B and C consider the patient's perspective, only Dr. C accepts his/her responsibility and acts to address the patient's need for information and guidance. Dr. C is altruistic, accountable, respectful, self-aware, and takes communication seriously as the medium through which effective relationships are sustained.

Physicians should help patients navigate the clinical system. The activated patient can be a partner in a mutually constructed fail-safe plan to prevent delay or lack of follow-up. For example, this physician could have asked the patient at the time of the biopsy about her preferences for hearing about the results. Although the physician may prefer to discuss information in person, as is recommended by most experts, the patient may prefer knowing sooner as compared to unavoidable waiting. This trade-off can be discussed and a plan agreed upon in advance and the patient empowered to call the practice if she does not hear from the physician in a timely manner.

The wisdom it takes to act professionally in every case is best cultivated through the habits of regular self-reflection and personal awareness.[44] Without these, the physician who feels uncomfortable sharing bad news or responding to patients' emotions may anticipate extreme responses as well as make uninformed or reactive assumptions about what is best for a patient.

Such a series of events, in turn, may lead the physician to avoid the patient, usurping the patient's role in decision making and therefore her autonomy. Such a response contradicts one of the primary principles of medical professionalism in the practice of relationship-centered care.[45,19]

Jo Anne L. Earp, Sc.D.
Professor and Interim Chair, Department of Health Behavior and
Health Education
Gillings School of Global Public Health, University of North Carolina

Beth A. Lown, M.D.
Assistant Professor of Medicine
Harvard Medical School

Adina Kalet, M.D., M.P.H.
Associate Professor of Medicine and Surgery
New York University School of Medicine

IMPROVING QUALITY OF CARE – PSYCHIATRY

A psychiatrist recently left her private practice and joined a practice in which she is employed by a managed care company. She has become increasingly concerned about several aspects of this new position. She feels that she is unable to provide the same quality of care to her patients as she did in her prior practice setting. Specifically, she is concerned that she has less time per patient, that she needs to see additional patients each day, and that the new contract her organization signed with a large employer group gives financial rewards for specific standards set by the employer group. She is also concerned about her practice arrangement in which she has been asked to provide medication management visits for patients who are seen by other mental health professionals in the community and at the company itself.

A Perspective from a Psychiatrist

Professionalism Considerations[46,47]

The professionalism dilemmas faced by this psychiatrist are multifaceted and very common in today's health care delivery system. Several questions stand out for discussion. Does this psychiatrist need to alter her professional and ethical values in this new position? Is it possible that she can deliver ethical care in this new treatment setting? Can she go along with proposals that may impact her care which are decided by non-medical individuals or groups? What are her ethical and professional obligations to her patients when she is doing only a part of the psychiatric treatment?

Let's start with the first question. This psychiatrist chose this new form of employment where she would derive a salary versus income from self-employment. While she changed the manner in which she earns a living, such a change does not obligate her to subjugate her professional values. If she believes that by working within the new system she can improve the quality of the care that her patients receive, she should and can aspire to work toward that goal. This setting – salaried and working in concert with other mental health care professionals – is not atypical for psychiatrists working in community health, prisons, or other public positions. If, no matter how much she works toward improved care in this setting, there is no improvement, then her option is to either learn to accept a professionally conflicted position or leave. She would need to think carefully whether the diminished time that she has with patients actually impairs their treatment, influences their outcome negatively, does not allow her to follow established practice guidelines or in some other way is harmful to her patients. If so, her professional obligation is to advocate for change based on ethical and scientifically valid information. If the concerns she has are more reflective of a style of treatment with little scientific backing, then this argument is weakened. It is possible to establish a good therapeutic relationship with a patient even during briefer sessions. The key issue is whether the time allotted suits the medical/psychiatric needs of the patients. If not, then she must advocate for improvement in that situation. Likewise, if the numbers of patients she is obligated to see impacts the quality of care that she can render, then she needs to advocate for improvement in the scheduling process.

The issue of financial rewards set by the employer group raises many complex issues of professionalism. First, the parameters of any medical/psychiatric standards or guidelines set must be developed by physicians and approved by current quality organizations that have representation by organized medicine and psychiatry. If the standards are more related to productivity or efficiency, then the concern is whether such standards and the financial incentives attached may threaten the quality of care that she can render. If so, she must object. Employer groups are looking toward managed care organizations and through them to respected physician organizations to set standards that are evidence-based and valid. Unfortunately, those standards are still in their developmental stages and some employer groups are pushing for incentives for measures that may not stand more rigorous scientific review or may have little to do with patient outcome.

Our psychiatrist's last dilemma – related to seeing patients for medication management – raises a number of potential professional pitfalls.[48] To protect both her patients and herself professionally, she should be assured of the credentials of the other mental health professionals and have open communication on an ongoing basis regarding their respective treatment of the patients. She should make sure that the other professionals are acting within the scope of their license and training and that she does not delegate any medical authority to them. Any medical/psychiatric decision made should be based on the personal assessment of the patient unless the other professional has some ability through his/her licensure to make such assessments and recommendations to the psychiatrist. This may be true in some states, where nurse practitioners have partial or full independent practice or are able to work under physician-approved protocols. This psychiatrist must make sure that she is not acting as a mere figurehead, writing prescriptions for many professionals, with an inadequate personal assessment of each patient. She has full ethical and legal responsibility for each patient even though she is only providing a part of their treatment.

Opinion

In summary, if the psychiatrist in the scenario can adapt her previous style of practice to these new arrangements with a sense that the quality of care she is providing is not harmful to patients or that by continuing in her position that she will be able to improve the care within the new practice, then she could feel comfortable remaining in her new position. However, if she finds the practice situation potentially harmful to patients or if she has no hope of improving their care, she must decide to accept that reality or leave. This is no easy decision, but it is one that many psychiatrists and other physicians must face in our changing health care system. Hopefully, as we have more evidence-based treatments coupled with valid outcome measures, this psychiatrist and other physicians will be on very solid footing in advocating for quality care. In the meantime, our psychiatrist will have to do her best to deal with what we know now and keep the needs of her patients first and foremost.

Jeremy Lazarus, M.D.
Clinical Professor of Psychiatry
University of Colorado, Denver School of Medicine

A Perspective from a Behavior Health Expert

The scenario highlights a psychiatrist who finds herself caught in a period of changing policy and practice – an experience that is likely to occur often in the lives of physicians for some time to come. One of these conflicting or unsettled policy areas is the balance between demonstrated effectiveness and our current capacities to measure that effectiveness. This is as true in psychiatry as in general health care. A second conflict is specific to psychiatry, as hybrid practice environments with multiple providers are a relatively new phenomenon for the specialty.

The reality of contemporary practice is that whether the setting is a private office or a large public clinic, payers are increasingly demanding evidence of both the efficacy and the efficiency of their expenditures. They expect to see evidence that patients are improving, and that the practitioner is not wasting scarce health dollars on practices that are not optimal. One of the legacies of a traditional private practice model was the lack of systematic assessment of interventions using standardized instruments. The psychiatrist may "feel" that she is not giving the same quality of care to her new patients, but she may also lack any sort of metric by which to gauge the difference.

The pressure for productivity and efficiency (more visits, less time per visit) almost inevitably leads to some negative consequences for both psychiatrist and patient, because it focuses on inputs (i.e., blocks of time spent with numbers of people) rather than outcomes (e.g., time spent differentially with patients based on acuity of need and clarity about preferred interventions).

And yet the goal is a laudable one. Problems arise, however, in the strategies used to achieve the goal. Dr. David Eddy, one of the champions of a more scientific approach to managing medical practices through the use of performance measurement, offers these sobering reflections: the "measures tend to be blunt, expensive, incomplete and distorting. And they can easily be inaccurate and misleading."[49] Hardly a ringing endorsement from a champion of the issue! The answer is not to abandon the search because the tools are weak or flawed, but to improve and refine the tools. We have an affirmative responsibility to improve services continuously and the only way to do that is to have reliable indicators of impact. In this scenario, the psychiatrist is caught in the middle of an effort to document – and strengthen – both efficacy and efficiency, using tools that can only serve as limited proxies for quality. At least that's the most positive interpretation.

Alas, too often external review and monitoring are driven not by a desire to improve quality through effectiveness or expand access through efficiency but by a desire to reduce costs – at all costs. When cost alone is the measuring rod, patients will ultimately be shortchanged and practitioners will feel diminished.

The psychiatrist similarly feels conflicted about engaging in a financial reward mechanism for achieving certain externally imposed standards. This arrangement probably challenges deeply held feelings about the altruistic nature of the practice of psychiatry, reducing her work to assembly line tactics. And yet many businesses are looking to this mechanism, often referred to as "pay for performance," to achieve desired health outcomes for their employees. This is a laudable goal but one that may appear to physicians as particularly indifferent to their clinical acumen and individual competencies. To this commentator, the scenario serves as a call for all practitioners to be actively involved in shaping the quality indicators by which their practices will be judged. It is unlikely that anyone currently in medical school will not experience some variant of the external review strategies identified in this scenario, and the wise physician-to-be will learn as much about the policy and administration of contemporary medicine as possible before launching into practice.

The final issue raised in the scenario – the concern about collaboration with other mental health care professionals – is even more complex. The devil, in this instance, will clearly be revealed in details not made explicit. The key will be whether or not the psychiatrist can establish smooth, integrated communication with his or her colleagues in the community and the company. Increasingly, psychiatry is best practiced in integrated systems of intervention, and if this arrangement is one of those, his or her patients are likely to be the beneficiaries. If, however, the psychiatrist is expected to serve as an automated prescription machine – without benefit of the insights and feedback of the other mental health professionals – then he or she is wise to be troubled.

Historically, we have done a poor job of preparing psychiatrists (and a host of other behavioral health professionals) for practice in the real world. Like it or not (and this commentator emphatically does not), health care in the United States has become a commodity. Unless and until that changes, it is essential that medical students learn much more than most currently do about the pressures that they will face and how to make limited health care expenditures go as far as possible while delivering as much good as possible.

John Morris, M.S.W.
Director, Human Services Practice, The Technical Assistance
Collaborative, Inc., Columbia, SC
Professor, Department of Neuropsychiatry and Behavior Science
University of South Carolina School of Medicine

IMPROVING QUALITY OF CARE – EMERGENCY MEDICINE

The emergency physician encounters an irate daughter of a seventy-five–year-old male patient in the emergency department (ED) waiting room. The daughter is upset about the eight hours that her father has been waiting to be seen for symptoms of a urinary tract infection (UTI). While awaiting treatment, the patient has developed shaking chills and has become less responsive. She insists that her father be attended to immediately.

A Perspective from an Emergency Medicine Physician

Clinical Background

Complaints suggestive of a UTI are very common among patients seeking ED care. The vast majority of UTIs are the result of ascending infections originating in the urethra, and therefore are much more prevalent in women. About 85 percent of UTIs are attributable to *E. coli*, with most of the remainder are due to *Staphylococcus saprophyticus*. Infections with other enteric pathogens are less common.

Most patients with UTIs can be treated as outpatients and recover quickly with antibiotics chosen empirically. Indications for hospitalization include poor medical compliance, vomiting, volume depletion, and pyelonephritis in children, men, pregnant women, and individuals with known urinary tract abnormalities. Admission is also generally warranted for patients with evidence of sepsis.

Professionalism Considerations

EDs are extraordinarily stressful environments for patients, families, and health care workers. From the physician's vantage point, many patients present with non-urgent complaints and can safely wait hours. Most ED patients, however, believe they have an important problem and need to be seen quickly; many are in pain or anxious. Physicians tend to dismiss discomfort and fear as legitimate concerns, particularly when confronted with other patients who have more pressing needs.[50,51]

There is a common misperception that the emergency physician is the "captain of the ship" and therefore vicariously liable for adverse events in all patients presenting to the ED – including problems arising from prolonged waiting times. In fact, most delays in emergency medical care are systems problems and largely out of the on-duty physician's control. EDs are highly complex and impersonal operations, and it is imperative that staff function as advocates for the well-being of their patients.

ED staff may become numb to complaints about long waiting times. It is tempting to label patients and families who complain as being difficult, leading to a cycle of further corrosion in physician–patient communication.[52] However, in this vignette there is danger in assuming that the initial triage decision was correct and that the seventy-five-year-old man is still a non-urgent patient. In light of the daughter's expression of concern, the ED staff is compelled to reassess the patient.

Practical considerations often make it difficult to expedite the care of a waiting patient. The logic of a triage system may be unclear to many patients, and they may become angry if they suspect that someone is receiving special attention. In this situation, it is wise to reassess the patient while he is still in the waiting room. If he is stable and the triage decision remains appropriate, he and his daughter can be reassured that the wait, while tedious and regrettable, appears to have caused no harm.

If the patient has deteriorated, the physician must act quickly to minimize the harm to the patient and the family's distress. The most professional and responsible action in this scenario is to acknowledge to the daughter that her father is sicker than he appeared on arrival, promptly evaluate the patient, explain the assessment and treatment plans, and offer tangible assurance that the remainder of his ED care will be expedited as much as possible. Expressing a clear understanding of the patient's problem is the single most important factor in recovering the confidence of the patient and his daughter.[53]

The physician may want to thank the daughter for intervening on her father's behalf. These actions affirm the daughter's role as the patient's advocate, mitigate her concern about further delays, and avoid creating the appearance that the ED staff is concealing an error. It is wise to apologize to the patient and his daughter. This further legitimizes their complaint and demonstrates personal concern for the patient's welfare. An apology is not an admission of negligence.

It may be tempting for physicians to adopt a defensive posture, offering excuses to the patient's daughter and denying responsibility for the adverse outcome. While legitimate circumstances contributing to delays can be related to the daughter, she is unlikely to be assuaged by excuses. A defensive attitude is likely to be counterproductive to the relationship between the patient, his daughter, and the health care workers. Furthermore, blaming an inefficient system for the delay is unlikely to reduce the possibility that the angry family will initiate legal action against the physician and the institution.

Many EDs have executed measures to minimize adverse outcomes related to prolonged waiting times. Periodic reassessment of waiting ED patients is now routine and actually required in many instances. Nurses should be empowered to override triage guidelines based on their gestalt, and the ED should foster a culture that encourages all personnel to voice concerns about a patient's condition.

Opinion

The emergency physician in this scenario should address the daughter's concerns for her father's health and see that the patient is re-evaluated in the waiting room. If the patient has deteriorated during a long wait, the physician should take all reasonable steps to expedite his care, acknowledge and apologize for the delay, and thank the daughter for her attentiveness to her father.

David J. Karras, M.D.
Professor of Emergency Medicine, Associate Chair for Academic Affairs
Department of Emergency Medicine, Temple University
School of Medicine

A Perspective from a Bioethicist and Emergency Physician

Receiving anger is always difficult, but especially when the anger is unjust. The daughter's anger in this case may seem unjust to emergency personnel who feel they are working as hard as they can to maintain patient flow and to ensure that the sickest patients are seen first. Yet there is much that can be done to avert such anger. Proper triage and the facilitation of patient flow are important (and presumably could have been improved in this case), but they are by themselves not sufficient to satisfy the ideals of medical professionalism.

The patient in this scenario has suffered harm from his eight-hour wait. Beyond the considerable inconvenience and physical suffering that occur when acutely ill people are forced to endure long hours in uncomfortable waiting rooms, this man has also experienced a potentially serious deterioration in his medical condition. His decrease in responsiveness may indicate the development of life-threatening sepsis. If he had received prompt medical attention, this dire situation might have been averted. Even if it were not possible to place him in a treatment room, urinalysis and culture could have been obtained during triage, and he could have been monitored periodically in the waiting room. When he deteriorated, his triage status should have been upgraded and treatment promptly instituted.

Given the obvious seriousness of her father's condition and his deterioration during a terribly long wait, the daughter's frustration is not only understandable, it is the inevitable result of humane filial concern. Sons and daughters are expected to be vigilant about caring for sick parents. Furthermore, the daughter is justified in thinking that her father should have received better treatment. In a society that strictly controls the practice of medicine (for instance, by forbidding lay persons with urinary tract infections from self-medicating with antibiotics), the emergency department is typically the only recourse for an acutely ill individual who needs prompt treatment. Because of their state-enforced monopoly on emergency services, hospital emergency departments incur an obligation of public responsiveness. Eight-hour waits for septic elders are not acceptable. Though the causes of emergency department crowding are diverse and not always under the control of hospitals,[54] the daughter has good reason to be angry.

The approach to preventing such unfortunate events begins with an attitude of loyalty in the medical staff. Physicians, nurses, and other medical personnel are beholden to a professional ideal of service. Medicine is a public enterprise, richly endowed for its task of healing – that is, of mitigating and ameliorating human suffering due to illness and injury. This service is the fundamental goal of medicine, and it is the cause that medical professionals are called to loyally serve.[55] The ideal is patient-centered in the sense that

(1) patients' suffering is the fundamental condition it seeks to address, and (2) the relief of suffering is always accomplished in the context of patient values (as both suffering and its relief are largely relative to patient motives and perceptions). Typically, family relations are an organic element of the experience of illness and recovery. Hence, medical professionals are also beholden to families.

The attitude of loyalty does not imply a "customer-is-always-right" mentality. To the contrary, patients and their families are not merely customers and they are certainly not always right. They are more than customers because the clinician–patient relationship, which centers on an ideal of healing, is more than a simple market arrangement, which centers on the ideal of exchanging commodities. Likewise, clinicians are not merely clinical "providers," they are also professionals beholden to professional ideals. For loyal clinicians, patient well-being trumps profit, provider convenience, ego gratification, and the other trappings of medical prestige. Embodying and projecting this attitude is the key to averting problems such as those exhibited in this scenario.

Several particular strategies suggest themselves to the loyal emergency department physician faced with the problem of long waiting times. First, it is important to recognize the clinical importance of minimizing waiting time. No available triage system is so efficient that it can always identify and avert potential medical disasters. Hence, when waiting time is excessive, patients are endangered. Further, the tedium and the feelings of being disrespected that characterize long waits are compounded by illness, thus exacerbating patient suffering.

Second, clinicians should communicate their concern to patients and those who wait with them. At a minimum, this requires an apology and some kind of an explanation for the long wait when clinicians greet patients at the bedside. Apologies need not be construed as admissions of guilt, but rather as acknowledgments that brief waiting times are crucial goals and that the medical staff is troubled that they are not being achieved. As an emergency physician, I have sometimes gone to the waiting room and addressed the waiting patients, offering a brief explanation for the long waiting time and inquiring if anyone has particular medical concerns that they think may have eluded triage. Such excursions to the waiting room are always brief, and always worth the time. Generally, patients will not speak out with trivial concerns. In every instance, they are appreciative. Further, this strategy facilitates the expeditious flow of patients by minimizing the time spent by other staff members addressing waiting room complaints.

Finally, emergency department physicians should do everything reasonable to insure that long waits are prevented. When emergency physician staffing is the problem, back-up physicians should be called in expeditiously. We should dispense with the ethos of protecting colleagues' time when it harms patients. In some cases, patients occupy emergency department beds long after they have been thoroughly evaluated by emergency department personnel – waiting for the arrival of a consultant or for the availability of a hospital bed. The latter are systemic problems that frequently need to be addressed at the level of hospital administration. Though advocacy for these ends can beget uncomfortable encounters, fidelity to patient well-being sometimes makes such encounters necessary.

Griffin Trotter, M.D., Ph.D
Department of Health Care Ethics and Department of Surgery,
Emergency Medical Division
St. Louis University School of Medicine

SUMMARY – COMMITMENT TO IMPROVING QUALITY OF CARE

The objectives of this summary are to present (1) issues regarding quality of care, (2) the rationale for engagement in quality improvement activities, and (3) meaningful strategies for quality improvement. The first part will provide an overview of quality improvement. Components include professional responsibilities to improve the quality of care, types and measures of quality, and evidence-based strategies to improve the quality of care. The second part will review themes from the case discussions in this context.

Background

Professional Responsibilities for Improving Quality of Care

In recent years, the need to improve quality of care has been increasingly emphasized as a professional responsibility of physicians. In 2002, the American Board of Internal Medicine (ABIM), American College of Physicians-American Society of Internal Medicine, and the European Federation of Internal Medicine released a charter on professionalism for physicians.[19] Included in the charter was the following:

> **Commitment to improving quality of care.** Physicians must be dedicated to continuous improvement in the quality of health care. This commitment entails not only maintaining clinical competence but also working collaboratively with other professionals to reduce medical error, increase patient safety, minimize overuse of health care resources, and optimize the outcomes of care. Physicians must actively participate in the development of better measures of quality of care and the application of quality measures to assess routinely the performance of all individuals, institutions, and systems responsible for health care delivery.

Physicians, both individually and through their professional associations, must take responsibility for assisting in the creation and implementation of mechanisms designed to encourage continuous improvement in the quality of care.

Other organizations have made similar recommendations. The American Medical Association's principles of medical ethics state that physicians should maintain competence and contribute to the improvement of the community and betterment of public health.[56] The American College of Graduate Medical Education (ACGME) requires all residents and the Joint Commission (JCAHO) requires all hospital medical staff to demonstrate competence in quality improvement as well as clinical competence.

As described in the endocrinology case discussed in this chapter, physicians have traditionally had a responsibility to study and remain current with knowledge and technical competence. While physicians were traditionally expected to do so independently, only recently has a requirement for public accountability and transparency been introduced. This applies not only to the demonstration of knowledge and technical competence, but to accountability for clinical decisions and quality of care. Many physicians will no doubt see this as an affront to personal autonomy, which in many ways it is. Physicians must keep in mind that the shift from personal autonomy to transparency and accountability is based on an expansive body of science demonstrating that the latter method results in better patient care. This section summarizes the issues depicted in the case vignettes, including the need for quality improvement, professional responsibilities for quality improvement, as well as non-professional reasons for quality improvement.

Background on Quality of Care

Although it is clear that the physician is responsible for quality of care, there is much debate concerning what constitutes quality and how to measure it. The cases presented in this chapter demonstrate many types of quality. This section will discuss the most common types of quality metrics and summarize how the U.S. health care system performs.

Population Health Indices. One way to measure quality is to look at population health measures, such as life expectancy and infant mortality. Despite being by far the most expensive health care system in the world, the United States trails many developed nations in population health and outcome measures.[57,58] Many have argued that these measures may not reflect performance of the health care system as other factors contribute to these numbers. A 2008 study measured mortality rates from causes considered amenable to health care in twenty countries in 1997–1998 and 2002–2003.[59] The United States had the highest amenable mortality rate of any country in

2002–2003 and showed by far the least amount of improvement between study periods. Although these findings demonstrate a need for improvement, the causes and solutions to measures such as national mortality rates are complicated and difficult for individual physicians to address.

Clinical Quality Measures. Clinical quality measures are more readily applied to an individual physician or system. Clinical quality measures are typically classified as process or outcome measures. Process measures gauge actions taken by the physicians such as performing screening mammographies. Outcome measures gauge clinical end points of treatment such as mortality rates, or intermediate end points such as the percentage of patients with controlled blood pressure. Process measures are directly controlled by physicians, but require clear scientific evidence and consensus to support their use. Outcome measures require less evidence, yet are criticized for being influenced by factors beyond a physician's control.

Numerous studies have demonstrated poor performance on quality measures. Comprehensive studies of the quality of care delivered in the United States have reported that adults receive 55 percent and children receive 47 percent of recommended care.[6,60] As the seminal Institute of Medicine (IOM) report *Crossing the Quality Chasm* reported: "Between the health care we have and the care we could have lies not just a gap, but a chasm."[61] Other studies, most famously the *Dartmouth Atlas*, have demonstrated significant differences in treatment patterns that cannot be explained by differences in patient preferences or severity of illness.[62] These studies have done much to challenge physician autonomy and increase the demand for transparency.

Attempts to measure quality have been catalyzed by these findings. Quality measures are designed and implemented by professional organizations, accrediting organizations such as the National Committee for Quality Assurance (NCQA), health plans, federal and state governments including the Centers for Medicare and Medicaid Services, and employers. Measures target individual physicians, hospitals, group practices, and health plans. Many measures are tied to financial payments, a practice known as pay-for-performance. Although in one study only 62 percent of physicians felt that their quality measures should be available to the public, this is happening with increasing frequency.[63] These measures will likely become more prevalent and be an integral component of clinical practice into the future.

Patient Safety. Patient safety addresses harm to patients caused by the medical system. Safety is closely related to quality, often overlapping in measures and underlying causes. The 1999 IOM report, *To Err Is Human*, catalyzed concerns about patient safety after reporting that nearly 100,000 patients may die each year and 1 million are injured due to preventable medical errors in hospitals alone.[64] Numerous studies have demonstrated that many errors occur in the outpatient setting as well.[65] Examples of safety concerns include medication errors, hospital-acquired infections, and falls.

Many hospitals have responded to these concerns with patient safety officers, committees, and policies. Legislators have responded through initiatives such as mandatory reporting of errors and near-misses in some states. Regulators such as JCAHO and the NCQA include patient safety measures in the accreditation process. Payers and purchasers are beginning to both reward practices that encourage safety such as computerized physician order entry (CPOE) systems and refuse payment for costs resulting from errors. Notably, Medicare stopped paying for eight types of preventable errors in October 2008, a policy which many private insurers are also adopting.[66]

Hospital-acquired infections (HAIs) have been a major focus for patient safety efforts due their prevalence, significant morbidity and mortality, and high costs. In 2006, Pennsylvania became the first state to publicize HAI data for all of its hospitals. For the 19,154 cases with an HAI, mortality rate was 12.9 percent and hospitalization cost was $185,260 per case, compared to 2.3 percent and $31,389 for cases without an HAI.[67] Studies revealed that discrepancies in mortality and costs were largely attributable to the infections themselves.[68,69] Most states have either adopted or are adopting similar reporting requirements.

Quality of the Patient's Experience. A final component of quality health care, which is more complex and poorly defined than other components, is quality related to the patient's experience. This includes service elements (wait times, friendliness of staff, etc.), adequate communication, emotional management, and involvement of patients in decision making. Measures of these elements are typically based on feedback from patients, such as the Press-Ganey survey and the Consumer Assessment of Healthcare Providers and Systems. Measures of communication and involvement of patients in decision making are sparse, yet some experts have proposed development of these measures.[70,71]

As discussed in the emergency medicine case in this chapter, many physicians consider patient experience quality to be of less importance than clinical quality and safety. As demonstrated in the emergency medicine, obstetrics-gynecology, and hospitalist cases in this chapter, inattention to the patient's experience resulted in significant distress for the patient, weakened provider–patient relationship, and even impacted clinical quality and safety. Emerging concerns for this component of quality reflects the shift from physician autonomy to physician transparency and patient autonomy, such that the patient has greater involvement in choosing the goals, treatments, and processes of care.

Strategies for Quality Improvement

Many strategies exist for quality improvement. Some have a wealth of evidence to support their use and others are relatively new. Key strategies include education, individual interventions, organizational interventions, and ensuring patient-centered care. The increasing demand for transparency requires that physicians not only engage in quality improvement activities, but they must be able to demonstrate these efforts and their results.

Education for Quality Improvement. Although physicians were always expected to keep current with medical knowledge and ensure the quality of care in their own practices, formal education programs have been lacking. Traditional methods of continued education such as continuing medical education courses and medical journals were felt to be inadequate as physician knowledge and performance declines over time.[17] In recent years, accrediting organizations have responded by creating requirements and programs to help physicians maintain competence and improve the quality of their practices.

In 2002, the American Board of Medical Specialties established the Maintenance of Certification program, requiring physicians to recertify periodically and demonstrate continued self-assessment during the interim. As discussed in the endocrinology case, the Maintenance of Certification is an efficient and effective method of continued education, and most physicians have chosen to participate.[72] In addition to the recertification exams, programs such as the ABIM's Practice Improvement Modules have helped physicians identify areas for improvement in their own practices.

Procedural specialists must maintain technical competence in addition to knowledge competence. Oversight for this aspect often falls on the hospital or physician practice. Several mechanisms can be used to ensure technical competence, as discussed in the gastroenterology case, such as ensuring performance of a minimum number of procedures, ensuring appropriate training, and the use of proctors when appropriate. The use of outcome measures has started to become a significant mechanism for measuring procedural competence.

As mentioned, the major accrediting organizations for residency programs, ACGME, and hospitals, JCAHO, now require that residents and medical staff demonstrate competence in quality improvement skills. Additional requirements, such as knowledge of health care systems and provision of cost-effective care, are integrally related to managing quality. Attention to these requirements will ensure that future physicians have the skill set they need for quality improvement.

Individual Interventions for Quality Improvement. Quality improvement efforts can be as simple as an individual physician focusing on her own practice. These projects often target measures that are part of a pay-for-performance or quality improvement program such as the LDL goals described in the primary care case. Strategies for quality improvement, as described in the case, include auditing data and providing feedback, reminder systems, physician and patient education, developing protocols, and others.

Individuals may similarly improve patient safety. Simply admitting an error and apologizing can be therapeutic both for the physician and the patient. A recent study of 3,171 physicians found that many suffered anxiety, sleep difficulties, and reduced job satisfaction from errors.[73] Physicians were nearly four times as likely to report significant distress over an error if they felt that disclosure was inadequate. Methods such as root-cause analyses and external review can help physicians identify safety concerns in their practice and develop strategies for improvement. Of course, this does not exempt them from following standard error-reporting policies set by their organization or regulatory bodies.

These systems are often inadequate. In a recent survey of 1,082 U.S. physicians, 70 percent of physicians felt that error-reporting systems were inadequate and relied on informal discussions with colleagues.[74] In one study, only 55 percent of physicians said they knew how to report an error and only 40 percent knew what kind of errors to report.[75] Another study found that only 53 percent of physicians had participated in a formal error-reduction program.[76] These results highlight the need for greater education and development of error-reporting systems.

Organizational Interventions for Quality Improvement. Most hospitals and physician practices are looking for formal methods to incorporate quality improvement activities into their organizations. Most hospitals and health systems have official positions such as chief quality officers to help manage quality. Many have made major investments in technology and management strategies to address quality. Central to these efforts is the need to facilitate teamwork.

Health information technology (HIT) has been championed as an important tool for improving quality and efficiency in health care. Many hospitals and physician organizations have adopted forms of HIT such as electronic health records (EHRs), computerized physician order entry (CPOE), and decision support tools, although only 23 percent of ambulatory physician practices used EHRs and 5 percent of hospitals used CPOE through 2005.[77] In 2006, President Bush declared "We will make wider use of electronic records and other health information technology to help control costs and reduce dangerous medical errors."[78] Financial support for EHRs is available from Medicare and other private groups for some physician practices. There is evidence that although EHRs are expensive to implement, they produce savings over the long run and can improve quality.[79] Recently the Veterans Affairs health system has been recognized for its exceptional performance on quality measures, credited in part to its comprehensive EHR.[80,81]

In addition to investing in the necessary resources, organizations have demonstrated quality improvement through effective management strategies. For instance, 108 intensive care units in Michigan were able to reduce their central catheter-related infections by up to 66 percent using a simple five-item checklist.[82] Other hospitals, such as Virginia Mason Medical Center, have adopted techniques from other industries, including the Toyota Production System and Six Sigma, to improve quality.[83] The Institute for Healthcare Improvement offers several educational programs and has launched campaigns to help spread proven strategies throughout the nation.[84]

Successful efforts to achieve quality improvement at the organizational level rely on teamwork. In the fourth year medical student case, elements of teamwork were discussed including leadership, mutual performance, and mutual trust (see the improving quality of care commentaries by Goyal and Holmboe in Chapter 2). Physicians are constantly required to work as part of a team, often as team leader, both in their practice setting and when carrying out quality improvement activities at the organization level. Physicians often work with colleagues such as consulting physicians, other health professionals such as nurses and residents, administrative staff, and third-party organizations such as health plans and disease management organizations. Effective teamwork is not automatic and requires constant attention.

An important element of teamwork is creating a conducive culture. Health care, particularly academic medicine, has traditionally been known for its hierarchical culture. As demonstrated in the two medical student cases illustrating quality of care in Chapter 2, this culture may have adverse effects on quality. Culture comes from the top and studies have demonstrated that cooperation between senior management and medical staff facilitates quality improvement efforts and results in hospitals and health care organizations.[85–90] As demonstrated in the emergency medicine case in this chapter, culture can be fostered in an organizational sub-unit, such as a department. All members of the team, particularly leaders, contribute to creating a culture compatible with quality improvement.

Improving Patient-Centered Care

Health care has traditionally been organized in a provider-centric manner. Practices are organized by provider type, often requiring multiple appointments for the same problem, schedules are set according to the provider's needs while patients often wait for hours, information is organized for the provider while patients often do not know what is happening, and goals and treatments are typically determined by the provider, often with little input from patients. Given these circumstances, the prospect of making care patient-centric is daunting. However, there are many strategies that providers can employ.

Several of these strategies were discussed in the case vignettes. In the obstretrics and gynecology case in this chapter, the importance of advanced planning for delivering of information and services was discussed, as well as the need for self-reflection to prevent erroneous assumptions. In the hospitalist case in this chapter, the need to keep the complexity and need to keep patients informed of their care was discussed, along with the devastating effects of failing to do so. In the emergency medicine case, the authors described the need to apologize and accept responsibility when the patient has a bad experience.

Other strategies are gaining favor and have shown promising results. The use of physician extenders such as nurse practitioners and physician assistants can provide high quality care that is convenient and cost effective.[91] Collaboration with third-party vendors such as disease management organizations can provide patient-centered care by coordinating care across providers. Practice innovations such as open-access scheduling and virtual visits can meet patients' needs and improve their satisfaction with care.[92] As pressure to improve patient-centered quality of care increases, providers will likely develop and invent effective strategies.

Review of the Cases and Commentaries

Using the information that has been presented as a framework, themes from the case vignettes will be discussed. The first section will address issues related to physicians' responsibility to improve the quality of their own care. The following sections will address the more daunting task of improving the quality of care delivered by others, including subordinates, superiors, peers, and quality at the population level.

Improving the Quality of One's Own Care

Several of the quality of care cases illustrated here demonstrate opportunities for the physicians to improve the quality of their own care. In the endocrinology case, the physician elected not to recertify. In a busy practice, the time requirements for recertification can make the process unattractive, particularly if the physician does not appreciate the benefits. As described, in addition to jeopardizing patient care, the physician may put himself in danger of being excluded by health plans, losing patients, or other consequences.

In the primary care and psychiatry cases, the physicians dealt with issues of quality as determined by outside parties, namely health plans and employer groups respectively. These cases presented the dilemma of resolving quality issues when external parties set standards that the physician may not agree with. Although physicians have a responsibility to ensure quality according to their standards, they cannot ignore metrics imposed by external parties. Physicians should determine whether these standards compromise quality in any way, using objective evidence. If it is determined quality is compromised, the physician should attempt to convince the external party to change the standard. These cases highlight the need for physicians to be aware of standards before signing contracts, and to proactively help create standards consistent with their professional values. Remember, these external parties develop standards because they have much at stake, and such standards will likely only increase in prevalence.

Another example of a physician's quality being judged by external parties is the case of lawyers and the courts adjudicating grievances or malpractice suits. Although physicians often feel that these non-health professionals are ill-equipped to judge quality, this process is necessary for settling legal disputes. As shown in the gastroenterology case, physicians must comply with the law, regardless of their professional standards. Thus, it is important for physicians to consider professionalism issues before agreeing to a legal settlement.

The obstretrics-gynecology and hospitalist cases demonstrated opportunities for physicians to improve patient-centered quality. In the obstetrics-gynecology case, the process was not described for receiving the results of a diagnostic test, leading to distress by the patient. A proactive approach by the physician to anticipate the patient's experience could have improved this situation. In the hospitalist case, a lack of communication with the patient and patient's family had severe effects on their experience. In the hectic hospital environment, physicians often focus on their tasks and neglect the communication aspect of care. Although this responsibility typically falls on the physician of record, all physicians involved in the patient's care have a professional responsibility to ensure that communication is adequate.

Improving the Quality Care Delivered by Others
The cases presented several opportunities in which physicians could impact the quality of care delivered by others. This includes trainees, staff, superiors, peers within one's organization, and care delivered across a broader population.

Trainees and Staff. Physicians often are responsible for oversight and thus the quality of care delivered by others, including physician trainees, other health professionals, and non-medical staff. The cases demonstrated several challenges physicians face in managing this aspect of care. In the psychiatry case, the physician felt uncomfortable with his responsibility for patients receiving care from other health professionals. In the emergency medicine case, the physician's oversight role was more complex, as the emergency department requires many variables and individuals to ensure timely, high quality care. In the medical student cases outlined in the quality of care vignettes in Chapter 2, although discussed from the perspective of the trainee, the attending physicians could have improved the quality of care by facilitating open expression of critical information by junior members.

Non-physician health professionals and other staff are critical to the delivery of efficient and effective care. Physicians must understand the scope of practice of other professionals with whom they work and strive to monitor quality through objective measurements. If physicians accept oversight responsibility without understanding the requirements of the role, they risk allowing poor quality and leaving themselves vulnerable to any consequences. These cases demonstrate the importance of fostering a conducive culture for teamwork and open communication to ensure delivery of high quality care.

Superiors. Improving the quality of care delivered by superiors can be very difficult as seen in the medical student cases in Chapter 2. Trainees and other members of the health care team may often feel that they must jeopardize their own relationship with a superior team member in order to advocate for patient care. The cases present several effective mechanisms for influencing other members of the team such as setting an example and simply speaking up. Having knowledge of the evidence for behaviors can also influence the team. Finally, if trainees are unable to influence the team, they should at least critically analyze the behavior of superiors to avoid developing the same faulty patterns of care.

Peers. Another challenge for physicians is improving the quality of their peers' care. As discussed in the primary care case in this chapter, a physician's responsibility to quality improvement involves the engagement of other physicians, particularly within the same organization. This task can be both uncomfortable and difficult, and is easier said than done. A recent survey found that 93 percent of physicians felt they should review peers, 96 percent felt they should report impaired or incompetent peers, and 93 percent felt they should report all significant errors. Yet only 56 percent had reviewed a peer's charts in the previous three years, 45 percent had not reported at least one impaired or incompetent peer, and 46 percent had not reported at least one significant medical error.[76]

The gastroenterology case discussed the challenges of reviewing a colleague's quality which is felt to be poor. Due diligence before forming partnerships with peers, as well as continuous monitoring of quality, can help prevent these situations, while improving quality overall. Managing patient-experience aspects of care delivered by peers can be particularly challenging. These issues were discussed in the emergency medicine case, where waiting on consultants may be one reason that delays and dangerous back-ups occur in the ED. The hospitalist case also demonstrated the challenge of monitoring the adequacy of communication between consultants and patients. Attention to these issues and the establishment of a patient-centered culture are crucial to improving quality amongst peers.

Population Health. In addition to improving quality within one's own practice and organization, physicians have a professional responsibility to improve quality for the population as a whole. This may include participating in the development of appropriate measures, sharing knowledge of quality improvement strategies, and conducting health services research. In the psychiatry and primary care cases, physicians felt that quality measures were imposed by external parties. These physicians should engage with external parties to find mutually agreeable quality measures that can apply to a broad population. There is a need for physicians to engage in measure development with their specialty societies, as a recent survey found that only 35 percent of these societies were currently developing measures.[93] If physicians do not participate in the process, they will be forced to accept measures that others propose.

Conclusion

This chapter discussed gaps in quality in the U.S. health care system and strategies to improve quality. The focus on quality improvement is a major shift away from traditional physician autonomy to a system of transparency and accountability. Physicians have a professional responsibility to improve quality for their own patients, across their organization, and for the population as a whole. In addition to professional responsibilities, with the increase in pay-for-performance incentives, quality ratings, and the high costs of poor quality, physicians who do not actively engage in quality improvement activities will likely lose patients, receive lower payments, face lawsuits, and risk exclusion from health systems.

David Nash, M.D., M.B.A.
Dr. Raymond C. and Doris N. Grandon Professor of Health Policy
Dean, Jefferson School of Health Policy and Population Health
Thomas Jefferson University

REFERENCES

1. AQA Web site. www.aqaalliance.org. Accessed June 24, 2008.
2. National Heart, Lung, and Blood Institute. National Institutes of Health. Third report of the national cholesterol education program (NCEP) expert panel on detection, evaluation, and treatment of high blood cholesterol in adults (adult treatment panel III); Publication no. 01–3670. May 2001.
3. Grundy S.M., Cleeman J.I., Merz C.N., et al. Implications of recent clinical trials for the national cholesterol education program adult treatment panel III guidelines. *J Am Coll Cardiol.* 2004;**44**(3):720–732.
4. Flynn J., Booth B., Portelli R. Professionalism and the quality framework. *Aust Fam Physician.* 2007;**36**(1–2):16–18.
5. Brennan T.A., Rothman D.J., Blank L., et al. Health industry practices that create conflicts of interest: A policy proposal for academic medical centers. *JAMA.* 2006;**295**(4):429–433.
6. McGlynn E.A., Asch S.M., Adams J., et al. The quality of health care delivered to adults in the United States. *N Engl J Med.* 2003;**348**(26):2635–2645.
7. Federman A.D., Adams A.S., Ross-Degnan D., Soumerai S.B., Ayanian J.Z. Supplemental insurance and use of effective cardiovascular drugs among elderly Medicare beneficiaries with coronary heart disease. *JAMA.* 2001;**286**(14):1732–1739.
8. Brown L.C., Johnson J.A., Majumdar S.R., Tsuyuki R.T., McAlister F.A. Evidence of suboptimal management of cardiovascular risk in patients with type 2 diabetes mellitus and symptomatic atherosclerosis. *CMAJ.* 2004;**171**(10):1189–1192.
9. National Committee for Quality Assurance. The State of Health Care Quality, 2005. ACQA Web site. http://web.ncqa.org/tabid/447/ItemId/741/Default.aspx. Accessed July 31, 2008.
10. Majumdar S.R., Lipton H.L., Soumerai S.B. Evaluating and improving physician prescribing. In: Strom B., ed. *Pharmacoepidemiology.* New York: John Wiley and Sons; 2005:419–438.
11. Jamtvedt G., Young J.M., Kristoffersen D.T., O'Brien M.A.,Oxman A.D. Audit and feedback: Effects on professional practice and health care outcomes. *Cochrane Database Syst Rev.* 2006;(**2**)(2):CD000259.
12. Soumerai S.B., Avorn J. Principles of educational outreach ("academic detailing") to improve clinical decision making. *JAMA.* 1990;**263**(4):549–556.
13. Thomson O'Brien M.A., Oxman A.D., Haynes R.B., Davis D.A., Freemantle N., Harvey E.L. Local opinion leaders: Effects on professional practice and health care outcomes. *Cochrane Database Syst Rev.* 2000;(**2**)(2):CD000125.
14. Bates D.W., Gawande A.A. Improving safety with information technology. *N Engl J Med.* 2003;**348**(25):2526–2534.
15. Planas R.I. *Museu Picasso: Guide Français.* Barcelona: Ajuntament de Barcelona, Institut; 1998.
16. Institute of Medicine. *Crossing the Quality Chasm: A New Health System for the 21st Century.* Washington, D.C.: National Academy Press; 2000.

17. Choudhry N.K., Fletcher R.H., Soumerai S.B. Systematic review: The relationship between clinical experience and quality of health care. *Ann Intern Med.* 2005;**142**(4):260–273.

18. Chassin M.R., Galvin R.W. The urgent need to improve health care quality: Institute of Medicine national roundtable on health care quality. *JAMA.* 1998;**280**(11): 1000–1005.

19. ABIM. Foundation. American Board of Internal Medicine, ACP-ASIM Foundation. American College of Physicians-American Society of Internal Medicine, European Federation of Internal Medicine. Medical professionalism in the new millennium: A physician charter. *Ann Intern Med.* 2002;**136**(3):243–246.

20. Institute of Medicine. *Performance Measurement: Accelerating Improvement.* Washington, D.C.: National Academy Press; 2004.

21. Baron R.J. Personal metrics for practice – how'm I doing? *N Engl J Med.* 2005;**353**(19):1992–1993.

22. Brennan T.A. Recertification for internists – one "grandfather's" experience. *N Engl J Med.* 2005;**353**(19):1989–1992.

23. Weisz G. *Divide and Conquer: A Comparative History of Medical Specialization* New York: Oxford University Press; 2005.

24. Stevens R. *American Medicine and the Public Interest.* New Haven: Yale University Press; 1971.

25. Ludmerer K.M. *Time to Heal: American Medical Education from the Turn of the Century to the Era of Managed Care* New York: Oxford University Press; 1999.

26. Ludmerer K.M. Learning to heal: The development of American medical education. 1985.

27. Angell M. *The Truth about the Drug Companies: How They Deceive Us and What to Do about It.* New York: Random House; 2004.

28. Kassirer J.P. *On the Take: How Medicine's Complicity with Big Business Can Endanger Your Health* New York: Oxford University Press; 2004.

29. Relman A.S. Assessment and accountability: The third revolution in medical care. *N Engl J Med.* 1988;**319**(18):1220–1222.

30. Kreimer S. Patient safety. fragmented care heightens error risk for surgical patients. *Hosp Health Netw.* 2007;**81**(6):32.

31. Suhonen R., Nenonen H., Laukka A., Valimaki M. Patients' informational needs and information received do not correspond in hospital. *J Clin Nurs.* 2005; **14**(10):1167–1176.

32. Hofer T.P., Hayward R.A. Are bad outcomes from questionable clinical decisions preventable medical errors? A case of cascade iatrogenesis. *Ann Intern Med.* 2002;**137**(5 Part 1):327–333.

33. Boosting Care Transitions Resource Room. Society of Hospital Medicine Web site. http://www.hospitalmedicine.org/ResourceRoomRedesign/RR_CareTran sitions/CT_Home.cfm. Accessed July 23, 2008.

34. Astrup K., Olivarius Nde F. Frequency of spontaneously occurring postmenopausal bleeding in the general population. *Acta Obstet Gynecol Scand.* 2004; **83**(2):203–207.

35. MacMahon B. Overview of studies on endometrial cancer and other types of cancer in humans: Perspectives of an epidemiologist. *Semin Oncol.* 1997;**24**(1 Suppl. 1):S1–122-S1–39.

36. Goldstein R.B., Bree R.L., Benson C.B., et al. Evaluation of the woman with post-menopausal bleeding: Society of Radiologists in ultrasound-sponsored consensus conference statement. *J Ultrasound Med.* 2001;**20**(10):1025–1036.

37. van Doorn H.C., Opmeer B.C., Burger C.W., et al. Inadequate office endometrial sample requires further evaluation in women with postmenopausal bleeding and abnormal ultrasound results. *Int J Gynaecol Obstet.* 2007;**99**(2):100–104.

38. Fallowfield L., Jenkins V. Communicating sad, bad, and difficult news in medicine. *Lancet.* 2004;**363**(9405):312–319.

39. Farber N.J., Urban S.Y., Collier V.U., et al. The good news about giving bad news to patients. *J Gen Intern Med.* 2002;**17**(12):914–922.

40. Arnold L., Stern D.T. What is medical professionalism? In: Stern D.T., ed. *Measuring Medical Professionalism.* Oxford, England: Oxford University Press; 2006:15–37.

41. Pellegrino E.D. Nonabandonment: An old obligation revisited. *Ann Intern Med.* 1995;**122**(5):377–378.

42. Institute of Medicine. *Crossing the Quality Chasm.* Washington, D.C.: National Academy Press; 2007.

43. Lown B., Kalet A.L. Patient advocacy: The clinician's experience: Incorporating advocacy into the 20-minute medical encounter. In: Earp J.A., French E.A., Gilkey M.B., eds. *Patient Advocacy for Health Care Quality: Strategies for Achieving Patient-Centered Care.* Sudbury, MA: Jones and Bartlett; 2007.

44. Epstein R.M. Mindful practice. *JAMA.* 1999;**282**(9):833–839.

45. Blank L., Kimball H., McDonald W., et al. Medical professionalism in the new millennium: A physician charter 15 months later. *Ann Intern Med.* 2003;**138**(10):839–841.

46. Lazarus J.A., Sharfstein S. Ethics in Mangaged Care: *The Psychiatric Clinics of North America.* Vol. **23**.; 2000.

47. Lazarus J.A. *Ethics in Entering Private Practice, A Handbook for Phsychiatrists.* American Psychiatric Publishing Inc; 2005.

48. Lazarus J.A. *Ethical Issues in Divided Or Collaborative Treatment in Psychopharmacology and Psychotherapy.* Arlington, VA: American Psychiatric Press; 1999.

49. Eddy D.M. Performance measurement: Problems and solutions. *Health Aff (Millwood).* 1998;**17**(4):7–25.

50. Iserson K.V. Understanding the incomplete text: Interpreting the emergency department patient. *Am J Emerg Med.* 1992;**10**(4):361–363.

51. Adams J., Murray R., 3rd. The general approach to the difficult patient. *Emerg Med Clin North Am.* 1998;**16**(4):689–700.

52. Harrison D.W., Vissers R.J. The difficult patient. In: Marx J.A., ed. *Rosen's Emergency Medicine: Concepts and Clinical Practice.* 6th ed. New York: Mosby; 2006:2972–2982.

53. Waitzkin H. Doctor-patient communication. Clinical implications of social scientific research. *JAMA.* 1984;**252**(17):2441–2446.

54. Asplin B.R., Magid D.J., Rhodes K.V., Solberg L.I., Lurie N., Camargo C.A., Jr. A conceptual model of emergency department crowding. *Ann Emerg Med.* 2003;**42**(2):173–180.

55. Trotter G. The loyal physician: *Roycean ethics and the practice of medicine.* 1997.

56. American Medical Association. Principles of Medical Ethics. http://www.ama-assn.org/ama/pub/category/2512.html. Updated 2006. Accessed April 26, 2007.

57. Hussey P.S., Anderson G.F., Osborn R., et al. How does the quality of care compare in five countries? *Health Aff (Millwood).* 2004;**23**(3):89–99.

58. Reinhardt U.E., Hussey P.S., Anderson G.F. Cross-national comparisons of health systems using OECD data, 1999. *Health Aff (Millwood).* 2002;**21**(3): 169–181.

59. Nolte E., McKee C.M. Measuring the health of nations: Updating an earlier analysis. *Health Aff (Millwood).* 2008;**27**(1):58–71.

60. Mangione-Smith R., DeCristofaro A.H., Setodji C.M., et al. The quality of ambulatory care delivered to children in the United States. *N Engl J Med.* 2007;**357**(15): 1515–1523.

61. Institute of Medicine, ed. *Crossing the Quality Chasm.* Washington, D.C.: National Academy Press; 2001.

62. The Dartmouth Atlas of Healthcare. The Dartmouth Institute for Health Policy and Clinical Practice Web site. www.dartmouthatlas.org. Accessed January 28, 2008.

63. Rowe J.W. Pay-for-performance and accountability: Related themes in improving health care. *Ann Intern Med.* 2006;**145**(9):695–699.

64. Institute of Medicine. To err is human. 1999. http://www.iom.edu/Object.File/Master/4/117/ToErr-8pager.pdf. Accessed May 2, 2009.

65. Moskowitz E.J., Nash D.B. The quality and safety of ambulatory medical care: Current and future prospects. *Am J Med Qual.* 2007;**22**(4):274–288.

66. Fuhrmans V. Insurers stop paying for care linked to errors. *The Wall Street Journal.* 2008.

67. Martin J. Hospital-acquired Infections in Pennsylvania 2005 – News Release. Pennsylvania Health Care Cost Containment Council Web site. http://www.phc4.org/reports/hai/05/nr111406.htm. Updated 2006. Accessed January 28, 2008.

68. Shannon R.P., Patel B., Cummins D., Shannon A.H., Ganguli G., Lu Y. Economics of central line – associated bloodstream infections. *Am J Med Qual.* 2006;**21** (6 Suppl):7S-16S.

69. Peng M.M., Kurtz S., Johannes R.S. Adverse outcomes from hospital-acquired infection in Pennsylvania cannot be attributed to increased risk on admission. *Am J Med Qual.* 2006;**21**(6 Suppl):17S-28S.

70. Wennberg J.E., O'Connor A.M., Collins E.D., Weinstein J.N. Extending the P4P agenda, part 1: How Medicare can improve patient decision making and reduce unnecessary care. *Health Aff (Millwood).* 2007;**26**(6):1564–1574.

71. O'Connor A.M., Wennberg J.E., Legare F., et al. Toward the "tipping point": Decision aids and informed patient choice. *Health Aff (Millwood).* 2007;**26**(3): 716–725.

72. Holmboe E.S., Lipner R., Greiner A. Assessing quality of care: Knowledge matters. *JAMA*. 2008;**299**(3):338–340.

73. Waterman A.D., Garbutt J., Hazel E., et al. The emotional impact of medical errors on practicing physicians in the United States and Canada. *Jt Comm J Qual Patient Saf*. 2007;**33**(8):467–476.

74. Garbutt J., Waterman A.D., Kapp J.M., et al. Lost opportunities: How physicians communicate about medical errors. *Health Aff (Millwood)*. 2008;**27**(1): 246–255.

75. Kaldjian L.C., Jones E.W., Wu B.J., Forman-Hoffman V.L., Levi B.H., Rosenthal G.E. Reporting medical errors to improve patient safety: A survey of physicians in teaching hospitals. *Arch Intern Med*. 2008;**168**(1):40–46.

76. Campbell E.G., Regan S., Gruen R.L., et al. Professionalism in medicine: Results of a national survey of physicians. *Ann Intern Med*. 2007;**147**(11):795–802.

77. Jha A.K., Ferris T.G., Donelan K., et al. How common are electronic health records in the United States? A summary of the evidence. *Health Aff (Millwood)*. 2006;**25**(6):w496–507.

78. Office of the National Coordinator: Mission. Health Information Technology Web site. http://www.hhs.gov/healthit/onc/mission/. Accessed January 28, 2008.

79. Miller R.H., West C., Brown T.M., Sim I., Ganchoff C. The value of electronic health records in solo or small group practices. *Health Aff (Millwood)*. 2005; **24**(5):1127–1137.

80. Asch S.M., McGlynn E.A., Hogan M.M., et al. Comparison of quality of care for patients in the Veterans Health Administration and patients in a national sample. *Ann Intern Med*. 2004;**141**(12):938–945.

81. Jha A.K., Perlin J.B., Kizer K.W., Dudley R.A. Effect of the transformation of the Veterans Affairs health care system on the quality of care. *N Engl J Med*. 2003; **348**(22):2218–2227.

82. Pronovost P., Needham D., Berenholtz S., et al. An intervention to decrease catheter-related bloodstream infections in the ICU. *N Engl J Med*. 2006;**355**(26): 2725–2732.

83. Pham H.H., Ginsburg P.B., McKenzie K., Milstein A. Redesigning care delivery in response to a high-performance network: The Virginia Mason Medical Center. *Health Aff (Millwood)*. 2007;**26**(4):w532–44.

84. Institute for Healthcare Improvement. www.ihi.org. Accessed January 28, 2008.

85. Bradley E.H., Holmboe E.S., Mattera J.A., Roumanis S.A., Radford M.J., Krumholz H.M. The roles of senior management in quality improvement efforts: What are the key components? *J Healthc Manag*. 2003;**48**(1):15–28; discussion 29.

86. Carman J.M., Shortell S.M., Foster R.W., et al. Keys for successful implementation of total quality management in hospitals. *Health Care Manage Rev*. 1996; **21**(1):48–60.

87. Joshi M.S., Hines S.C. Getting the board on board: Engaging hospital boards in quality and patient safety. *Jt Comm J Qual Patient Saf*. 2006;**32**(4):179–187.

88. Weiner B.J., Alexander J.A., Baker L.C., Shortell S.M., Becker M. Quality improvement implementation and hospital performance on patient safety indicators. *Med Care Res Rev*. 2006;**63**(1):29–57.

89. Weiner B.J., Alexander J.A., Shortell S.M., Baker L.C., Becker M., Geppert J.J. Quality improvement implementation and hospital performance on quality indicators. *Health Serv Res.* 2006;**41**(2):307–334.

90. Clough J., Nash D.B.. Health care governance for quality and safety: The new agenda. *Am J Med Qual.* 2007;**22**(3):203–213.

91. Hansen-Turton T., Ryan S., Miller K., Counts M., Nash D.B. Convenient care clinics: The future of accessible health care. *Dis Manag.* 2007;**10**(2):61–73.

92. Valko G.P. Open access scheduling. In: Nash D.B., ed. *Practicing Medicine in the 21st Century.* Tampa, FL: American College of Physician Executives; 2006:243.

93. Ferris T.G., Vogeli C., Marder J., Sennett C.S., Campbell E.G. Physician specialty societies and the development of physician performance measures. *Health Aff (Millwood).* 2007;**26**(6):1712–1719.

Commitment to Maintaining Trust by Managing Conflicts of Interest

Cases and Commentaries

MANAGING CONFLICTS OF INTEREST – PRIMARY CARE

A family physician becomes increasingly frustrated with his medical practice. He notes that his income has decreased, relative to inflation, over the past twenty years. He also notes that the time he is able to spend with patients had decreased – now thirty minutes for new patients and about ten minutes for established patients. Two of his long-standing patients are also frustrated with his practice. They complain about the long wait to see him and the decreased time for the visit. Both of these patients suggest that the family physician consider starting a retainer or "boutique" medical practice. This type of practice would increase the physician's income by requiring patients to pay a retainer fee and would allow him to spend more time with his patients. The physician considers this change.

A Perspective from a Family Physician

Control of today's typical primary care practice has passed to third parties including Medicare, Medicaid, HMOs (health maintenance organizations), PPOs (preferred provider organizations), and employers since they, not patients, control the ever diminishing flow of funds to physicians and other providers of health care. Patients are churned, one problem at a time, with brief visits, to maximize ever shrinking third party per-visit revenue. After-hours and hospital care is shunted to the emergency department and to hospitalists. The former financial and personal rewards of practice are now replaced by frustration and bureaucracy. As a result, primary care, the indispensable backbone of our profession, is crumbling.[1] Concierge medicine is the rational reaction to these realities.

Rather than continuing to play the Medicare and managed care game the concierge doctor has returned to focusing on serving and pleasing patients.

Millions of patients are or would be happy to pay a premium for an attentive, available, consumer-focused primary physician. They are sincerely embarrassed by how little Medicare and insurance pay their doctor. When my own active patients were polled in 2005, 33 percent said they would gladly pay extra for such service, but most physicians have no mechanism to accommodate them.

Some doctors, often those who have not experienced the private practice environment, actually believe that such singular care would be unjust. Concierge physicians, in contrast, firmly believe that in America a mechanism must exist to serve patients seeking such singular care and that in fact such care could be the standard by which all primary care is judged. We further believe that it is possible for most Americans, regardless of income level, to eventually have this kind of "medical home." This is the care Americans say they want and it translates, we believe, into better outcomes.[2]

Retainer practice (also referred to as concierge medicine or direct practice) strongly resembles the "medical home" advocated by various academies and study groups.[3] Adequate funding is the key to any such design, but when that funding comes from third parties or government it tends eventually to become insufficient since control of the level of funding is determined by a third party payer uninvolved in the actual value transaction. And that third party payer fails to see the appropriate value. Therefore, concierge doctors believe the funding must come directly from patients. Only the actual consumer appreciates the real value of any service.

Retainer practice provides sufficient income to allow extended, same day, or next day visits with almost no waiting. It offers a rested, cheerful physician willing to be available 24/7 to this selected group of patients. All issues that concern the patient are covered at each visit, greatly reducing the number of visits necessary later. Care the physician was trained to deliver is actually done on site and at the time rather than deferred or referred due to lack of time or economics. Patients are followed by their own doctor when hospitalized. The patient's concerns, time, and convenience are paramount, not the insurance company's.

Once a physician concludes that he or she must make this transition, as did I, several ethical concerns must be addressed. The first issue is abandonment. In my own situation, the year of transition was instructive. My demographic files contained 7,000 verifiable patient names. I attended 1,500 different individual patients in the previous twelve months and 2,500 in the previous twenty-four months. All 7,000 patients in my files were offered participation in my redesigned practice and advised that the practice size, being dominantly geriatric, would be limited to 600.[4] By the launch date about 500 had enrolled, so clearly, and as expected, most patients chose not to join. I had clear obligations to those non-joining patients.

It was mandatory to identify several comparable doctors in the community willing to accept patients not joining the retainer practice. It was necessary to provide emergency care to all patients until such time as they were firmly established with that new doctor. Records must be transferred at no charge and smooth transition must be ensured.

The offer to join the retainer practice must be made to patients months in advance of launch date, free of undue pressure and with clear terms, conditions, and contracts. It must include usable information about alternatives, an effective system to assist in transition, and declination forms to sign for patients who choose not to join, linked to the smooth transfer of care to a new doctor.

Of course, thousands of patients, most in fact, never responded at all. When those patients later called, they had to be cared for until they were officially and smoothly directed elsewhere for follow up and future care. While abandonment is the most important concern, it is not the only ethical issue facing physicians launching or converting to retainer practice.

Critics of retainer medicine claim it removes doctors from the overall pool needed to care for everyone else. This is a false allegation. Concierge physicians usually have no trouble identifying comparable, local physicians willing to assume the care of non-joiners. Further, the actual number of concierge doctors is insignificant.[5] At this writing there are probably fewer than 2,000 concierge physicians nationwide while there are 900,000 doctors.

Furthermore, though some recently trained physicians do start retainer practices, most are rather senior. Many would have retired, had they not converted to a retainer model, leaving all their patients in need of a new physician. In contrast, once converted, the concierge doctor, though still quite busy, is usually very happy with practice and negative thoughts about the practice of medicine fade away.

In fact, I have never met a more positive group of physicians than at a concierge practice society meeting. They work only for patients, determine their own compensation, control the quality of their care and have a strong sense of professional fulfillment. They rarely think about early retirement. Thus, conversion to concierge medicine preserves these physicians in practice perhaps decades longer and may actually expand the pool.

Concierge medicine could serve most Americans. About 300,000 physicians now do primary care. That number of physicians could serve 240 million patients in an 800-patient retainer model, even without extenders. The fee to be in such a practice should be about $100 per month, often less. The majority of Americans can easily afford such a fee.

Charity care is an ethical issue. Typical retainer practices have about 10 percent charity cases. Most concierge doctors believe they have no absolute obligation to extend charity except in emergencies, but do so because they want to and can afford to. The AMA's statement on the ethics of retainer medicine,[6] as well as our professional society's statement on ethics[7] address this issue explicitly. Sadly, many primary care doctors in today's typical practices cannot afford to extend charity care at all for lack of time and fear of further economic damage.

In summary, retainer medicine, seen first in 1997, is growing slowly. It will further evolve to serve varied population groups as consumer-directed health care expands and empowers patients. Preliminary impressions suggest retainer or direct practice saves money by preventing and shortening hospitalizations, limiting ER visits and practice errors and providing exceptional preventive care.[2] Lives are probably saved and prolonged, but empirical studies are lacking. Research on the impact and efficacy of the concierge medicine issue is needed. I would argue that concierge medicine is an ethical mode of practice; indeed, it could well be the salvation of our now critically ill primary care system.

Thomas W. LaGrelius, M.D., FAAFP
President, Society for Innovative Medical Practice Design
Clinical Instructor of Family Medicine, USC Keck School of Medicine

A Perspective from a Primary Care Physician

Luxury or Concierge Primary Care: Background
Luxury care (also known as concierge care, retainer practice, and boutique medicine) has been flourishing over the last few years in the United States.[8-10] In such practices, patients are charged an average fee between $2,000 and $4,000. They may be indulged with perks such as valet parking, buffet meals, and massages.[8,9] Subspecialty referral appointments occur on the same day as the general physical exam. Vaccines in short supply elsewhere are readily available. Physicians are available by cell phone or pager year-round; some make house calls. Waiting times for an initial appointment are short, and patient–physician ratios are between 10 percent and 25 percent of typical managed care levels.[8-10]

Most luxury care patients are asymptomatic, fairly healthy, and of high socioeconomic status. They are disproportionately white men.[8,9] Ironically, lower socioeconomic status patients have the worst health outcomes and most need efficient, comprehensive health care.[8,9,11]

Luxury practice physicians make substantially more money, have smaller patient panels and care for fewer African-Americans, Hispanics, and Medicaid patients than non-luxury practice physicians.[5,8,9,12] Doctors who convert to a luxury practice keep an average of only 12 percent of their former patients.[5] Most concierge physicians conduct charity care, although the nature and amount of such care is unknown.[5]

Luxury practice doctors often cite the desire for greater autonomy and more independence in decision making, increased time to spend with their families or on altruistic endeavors, and the satisfaction of getting to know their patients more intimately. Such motivations are understandable, even laudable, and an unfortunate consequence of the current U.S. health care system. Even so, increased financial compensation is likely an important motivating factor for some concierge physicians.

Legal risks of operating luxury practices in the United States include violations of Medicare regulations, the False Claims Act, provider agreements with private insurance companies, state insurance laws, the anti-kickback statute and other laws prohibiting payments to induce patient referrals, and potential liability for the abandonment of existing patients. Some hospitals have used economic credentialing to deny hospital privileges to physicians practicing concierge care. Certain states have investigated the payment mechanisms of concierge practices; New Jersey and New York place limits on such practices.[8,9]

Luxury Care and the Erosion of Science and Medical Ethics

There is no evidence documenting a higher quality of care in concierge practices, and little data to support the clinical- or cost-effectiveness of many tests offered to their asymptomatic clients. Examples of such tests that are inappropriately used include percent body fat measurements, chest X-rays in smokers and non-smokers aged thirty-five and older to screen for lung cancer, electron-beam computed tomography (CT) scans and stress echocardiograms looking for evidence of coronary artery disease, and abdominal-pelvic ultrasounds to screen for ovarian or liver cancer.[8,9] Ironically, this over-testing occurs despite the well-documented under-utilization of validated, beneficial interventions in both uninsured and insured patients.[8,9,13] While clients pay for these procedures, technicians and equipment time are diverted to produce immediate results. Since patients jump the queue, tests may be delayed on other patients with more appropriate and urgent needs. Furthermore, certain tests, such as whole body CT scans to screen for subclinical malignancies, expose patients to dangerous levels of carcinogenic radiation.[14]

False-positive results may lead to further unnecessary investigations, additional costs and anxiety (for patients), and increased profits (for physicians). True-positive results can lead to the over-diagnosis of conditions that would not have become clinically significant, resulting in further unnecessary (and potentially harmful) interventions and possibly impairing future insurability. The use of clinically unjustifiable tests erodes the scientific underpinnings of medical practice and runs counter to physicians' ethical obligations to responsibly manage health care resources.

The general public contributes substantially, through state and federal taxes, to the education and training of new physicians. Even so, many physicians who staff luxury primary care clinics limit their practices to the wealthiest fraction of our citizenry.[8,9] Given their investment in the training of physicians, the public might object to physicians limiting their practices to the wealthy or refusing to care for Medicaid or Medicare patients. On the other hand, doctors might justify limiting their practices to the wealthy by claiming a need to repay large educational debts or the right to determine the nature of their practices.

The trend toward luxury primary care has been occurring at a time of increasing injustice in health care in the United States and worldwide, and during a period of increasing dissatisfaction and cynicism among patients, practicing physicians, and trainees.[8,9] In 2007, 45 million Americans lacked health insurance. Millions more are underinsured, remain in dead-end jobs to maintain their health insurance, or go without needed prescriptions because of skyrocketing drug prices. The proportion of physicians providing charity care has declined over the last decade.[15] The development of luxury care has diverted attention from these issues without improving health outcomes at the population level.

Despite spending a larger proportion of its gross domestic product on health care than any other industrialized nation, U.S. population health outcomes compare unfavorably.[8,9,11,13] Disparities have grown in wealth, access to care, and morbidity and mortality between rich and poor and whites and non-whites.[8,9,11,13] Basic preventive services at recommended frequencies are commonly missed or delayed owing to time and financial constraints.[8,9,11,13] Some doctors offer varied levels of testing and treatment based on patients' abilities to pay. Luxury care will likely worsen these problems.

Medical schools and professional societies have been relatively quiet on the subject of luxury primary care, no doubt in part to avoid drawing attention to their support of profitable enterprises. To compete financially, many academic medical centers have established luxury primary care clinics. Little is known about the participation of medical students and residents in such clinics, start-up costs, degree of profitability, or whether financial resources from these clinics are diverted to indigent care or educational programs.[8,9] Given widespread disparities in health, wealth and access to care, as well as growing cynicism and dissatisfaction with medicine among trainees, the promotion by academic centers of an overt two-tiered system of care which exacerbates inequities and injustice erodes fundamental ethical principles of medicine such as equity and justice.

Conclusions

While I appreciate the concerns of the physician in this vignette, I suggest other ways he might enhance his career satisfaction, such as teaching, considering the financial and time benefits of coordinating care with a nurse practitioner and/or physician's assistant, and political activism (along with his patients) to change those aspects of medical practice which he finds troubling. More broadly, the medical profession should divert its intellectual and financial resources away from luxury care and toward more equitable and just programs designed to promote individual, community, and global health. The public and its legislators should in turn provide adequate funds to facilitate these efforts.

Martin Donohoe, M.D.
Department of Community Health
Portland State University

MANAGING CONFLICTS OF INTEREST – GENERAL INTERNAL MEDICINE

A patient with a history of coronary artery disease, congestive heart failure, hyperlipidemia, and without a prescription plan expresses concerns to his family physician about difficulty affording medications. In particular, the patient had difficulty paying for the simvistatin-ezetimibe (Vytorin), telmisartan (Micardis), and nebivolol (Bystolic) that was recently prescribed. The patient also comments about the two drug representatives that he saw in the office a few minutes earlier, the drug-sponsored pens that the physician is using, and the drug-company sponsored clock and calendar that are in the examination room.

A Perspective from an Internist

Clinical Background

The medical patient enters the physician's office in an era when there are new, highly effective drugs with solid evidence of life-saving and life-improving benefits such as the statin for primary or secondary prevention of myocardial infarction, and the beta-blocker and angiotensin enzyme inhibitor for the patient's congestive heart failure. The benefits of new drugs to the patient have changed forever the devastating impact of many high impact diseases such as congestive heart failure, diabetes, asthma, and rheumatoid arthritis. However, the "class" benefits of such exciting drugs may or may not apply to every newly patented, expensive product within that class. The newer drug is almost always more expensive than the older drugs, often with surprisingly less added value over the drug whose patent protection expires, or a much less expensive drug within the same class of medications.

Professionalism Considerations

This is a much more complex era which the young physician enters today. The young physician dons the white coat, completes his or her professional training and deservedly or not becomes a moral agent in the lives of their patient. One might propose that it is the magic of the white coat that confers this power, or simply the expectations generated in the profession as a whole; but in either case the patient trusts the physician to be guileless, dependable, and to always put their interest first.[16] This trust arrives through grace – whether deserved or not. The power of that trust extends a halo of endorsement, sometimes unwittingly, to all we do, say, wear, or associate with as a physician. It is the presence of the pharmaceutical representative whose understandable interest is selling a product and advertising in this milieu which by definition creates a conflict.

Why is there such interest in getting advertising in front of physicians, in the office and directly to the patient? There were forty blockbuster newly released drugs in 2002 which accounted for combined global sales of $89.3 billion for eleven companies. Of 415 of these new blockbuster drug products released between 1998 and 2002, for which pens, pads, clocks and free samples abound, fewer than one-third were new molecules, and only 14 percent were judged by the FDA to be "a significant improvement" over older and sometimes significantly less expensive drugs. These in essence were "me too" drugs that provide similar benefits at greater costs, and often without formulary or generic benefits.[17] The patient, however, often enters that office without a perceived need for the drug, and without a demand actually to consume that drug in an economic market. The economics of free samples and new drug advertising is not surprisingly complex, but at times it is a bit troubling in its transparency.

The physician has the power to create a demand, by recommending a particular drug as beneficial or even essential to the patient's welfare. Nonetheless, when the physician recommends a specific drug, he or she brings the weight of the physician's moral agency and the unspent trust invested by the patient to that recommendation. Often the young physician may be unaware of that power which he or she exerts by their very presence and implied endorsement with certain products. It seems ironic that even the unspoken endorsement of a drug on a ballpoint pen, a notepad, or a clock wields that same power.

A survey of medical students' attitudes toward the influence that pharmaceutical marketing might have through gifts, meals, pens, or calendars indicates a naiveté in understanding influence that advertising might have on practice patterns. The results disclose that the students think that influence would be bad, but they generally over-estimate their ability to resist such influences (Shashaty E, Fisher C, Chiazzi L, Georgetown University – unpublished). Most other data, as outlined in the commentary by Dana, would also suggest this lack of accurate insight, and support the concept that the influence of such contact is more subtle and effective on the judgment of the physician than most might think. Importantly, these data do not deal with the unwitting influence that association with such marketing might have on our patients without our insight.

Opinion

This case illustrates that the very presence of such advertisement in our practice environment wraps these products in that sacred cloak of patient trust – often unwittingly. The physician must respect the influence that moral agency of the profession brings. This halo of trust can empower even those commercial influences that fall within the environment of practice.[18]

There will fortunately continue to be new drugs with revolutionary benefits to those patients, and those drugs as they emerge will likely be expensive with or without co-pay prescription plans. We must, as physicians, remain aware of the evidence and foundation for their rational and cost-effective use. Many institutions have extended this logic to the free samples we distribute by using resources to buy generic and cost-effective bioequivalent drugs that can be sustained independently of the sampling/retail cycle. As educators, we must give young physicians the evidence-based tools to use to provide the newest highly effective therapies based on evidence, not marketing. We must never lose sight of the profound influence that our presence, our endorsement, and our prescription of therapies will have on our trusting patients. We must be aware of the accurate, ethical, and strategic use of this power, even unwittingly, in the best interest of the patient's welfare.

Stephen Ray Mitchell, M.D., FACP
Dean for Medical Education
Georgetown School of Medicine

A Perspective from a Psychologist

This physician's treatment choices appear to be driven more by marketing than by research, to the patient's detriment. Inexpensive diuretics and beta-blockers are effective first-line treatments for hypertension and heart failure. However, this physician favors more expensive, non-generic angiotensin receptor blockers and beta-blockers. For primary care physicians treating hypertension, this prescription practice has been linked to contact with pharmaceutical representatives.[19] Unfortunately, the problematic influence of pharmaceutical representatives is not limited to hypertensive therapy.

Contact with pharmaceutical representatives and acceptance of gifts are generally associated with costly and inappropriate treatment choices.[20]

Some physicians may take umbrage at the suggestion that their objectivity can be compromised by accepting such trinkets as clocks, calendars, and pens. Keep in mind, however, that pharmaceutical companies are profit-minded entities and that the pharmaceutical industry in the United States has enjoyed great success. The sheer ubiquity of these trinkets strongly suggests that they do influence prescribing behavior. Further, there are other reasons why gifts can be influential besides compromised integrity.

Ample social science research has shown that decision makers often fall prey to an unwitting and unintended self-serving bias.[21] Individuals consistently rate themselves above average on a variety of tasks;[22] for instance, one study found that 90 percent of automobile drivers rated themselves above average.[23] When people allocate wages for effort they inevitably gravitate toward rules that favor themselves.[24] This bias persists even when it conflicts with a person's self-interest. For example, participants in simulated legal disputes cannot adopt an objective view of a fair settlement amount when they know their role of plaintiff or defendant before (but not after) reading the case materials.[25] As a result, they suffer costly failures to settle. This bias is so insidious that when people are taught about it, they tend to recognize it in others, but not themselves.[25,26] Thus, even well-intentioned individuals may be inclined to reach conclusions (such as what therapy is best) that favor their self-interest, despite believing that they do not. Small gifts can be sufficient to induce this self-serving bias, as well as implicit pressures to reciprocate, so that even pens cannot be considered harmless.[27]

Alternatively, this physician may simply be unaware of the subtle influence of marketing. Many of us greatly underestimate the influence of marketing on our choices. This physician may believe that the support for choosing these therapies comes from research literature or clinical experience, when it actually comes from marketing sources and effective branding.[28] These basic facts of human cognition are cause to avoid gratuitous contact with industry, regardless of how objective or ethical physicians feel themselves to be.

Even if this physician's contact with pharmaceutical representatives has no negative impact on prescribing, he or she should consider the impact that these relationships have on patient trust. The patient is already concerned about the costs of his treatment and has made it a point to mention the gifts and the presence of the representatives. Articles in popular press outlets have highlighted some of the worst abuses and raised awareness of the issues surrounding gifts from industry. This issue could damage patient trust and, combined with financial hardship, could ultimately lead to dangerous non-compliance. These interactions are not worth the cost of negative patient perceptions. Objectivity must be maintained not only in fact, but also in appearance.

Jason Dana, Ph.D.
Assistant Professor, Department of Psychology
University of Pennsylvania

Editor's note: As of 2008, the Pharmaceutical Research and Manufacturers of America, the industry trade group that represents pharmaceutical companies in the United States, recommended that pharmaceutical companies not give to physicians "non-educational items" such as pens, note pads, mugs, and similar reminder items with company of product logos.

MANAGING CONFLICTS OF INTEREST – OBSTETRICS AND GYNECOLOGY

A gynecologist considers how to increase the revenue of her practice and hires a marketing consultant. The consultant recommends that she advertise her practice through mass mailings, the yellow pages, and the Internet. The consultant also recommends that the doctor consider offering Botox injections and selling health care products in the office. The gynecologist is concerned about the ethics of these proposals.

A Perspective from an Obstetrician and Gynecologist

Professionalism Considerations

There is no question that it is becoming difficult to sustain a private practice in gynecology. More and more patients are enrolled in some form of "managed" care. Insurance companies, exempt from antitrust legislation, continue to lower reimbursements while office overhead continues to rise. It is no wonder that physicians are looking for ways to increase their practice income. So when a consultant suggests we advertise our practice, sell products, and learn cosmetic procedures such as Botox how do we determine what is ethical?

The American Medical Association clearly states that advertising is ethical as long as it is truthful and not misleading by commission or omission.[29] Thus an advertisement that states a physician's background and interests is ethical. Claims of special expertise or a unique skill could be misleading if they falsely imply that the physician is the only one providing a skill that is readily available in the geographic area. Testimonials can be misleading if they imply a result that is not typical of what can be expected. Nevertheless, there is nothing unethical about tasteful advertising.

The ethics of product sales by gynecologists has also been well defined by the American College of Obstetrics and Gynecology.[30] They clearly state "Sale or promotion of products by physicians to their patients is unethical, with some exceptions . . . "

Let's first look at the exceptions. It is ethical to sell drugs or devices that must be administered by the physician. Such examples would be the insertion of an intrauterine contraceptive device, or administration of a vaccine. In these situations it is ethical to charge for the direct cost of the device or medication, and the overhead costs of ordering, storing, and administering the product. Similarly it is reasonable to supply products, at cost plus overhead, that are difficult to obtain elsewhere. An example of such would be a pessary for uterine prolapse, which is not stocked in pharmacies and can be difficult for a patient to order directly. There are other minor exceptions that are not relevant to this discussion.

In contrast to the above examples, the sale of health care products poses a clear conflict of interest. The primary purpose of selling these products is to increase the income of the physician rather than to provide a medically indicated service. The fact that the physician is selling a product also implies that she has selected the product and is endorsing it. This is in conflict with the physician's fiduciary duty to the patient, which requires that she puts the best interest of the patient before her own financial gain. While it is easy to rationalize that it is more convenient for the patient to obtain products from the physician than having to go to a pharmacy, the conflict of interest clearly overrides any gain in convenience.

Botox injection is just one of many cosmetic procedures being marketed to gynecologists. Ads for courses in liposuction, skin resurfacing, cosmetic breast surgery, "vaginal rejuvenation" and assorted other cosmetic procedures fill the classified ad sections of gynecologic publications. The one element common to all of these treatments are that they are paid "cash" rather than by insurance. I could not, however, find any offerings for courses in general skin diseases, how to do breast biopsies, or similar treatments that are reimbursed by insurance. Is it ethical for a gynecologist to decide on what surgical procedures to learn based solely on reimbursement?

With appropriate training most medical school graduates have the potential to learn dermatology, plastic surgery, and even cardiac or neurosurgery. Although it is questionable whether a weekend course is adequate for many of these procedures, I will assume for the sake of argument that our gynecologist is reasonably trained in Botox injection. Since she is also running a full-time practice in gynecology, it is questionable, however, whether she will develop and maintain the skill level of someone whose sole practice is doing cosmetic procedures.

Even more troublesome is the major conflict of interest between her responsibility to the patient and her own financial gain. Today cosmetic procedures are a commodity. Advertisements for cosmetic surgery are all around us. As the trend toward directing medical practices away from treating medical problems to cosmetic surgery continues, it is becoming increasingly more difficult to find a dermatologist who will care for skin diseases, or to find a plastic surgeon who will do non-cosmetic reconstructive surgery.

Opinion

A common argument for the gynecologist to do cosmetic procedures is that if the patient wants it then the gynecologist might as well be the one to do it. But the gynecologist should be the one to provide impartial advice to the patient. Television bombards women with plastic surgery promotion, as does the Internet and printed media. Many women desire cosmetic surgery because they mistakenly believe they are not normal, or that their life will be improved if they have larger breasts, smaller labia, or fewer wrinkles. Women are in a more vulnerable position with the gynecologist than with a cosmetic surgeon, as the gynecologist has usually developed a physician–patient relationship based on intimate trust, while the plastic surgeon is "selling" a procedure. It is far less lucrative to take the time to explain to patients the wide variation in normal anatomy or to try to track down the real cause of low self-esteem than it is to schedule the patient for a cosmetic procedure. The mere announcement by the gynecologist that she is doing these procedures legitimizes and promotes them. The fact that she does Botox injections makes a statement that she endorses them. She will make hundreds of dollars if she does the Botox, but will not be reimbursed at all if she discussed the normal aging process and help her patient to accept it. If this isn't a conflict of interest I don't know what is!

Paul D. Indman, M.D.
Private Practice, Gynecology
Los Gatos, CA

A Perspective from an Attorney and Ethicist

The marketing consultant in this case has raised several very different ethical issues for the gynecologist – but each of the consultant's recommendations may, if the doctor takes it, have a significant impact on the trusting relationship she currently enjoys with her patients.

First, there is the issue of advertising. In the United States, our First Amendment law protects freedom of commercial expression, and antitrust law largely prevents professional associations from controlling (as they once did) professionals' choices of advertising methods and approaches. The law and professional ethics rules basically demand only that advertising be truthful and non-deceptive; they say nothing about taste. Nonetheless, the gynecologist ought to think carefully about the way she wants to present herself and her practice to the public. Her methods of advertising will affect the public's view of her and her motives. A crass or aggressive advertisement may be attention grabbing, but may also make her seem less trustworthy. She should choose her words and images with care, as they may in some small way affect the public's trust not only in her, but in physicians more generally.

Second, there is a nest of ethical issues connected with the consultant's recommendation that she offer Botox injections as a way to earn extra money. The extensive debate about the ethics of offering enhancement therapies, as opposed to medical treatments, is left aside here; significant ethical questions arise even if we assume that offering enhancements to those who want them is ethically fine. One question is that of competence: Does she understand how to administer Botox in a safe and effective way? Or can she find adequate professional training in its administration, so that she can meet her ethical duty of competence? Can she inform her patients adequately of its risks and benefits, so that their decisions will be well informed? Additionally, there is the difficult question of marketing the new service – which is not an ordinary part of gynecological practice – to her existing patients. It may be difficult, or even offensive, to raise the option of cosmetic treatment with patients who haven't thought about it before, and who certainly aren't expecting their gynecologist to broach the question. Wall posters or information sheets in the waiting room may avoid the awkward conversation, but the gynecologist has to think carefully about the impression such marketing materials might make. What effect will her offering a cosmetic procedure have on her patients' understanding of her goals and trustworthiness as a physician? Rightly or wrongly, Botox is associated with "celebrity medicine." Is this an association she wants to court in her practice?

Finally, there is the question of selling products to patients. Such sales can undermine the patient-physician relationship in several ways. The aim of selling products to the patient creates an intrinsic conflict of interest. When the physician is selling her own medical skills to the patient, that sale is in the physician's financial interest, but also – if the physician is doing her job correctly – in the patient's best medical interest. In contrast, when a physician is selling a product to a patient that the patient could purchase elsewhere, the physician's interest in the sale and the patient's interests are often out of alignment. A patient who is overawed by the physician's authority may be misled into making a purchase; a patient may feel forced into making a purchase in order not to undermine her relationship with the physician. For these reasons and more, the American Medical Association's Council on Ethical and Judicial Affairs has issued two ethics opinions designed to sharply curtail the sale of products to patients.[31] The first opinion (Opinion 8.062, "Sale of Non-Health Related Goods from Physicians' Offices") is a general prohibition on the sale by physicians to their patients of non-health-related goods; it includes a narrow exception designed to permit occasional in-office sales of such items as Girl Scout cookies or raffle tickets for some worthy local cause. The second opinion (Opinion 8.063, "Sale of Health-Related Products from Physicians' Offices") deals with sale or endorsement of health-related goods by physicians (e.g., skin creams by dermatologists, or bicycle helmets by pediatricians). That opinion insists that physicians sell only health-related goods whose health benefits are well established scientifically; that they sell only products that address their patients' immediate and pressing health needs; and that they fully disclose their financial interests in the sale of any products. Further provisions deal with the free distributions of goods from physician's offices, and prohibit physician participation in exclusive health-product distributorships. These opinions – as well as, importantly, the reports on which they are based, and which contain all the underlying arguments about the threat posed by sales of goods to the trust relationship between physician and patient – are available at the AMA's website.[31] The gynecologist should read these opinions and reports carefully, and think about the importance of maintaining her patients' trust.

Stephen Latham, J.D., Ph.D.
Deputy Director, Yale's Interdisciplinary Center for Bioethics
Yale University

MANAGING CONFLICTS OF INTEREST – PEDIATRICS

A pediatrician in private practice agrees to participate in a Phase III study of a new class of antibiotics for the treatment of acute otitis media conducted by a contract research organization. It is a randomized, double-blind study whose active control is azithromycin. The pharmaceutical company is seeking to enroll 2,000 children between the ages of six and seventy-two months. The primary outcome measures include clinical cure at the posttherapy visit. Physicians will be paid $100 for each subject enrolled and an additional $300 for each subject who completes the study and for whom "clean" data are submitted. The consent form does not disclose these payments. The study has been approved by an independent Institutional Review Board (IRB). The pediatrician is excited to participate in clinical research and earn extra money to defray her student loans.

Several weeks later, the pediatrician sees a toddler whose mother reports that he has been warm to the touch and pulling on his right ear since the previous night. The physician mentions the study to her and she says that she would be happy to take part if that is what is best for her son. While looking into the child's ear, the pediatrician is not sure whether the tympanic membrane is bulging.

A Perspective from a Pediatrician

Clinical Background

An important aspect of medical professionalism is a commitment to scientific knowledge.[32] As clinical trials are increasingly being performed outside of academic medical centers, physicians in private practice have the opportunity to promote research. Fulfilling this component of professional obligations requires a basic understanding of study design, statistics, research ethics, and the research topic.[33] In this vignette, the research is a Phase III active control study of treatment for acute otitis media. In terms of study design, one should be able to differentiate between Phase III and Phase IV trials. If this was a Phase IV, post-marketing surveillance trial, one would need to consider whether it was primarily being conducted to monitor side effects or to increase market share. Ethically, potential investigators would need to confirm that the publication of results of the study would not be unduly delayed or obstructed. In terms of the research topic, one might question the use of azithromycin as the control. If an antibiotic is used, the American Academy of Pediatrics recommends high-dose amoxicillin. Azithromycin is only recommended as the initial antibiotic in children with type I hypersensitivity reactions to amoxicillin.[34]

Professionalism Considerations

The commitment to scientific knowledge may conflict with the primacy of patient welfare. Parents may not understand the difference between research and clinical care or they may feel obligated to participate. The mother's response in this case may suggest such a misunderstanding. She may mistakenly interpret the study drug as cutting-edge treatment rather than one of unproven efficacy. Moreover, one might question whether the patient benefits from participation, given effective treatments for acute otitis media already exist. In addition to making the experimental nature of the treatment clear, the description of the study should reinforce that participation or lack of participation will not affect future care. Having someone other than the treating physician review the consent document with potential subjects may protect against such misunderstandings.

Financial incentives may represent additional sources of conflict. On the one hand, clinicians should not be expected to bear the cost of research. They may legitimately be compensated for the costs of participation in research, consistent with their usual professional fees. (Additional costs of study participation should not be billed to the patients or their insurance companies either.) On the other hand, fees paid to physicians simply for referring patients to clinical trials are unethical because such activity requires little additional effort beyond routine clinical care. Bonuses for fulfilling quotas within a deadline would also be inappropriate. Physicians should also not accept excessive fees that potentially generate a conflict between their economic self-interest and the primacy of patient welfare or the commitment to scientific knowledge. In this case, might the promise of remuneration influence, consciously or unconsciously, the physician's diagnosis of otitis media in marginal cases? While it may be difficult to determine when such payments become an undue incentive, clearly excessive payments may constitute kickbacks and be illegal.[35] (Alternative financial conflicts, not illustrated by this vignette, include owning stock in the company developing the medication or holding the patent on the device or agent being tested.)

Medical professionalism entails a commitment to maintaining trust by managing conflicts of interest. One way in which such conflicts can be addressed is disclosure, not only to oversight bodies, but also to subjects. Disclosure is congruent with the fundamental principle of patient autonomy and the commitment to honesty with patients. In this case, disclosure of the financial arrangements would allow potential subjects to consider such payments in their decision making. Disclosure, however, may not provide sufficient protection. In their interviews of patients enrolled in cancer trials, Hampson and colleagues found concerns about health superseded worries about financial ties between researchers and drug companies. They also found that a large majority of patients were confident about the existence of an oversight system.[36] These findings suggest that, in addition to requiring disclosure, IRBs could attempt to limit the payment to reimbursement for the costs of study participation and seek to prohibit clearly excessive payment. Potential conflicts of interest might also be managed by prohibiting direct, personal payment in favor of other payment mechanisms.

Opinion

Physicians have multiple professional responsibilities and these may, at times, conflict. The primacy of patient welfare is a fundamental principle which personal interests should not compromise. Both personal virtue and institutional oversight are necessary to protect patient welfare and maintain the public's trust in the medical profession.

Armand Antommaria, M.D., Ph.D.
Assistant Professor of Pediatrics
University of Utah School of Medicine

A Perspective from a Parent

I have come to my pediatrician's office having been up most of the night with my two-year-old son who has been fussy and warm to the touch. I tried treating him with Tylenol but he was still not himself this morning. I think that my son probably has an ear infection. I have read that sometimes doctors do not like to give antibiotics for ear infections, preferring to wait to see if the symptoms will go away without treatment. I wonder if I should wait to see if he will get better without medicine but my pediatrician brings up the possibility of participating in this study. I know there have been some concerns about new strains of "bugs" and I am concerned about not having new drugs to treat them.

As I consider whether I should be part of this study, my highest priority is that my son not suffer any longer than necessary. I would not want to participate in the research if the test medicine is less effective or if it could possibly risk his health. The proposed treatment sounds reasonable and, if my pediatrician thinks that it is safe and good care, I would be willing to participate. I have a few concerns, however.

My first concern is whether my doctor's judgment is affected by the compensation received from the company sponsoring the research. I understand that some doctors are paid to recruit patients for research studies. I have mixed emotions about this. While I would not expect my pediatrician to participate in research if it meant losing money, I might wonder about her real motivations if she is paid a lot. I would like to assume that, as a professional, my doctor is above that, but I also know that anyone can be tempted by monetary advantages. If she is making more than a standard amount for enrolling subjects in the study, I would want to know. I do not think that she should be prohibited from doing this, but it would make me think twice. I would hope that there is some form of oversight of this process, and I think it would be valuable to have parents like me participate in such an oversight process.

My second concern is about the financial costs of my participation in the study. I do not know if my insurance should be expected to cover the costs of the visit or if the pharmaceutical company will pay for it. For example, who is going to pay for today's visit? When I come back for the scheduled follow-up, will I be responsible for an additional co-pay? What if problems arise? The possibility of getting the medicine for free is appealing. I have also heard that sometimes participants are paid to take part in research studies. If my pediatrician is being paid, will my son and I be compensated for coming back?

While I had different plans when I came into the office, I am willing to consider participating in the study. I trust my doctor to recommend what she thinks is best for my son. I just want to make sure that he will not hurt any longer than he would otherwise. Finally, in making my decision, it is important that my rights as a parent and your responsibilities as a physician are understood.

Kathy Jensen
Salt Lake City, Utah

MANAGING CONFLICTS OF INTEREST – SURGERY

An orthopedic spine surgeon has had a long-standing relationship with a device manufacturer. He has participated in several clinical trials sponsored through this company and has received honoraria for work through his role on the company's scientific advisory board and their sponsored continuing medical education (CME). Although he regularly completes disclosure forms when preparing for talks or writing publications, he is increasingly concerned about his conflict of interest with this work, particularly after attending a recent talk on conflicts of interest at the American Orthopedic Association annual meeting.

A Perspective from an Orthopedic Surgeon

Background

Interactions with industry are commonplace in all branches of medicine. These interactions constitute the basis for technology transfer and are key to future developments that are rapidly changing the nature of orthopedic surgery.[37] They may also spawn major conflicts of interest that are intimately tied to the actions and character of individual physicians and to the practices of the implant manufacturing industry.

In my own experience, I witnessed the development of an orthopedic implant through a number of stages. It begins as an idea conceived by a surgeon, often in collaboration with an engineer or a basic scientist. It is then developed by the team in a research environment and eventually may lead to a new material, a new design principle, or a specific new implant. At this juncture, the researchers typically discover that they cannot advance the project further without the participation of industry. A patent becomes an important tool. The protection afforded by the patent that grants inventors the right to prevent others from making, using, or selling their inventions is critical for the potential involvement of industry.[38] Eventually, the surgeon and his collaborators will enter into an agreement with an implant manufacturer.

Next, a development team is assembled where members of the industrial outfit work with the investigators in the design of the device and all the other elements necessary to bring it to the marketplace. In addition to the development of the implant, this work includes refining and standardizing surgical techniques, and designing the educational activities needed to train and instruct surgeons, operating room personnel, and others in the proper use of the device. There may also be clinical trials required for regulatory approval. At some point, the device may be approved by the regulatory agencies and will enter the marketplace. A licensing agreement generally involves a flow of royalties to the developers and to their home institution as well. Thus, substantial financial benefits may accrue to both, with resulting conflicts of interest.[39]

Professionalism Considerations

The developer surgeons are typically involved in almost all of the activities mentioned above. These practices are in my opinion appropriate although they can be extremely damaging in the absence of proper ethical behavior.

A number of questions can be raised regarding the orthopedic surgeon in this vignette. Is intellectual property involved in his interactions with industry? In all probability it is not, as he is neither the inventor nor the developer of the spinal implants. This surgeon, on the other hand, participates as a consultant in clinical trials, advisory boards, and CME activities, and uses the implants in his practice. His input can be valuable by providing feedback from his clinical experience and may also be constructive in the education of surgeons. He should be paid a consultant's fee for this work that is commensurate with the time and efforts invested.

As with the developer surgeons, ethical behavior of the surgeon collaborating with industry is critical. Is his judgment affected in any way by the financial benefits that result from his involvement with industry? Is there bias in the reporting of results at lectures or in his publications? If the answers to these questions are yes, then the impact of such bias can influence the use of the implants by the orthopedic community at large regardless of whether the benefits justify their selection. The appearance of bias may not always be the product of dishonesty. It is not uncommon for the developers or the early users of a device or surgical procedure to have better results than other surgeons simply because they are more familiar with the relevant principles and surgical technique. However, honest reporting of results and complications is to be expected and should be the guiding norm for every surgeon involved in these matters.

One could also ask if this surgeon is really functioning as a consultant or whether this is just a mechanism to help promote devices. Or of more concern, is this a way for the manufacturer to secure the almost exclusive use of these particular implants on his patients? These types of questions have led to an ongoing investigation by the Department of Justice of the relations between the orthopedic industry and its consulting surgeons.[40]

Implant manufacturers have developed a great deal of sophistication in their research, development, and manufacturing capabilities. Their research laboratories compete today with some of the best that academia has to offer. In partnership with academic entities they can produce materials, implants, and innovations to advance the state of the art and thus offer cures and solutions not possible otherwise.

At the same time, industry has developed sophisticated marketing capabilities. The ultimate fiduciary responsibility of these companies is to the stockholders and profit plays the major role. The ability to engage prominent surgeons as opinion leaders on behalf of their products is an important marketing tool. Thus, knowingly or unknowingly our spinal surgeon becomes a significant element in a company's marketing plan.

There are many policies designed to deal with conflicts of interest. The American Medical Association, the American Academy of Orthopedic Surgeons, the individual academic institutions, the scientific journals, industry, the federal government, all have developed specific guidelines. These policies and documents set up a framework that should have the capacity to prevent or resolve most conflicts of interest. However, from a practical viewpoint, problems still arise with disturbing frequency.[41]

Opinion

Intellectual honesty and ethical character are two critical qualities that can only be exercised by the individual physician and are difficult or impossible to legislate. The ideal model to follow is one that allows productive collaborations without the hint of real or perceived misconduct. Conflicts of interest can be prevented by the zealous application of the appropriate ethical practices. Our surgeon should engage in a critical review of his industry-related activities to understand the difference between what may be legitimate consulting or educational efforts in contrast to strategies used strictly to promote the utilization of the spinal implants. This should help him resolve his concerns and allow him to continue a productive and ethically justified collaboration.

Jorge Galante, M.D., DMSc
Professor, Department of Orthopedic Surgery
Rush University Medical Center

Another Perspective from an Orthopedic Surgeon

This industry routinely violated the anti-kickback statute by paying physicians for the purpose of exclusively using their products. Prior to our investigation, many orthopedic surgeons in this country made decisions predicated on how much money they could make – choosing which device to implant by going to the highest bidder. With these agreements in place, we expect doctors to make decisions based on what is in the best interests of their patients – not the best interests of their bank accounts.[42]

"U.S. Attorney Christopher Christie," September 28, 2007

The clinical relationship between patients and treating physicians rests on a foundation of trust.[43] Patients share sensitive information with physicians, rely on information provided by the physicians, and comply with treatment recommendations of their doctors. In turn, patients expect undivided loyalty. At a time when they are most vulnerable, anxious patients yearn to believe that their doctor is a caring professional, maintaining the well-being of patients ahead of self-interest or the interests of any third party.[43] Financial conflicts of interest risk breach of loyalty to patients.

The spine surgeon in our case is wondering about the potential for several conflicts of interest. Simply by having sufficient concern to attend a symposium on the topic, listening to the debate, and trying to apply the new knowledge to his own situation, our surgeon is already well on his way to successfully resolving his concerns. Like most physicians, he wants to do the right thing. Regardless of how far removed we sometimes may get from our ideals, there remains some of the original altruistic inspiration that led to a career in health care. It must be extremely rare that a practicing physician consciously deviates from established standards of medical research or clinical practice in order to satisfy personal financial gain; such fraudulent behavior is hard to hide and is not sustainable. The more dangerous threat to the values of our profession is ignorance or denial of the insidious ways in which self-interest can creep into the decisions we routinely make in our daily clinical practice.

True innovation in modern medicine is rare. Most products approved as new by regulatory agencies are minor modifications of drugs or devices already marketed.[44] In this context, real innovation deserves rich rewards. Innovators who see their novel ideas complete the prolonged, expensive, and complicated journey from concept to prototype to investigational device to approved device have duly earned their fair-market financial returns, no matter how exorbitant.[45] However, only a handful of orthopedic and neurosurgeons could claim such credit. Mostly, device manufacturers have learned to boost the egos of opinion leaders in local communities and recruit them to advance marketing goals, veiling financial rewards as scientific consulting activity.[46] These types of consulting arrangements with surgeons have been common. The agreements usually have not specified the nature of the required scientific work nor provide justification for disproportionately high payments. The U.S. Department of Justice in 2007 appropriately condemned these arrangements as nothing more than bribes to surgeons for using specific products.[42]

How could orthopedic surgeons go so far into unethical waters and stay there comfortably for so long? What did we as individual surgeons fail to see, and what did our self-policing professional organizations fail to point out? In hindsight, why did it take a criminal fraud investigation to make us realize the obvious?

The answers can be gleaned in part from social sciences research. Self-interest affects choices indirectly.[21] We have difficulty maintaining a neutral, objective perspective when we have a personal interest in a specific conclusion.[21] When we have a stake in reaching a particular outcome, we tend to weigh arguments in a way that favors that outcome.[21] Human frailty allows us to unconsciously succumb to self-interest, even when we know about it and are on alert against it.[21] In many situations, multiple notions of fairness may apply; we tend to favor those interpretations that serve our interests best.[21] Physicians tend to believe that our education and training give us control against bias, while at the same time we believe that colleagues around us with similar education and training remain susceptible to bias.[21]

The drug and device industry knows these human weaknesses well; their salespersons are forbidden from accepting gifts of any size while they themselves dole out payments, trips, and perks to highly educated physician clients absorbed in a sense of entitlement from inflated self-perception and paralyzed by unreal confidence in self-control over bias.

Although disclosing conflicts of interest can be one solution for dealing with such a challenge, disclosure can have perverse, unintended effects.[21] The goal of financial disclosure is to allow the audience to discount the received information by some amount proportional to the perceived intensity of the conflict. However, terminology used in disclosures is frequently vague. Without clarity, disclosure in scientific presentations can be portrayed as a burdensome obligation that, once completed, somehow removes risk of bias. The settlement agreement between the Justice Department and orthopedic device manufacturers requires that payments to consultants also be disclosed to their patients,[42] but patients' expectations of clinical fidelity may persist despite cognitive information to the contrary.[43]

Professional institutions must also adopt policies self-consciously biased toward interests of patients. Translational research depends on collaboration with industry.[47] In fact, industry spends more on biomedical research than public funds ($60 billion compared with $25 billion in 2000).[48] Investigators, however, must be clear about differences in publicly funded and industry-sponsored research (Table 9.1). Academic institutions, whose mission is to create, disseminate, and preserve knowledge, can mediate physician–industry research collaborations. They can formalize terms of research agreements prior to project initiation, safeguard scientific integrity, provide public transparency, and maintain some distance between investigators and their

Table 9.1. Comparison of federal and industrial research funding sources[21,48,50]

Consideration	Federal funding	Industrial funding
Annual research budget[48a]	$25 billion	$60 billion
Subject of research	Fundamental questions	Product development
Application process for funding	Complex	Simple
Application review process	Peer review	Business review
Degree of difficulty in obtaining funding	Intense competition	Non-competitive
Response time to funding application	Prolonged	Rapid
Contact between sponsor and researcher	Rare	Close
Timing for producing research data	Important but not specified	Critical and specified
Access to all research data for all study sites	Unrestricted	May be restricted
Relationship of sponsor to research findings	Generally disinterested	Invested
Timing of publication of results premature or delayed	As soon as possible	May be premature or delayed
Considerations for investigator	Funding provides protected provide time, salary, prestige, and academic promotion	Funding may not provide protected time, salary, or credit towards promotion

Note: [a] Contract Research Organizations received approximately 60% of grants from pharmaceutical companies and academic centers received 40%.[21]

industry sponsors.[49] Industry support of continuous medical education can similarly be managed disinterestedly through academic institutions.

The existence of a clinical relationship merits special respect for patients' expectations of loyalty and fears of betrayal.[43] Physicians must refuse gifts and personal benefits from medical industry. Medicine's professional status depends on its capacity to keep faith with patients.

Sohail K. Mirza, M.D., M.P.H.
Vice Chair, Department of Orthopedics
Professor, Dartmouth Medical School and
The Dartmouth Institute for Health Policy and Clinical Practice

SUMMARY – COMMITMENT TO MANAGING CONFLICTS OF INTEREST

This summary discusses issues related to financial conflicts of interest commonly encountered in medical schools and teaching hospitals. The first three parts provide a conceptual background for the discussion and a summary of considerations relative to two major classes of relevant financial conflicts of interest: those encountered in the conduct of human subjects research, and those encountered in the context of medical education. The fourth part will comment on the case discussions that illustrate several of these matters.

Background

The Physician Charter was published in 2002 by the American Board of Internal Medicine Foundation, the American College of Physicians Foundation, and the European Federation of Internal Medicine.[32,51] The Charter sought to articulate the principles and responsibilities of professionalism for physicians in the new millennium. The effort was prompted by a concern that contemporary realities of medical practice were undermining the commitment of individual physicians to maintain the ethical standards required to fulfill medicine's "social contract." Of particular concern was the threatened erosion of public trust in the medical profession prompted by the onslaught of frank commercialism into heretofore sacrosanct realms of professional responsibilities. Commercialism's appeal to self interest, with its motto of *caveat emptor* – buyer beware – is the very antithesis of medical professionalism's call for self sacrifice, with its motto of *primum non nocere* – first, do no harm.

The Charter identified three overarching principles of medical professionalism – the primacy of patient interest, patient autonomy, and social justice – and ten categories of responsibilities to guide physicians' actions (see Table 9.2). Arguably chief among these responsibilities is maintaining trust by managing conflicts of interest. For it is conflicts of interest, particularly financial conflicts of interest, that are the most frequent challenges to professionalism, and hence, the most frequent reminder of how easily an era rife with commercialism can undermine the ethical foundations of the profession.

Medical educators have no greater responsibility then to educate medical students about the potential sources of conflicts of interest and to bolster students' resolve to prevent potential and real conflicts from compromising their commitment to professionalism. Students must understand that conflicts of interest are an inevitable feature of professional life. We all have them. When there are multiple notions of what "the right thing to do" is, as is often the case, social science research reveals that individuals tend to

Table 9.2. Categories of doctor responsibilities required to sustain professionalism[1,2]

Maintain professional competence
Be honest with patients
Respect patient confidentiality
Avoid inappropriate relations with patients
Advance scientific knowledge
Fulfill the obligations imposed by membership in the profession
Improve quality of care
Improve access to care
Promote the just distribution of resources
Maintain trust by managing conflicts of interest

default to those notions that favor their personal interests.[21] Even when taught about this reality, individuals are typically not aware of their personal biases. For example, individuals have a strong tendency to reciprocate in some way when given a gift, even when the gift is small and even when it is not tied to an explicit demand. Bias can be, and often is, unconscious and unintentional, but real.

Although some sources of conflicts of interest can and must be eliminated, most cannot be simply abolished; they are intrinsic to a doctor's ordinary work. The challenge is twofold: first, to recognize the ever-present opportunities to pursue self-interest at the expense of professional obligations and, then, to stifle the natural tendency to yield to temptation in order to maintain the primacy of patient interest. Examples of such opportunities abound: how soon to schedule a patient for a return visit; whether to recommend a fee-generating procedure; whether to care for an uninsured patient who cannot afford to pay; whether to accept a "consultant's" fee for merely attending an industry-sponsored conference; whether to accept a gift from a representative of a pharmaceutical company that produces drugs you might prescribe.

Although the formal curriculum (e.g., lectures, seminars, problem-based discussions) offers crucial opportunities to elucidate issues surrounding this topic, medical students undoubtedly learn the most enduring lessons about conflicts of interest from what they observe as "normal" in the real-world clinical environments in which they are immersed. Unhappily, the learning environments experienced by today's medical students are often rampant with commercialism. Students who observe respected faculty paying only lip service to medicine's lofty principles while openly pursuing their personal financial self-interest are likely to learn an indelible lesson, not in professionalism, but in cynicism. Medical school faculty, and the institutions in which they work, have a unique responsibility to prepare students to resist the inevitable temptations of the commercial marketplace in which they ultimately will find themselves. But, they can do so only by maintaining a culture of professionalism in which financial conflicts of interest are routinely monitored and managed effectively.

Two classes of financial conflicts of interest are of particular importance for medical schools and teaching hospitals to acknowledge and control: those arising in the conduct of human subjects research and those arising in the conduct of medical education.

Financial Conflicts of Interest in Human Subjects Research

Medical schools and teaching hospitals play a major role in advancing medical knowledge through the conduct of human subjects research. Advances in our understanding of the fundamental biology and of the effective treatment of many human ailments depend entirely on our ability to perform carefully designed studies on normal volunteers and/or patients who consent to be research subjects. In our capitalist economic system, major commercial entities – notably pharmaceutical companies and medical device manufacturers – also play an important role by exploiting advances in medical knowledge to develop and disseminate useful products and services to the public.

The public has dual, and potentially competing, interests in human subjects research; on the one hand is the strong desire to accelerate advances in the prevention, diagnosis, and treatment of disease, and on the other hand is the imperative to safeguard both the welfare of human subjects and the integrity of science. Financial incentives from industry to conduct human subjects research in academic settings have proven effective in hastening the translation of new discoveries into beneficial commodities.[52] By the same token, however, such financial incentives have raised understandable public concern that investigators who stand to benefit individually from their research may take shortcuts or otherwise jeopardize the safety of human subjects or the validity of the research results.[53,54]

In balancing these two competing public interests, it would clearly not be desirable for medical school faculty to be prohibited from having any financial dealings with industry, nor would it be desirable for faculty to be permitted to have unfettered financial dealings with industry. Thoughtful guidance for striking this balance has been provided and is based on the principle of rebuttable presumption.[55,56] In accordance with this principle, investigators are presumed to be ineligible for conducting human subjects research if they have a significant financial interest in the outcomes. This guidance tilts strongly toward prohibition but recognizes that exceptions may be warranted if a strong case (i.e., a rebuttal) can be made to a duly authorized, independent body that

circumstances justify doing so. For example, if the research could not otherwise be conducted as safely or as effectively, or if the risks to human subjects
are truly negligible, the conflicted investigator might be allowed to proceed,
but only under rigorous oversight by a disinterested party and with full disclosure of the financial conflict to all interested parties, including the subjects of
the research.

Medical students are routinely aware of, and often assist in, human subjects research conducted by their faculty. Institutions that have implemented
comprehensive policies for the effective management of financial conflicts of
interest in human subjects research are well positioned to model this aspect
of professionalism for the learners in their midst.

Conflicts of Interest in Medical Education

It would appear axiomatic that medical educators should be scrupulous in
avoiding even the appearance of bias and be assiduous in basing all of their
teachings on available scientific evidence. Yet, over the past several decades,
wittingly or unwittingly, medical educators have allowed commercial entities
within the health industry to play an increasing role in medial education at all
levels – undergraduate, graduate, and continuing. The undeniable (and understandable) intent of the health industry – notably pharmaceutical firms
and device manufacturers – in accessing medical education venues is to
influence the decision making of physicians, who after all are the prime
marketing target for their products and services.

The ways in which commercial entities have sought to influence the current and future prescribing patterns of students, residents, and faculty physicians are manifold. They include gifts both large and small; "free" meals;
payment for invited speakers; reimbursement for travel expenses to meetings
for students, residents, and faculty; payment for attending lectures, conferences, and online presentations; payment of faculty for participating in
speakers' bureaus; drug samples; and sham "consulting" fees for faculty.

The effectiveness of these practices is reflected in the huge sums that industry expends on marketing activities aimed at physicians. Studies reveal
that approximately 80 percent of medical school department chairs receive
some sort of support from industry for education-related activities.[57] In 2006,
medical schools received an estimated $275 million in aggregate to support
continuing medical education, and physician membership organizations
received an additional $380 million.[58]

Allowing commercial entities to influence the core educational mission of
medical schools and teaching hospitals can never be justified. Tolerating the
obvious conflicts of interest inherent in this practice signals to the public that

physicians have divided loyalties, and cannot be trusted to place patients' interest uppermost. Moreover, it undermines the profession's commitment to evidenced-based information and to cost-effective prescribing. Equally important, it validates and reinforces the "entitlement mindset" that is all too common among fully trained physicians: that is, a belief that physicians are somehow entitled to have someone else pay for their continuing education.

As with the case for financial conflicts of interest in human subjects research, thoughtful guidance has been provided for those medical schools and teaching hospitals that wish to strengthen institutional policies governing their interactions with industry.[59–61] Table 9.3 lists some of the steps academic institutions can take to minimize the conflicts of interest that can compromise the integrity of their medical education programs.

Several national organizations have been particularly active in encouraging their members and the medical profession at large to discontinue those interactions with industry that threaten the integrity of the profession and risk undermining public trust in medicine. Following are some examples:

- The Association of American Medical Colleges has proposed sweeping changes in the way medical schools and teaching hospitals manage their relationships with industry.[61]
- The American Medical Student Association inaugurated a "PharmFree Campaign" in 2001; the campaign advocates a ban on all pharmaceutical company sponsorship of educational programs, has launched a "Counter Detailing Initiative" to provide physicians with objective information about pharmaceutical agents, and has developed a "score card" to access the degree to which medical schools have implemented policies to minimize "conflicts of interest caused by pharmaceutical industry marketing."[62]
- No Free Lunch is an organization of health care providers "who believe that pharmaceutical promotion should not guide clinical practice." Its mission is "to encourage health care providers to practice medicine on the basis of scientific evidence rather than on the basis of pharmaceutical promotion." It discourages "the acceptance of all gifts from industry by health care providers, trainees, and students."[63]

Review of the Cases and Commentaries

Conflicts of Interest in Human Subjects Research
Two of the cases in this chapter involve physicians with financial interest in the conduct of human subjects research.

Table 9.3. Recommendations to minimize conflicts of interest in medical education[11]

Prohibit all gifts, large or small (including "free" meals)
No direct support for physician travel to meetings
Do not permit manufacturers to provide direct support for CME even through subsidiaries
Eliminate direct provision of drug samples
Consulting arrangements and research support must be transparent
Prohibit "no strings attached" grants to faculty
Physicians with financial ties to drug companies should not be members of formulary
  committees
Faculty should not participate in industry speakers' bureaus
Prohibit "ghost writing" by industry employees

1. The general pediatrician who has contracted with a pharmaceutical company to enroll patients in a clinical trial poses two ethical issues. The first is whether accepting payment for enrolling patients is, itself, a deviation from ethical norms. The guiding principle here is whether the payment exceeds the market value of the service being provided. In this case, being paid $100 for the initial enrollment does not seem excessive, given that the physician must spend time speaking to the patient's mother about the study, obtaining the mother's informed consent, and filling out the necessary enrollment forms. So far, so good. However, the failure of the enrollment process to fully disclose the financial arrangements to the mother is unacceptable.

   The second ethical issue posed by this case relates to the offer of $300 for "each subject who completes the study and for whom 'clean' data are submitted." This level of payment could be a sufficient inducement to tempt the physician to serve her own interests by enrolling ineligible patients in the study and/or being less than dutiful in determining that submitted data were, in fact, "clean." This dilemma is illustrated by the decision she must make about whether to enroll the sick child who lacks clear-cut evidence for the condition (i.e., an ear infection) for which the study is designed.

2. The orthopedic surgeon who has multiple financial dealings with a manufacturer of an implantable device is, unfortunately, illustrative of common ethical lapses that have received much media attention.[64] This surgeon conducts clinical trials of devices manufactured by a commercial entity in which he has a significant financial interest. Moreover, he is paid for participation in the company's speakers'

bureau. Both of these activities are proscribed by widely accepted ethical standards.[55,56]

The surgeon's disclosure to patients in whom he implants the device that he has financial ties with the company illustrates another important ethical point. A common misconception is that disclosure alone is all that is required to "cure" a conflict of interest. Although full disclosure of such financial ties is unquestionably necessary, it is never sufficient to immunize the physician from the potentially adverse effects of a conflict of interest. Nor is disclosure of a conflict of interest sufficient to reassure a patient, a journal reader, or a lecture attendee that the surgeon, author, or speaker, respectively, is unbiased and unaffected by the conflict.

Conflicts of Interest in Medical Education

Three of the conflicts of interest cases illustrate ways in which "medical education" can be distorted by the contaminating influence of commercial interests.

1. The student who attended the pharmacology lecture is entitled to be in a quandary (see the first Managing Conflicts of Interest vignette, Chapter 2). The student notes that the faculty member who delivered the lecture has financial interests in the company that manufactures the drug he discussed, and presumably touted. What is the student to believe? Having disclosed his financial interest clearly does not provide assurances that the information the faculty member communicated was unbiased. Whether conscious or unconscious, potential bias resulting from a financial interest does not evaporate merely by disclosing it.

    As a matter of principle, members of a medical school faculty have a primary obligation to the truth. They must not be, nor appear to be, spokespersons for commercial entities with ulterior motives. For this reason, stringent ethical guidance calls for prohibiting faculty members from participating as paid speakers for pharmaceutical or medical device companies.[59] Whether, as is presumably the case here, faculty who receive legitimate consulting fees from a for-profit company should also be prohibited from lecturing to students about that company's products is less certain. Clearly, the safest course of action in preserving optimal objectivity would be to utilize a lecturer who did not have even the appearance of a conflicting interest.

2. The third year students engaged in a discussion about the ethics of receiving lunches and gifts from pharmaceutical companies raises several important issues (see the second Managing Conflicts of Interest vignette, Chapter 2). First, we must dispel the notion that students who are not yet in a position to prescribe drugs are somehow insulated from the adverse effects of commercial marketing activities. Abundant evidence exists that marketing efforts directed at students do, indeed, affect future prescribing habits.[62,65] Suffice to ask: Why else would industry spend millions of dollars each year on such activities?

Students understandably welcome the gifts proffered by commercial entities. Unfortunately, students are typically unaware of the unconscious effects that these gifts have, even those that appear of trivial value.[65] The evidence is overwhelming that gifts of any size engender a tendency to reciprocate, to return "the favor" to the gift giver.[21] Once again, it suffices to ask why industry would spend such large sums on gift giving to students, residents, and practitioners. In theory, it could be in gratitude for all the hard work that doctors do. In reality, though, it is clearly in the hope of currying favorable views of company products.

Students also understandably welcome the "free" lunches provided by industry at educational sessions. Institutions that permit lunches (and gifts) to be "donated" by pharmaceutical companies are, no doubt unwittingly, functioning as co-conspirators in an unbridled attempt to bias the decision making of future physicians toward the products of a particular commercial firm. To avoid being co-opted in this way, institutions should prohibit all industry gifts to students, residents and faculty, and should allocate the necessary resources to defray the cost of meals (if necessary) at educational sessions.[59]

3. One could hardly avoid feeling sympathy for the patient who could barely afford the drugs prescribed by the doctor whose office was strewn with logo-laden drug company paraphernalia. This vignette is a disturbing reminder to students that the intrusion of commercial interests into the sanctity of the doctor–patient relationship is fraught with serious risk of undermining the trust that sustains medicine as an ethical enterprise. Entering a doctor's office should provide comforting assurance to patients that all concerned are focused on their interests alone. Offices that reek of commercialism provide discordant reminders that other interests can conflict with the doctor's primary obligation and, in this case, evidently have.

Conclusion

This chapter summarizes the multiple ways in which individual and institutional financial conflicts of interest can jeopardize patient safety and scientific integrity in human subjects research, can bias information communicated to students by medical educators, and, most important, can undermine public trust in doctors and the medical profession. Medical schools have a critical responsibility to educate medical students about the potential sources of conflicts of interest and to bolster students' resolve to prevent potential and real conflicts from compromising their commitment to professionalism.

Jordan C. Cohen, M.D.
President Emeritus, Association of American Medical Colleges
Professor of Medicine and Public Health,
George Washington University
Chairman, Board of Trustees, The Arnold P. Gold Foundation

REFERENCES

1. American College of Physicians. The impending collapse of primary care medicine and its implications for the state of the nation's health care. 2006.
2. MDVIP. MDVIP Web site. http://www.mdvip.com/NewCorpWebSite/index.aspx. Accessed August 5, 2008.
3. Davis K, Schoenbaum SC, Audet AM. A 2020 vision of patient-centered primary care. *J Gen Intern Med.* 2005;**20**(10):953–957.
4. Highlights and Details. Skypark Preferred Family Care Web site. http://www.skyparkpfc.com. Accessed August 5, 2008.
5. Alexander GC, Kurlander J, Wynia MK. Physicians in retainer ("concierge") practice. A national survey of physician, patient, and practice characteristics. *J Gen Intern Med.* 2005;**20**(12):1079–1083.
6. American Medical Association. Retainer Practice Ethics Guide. American Medical Association Web site. http://www.ama-assn.org/ama/pub/category/11967.html. Accessed August 5, 2008.
7. Society for Innovative Medical Practice Design. SIMPD Ethics Guide. SIMPD Web site. http://www.ama-assn.org/ama/pub/category/11967.html. Accessed August 5, 2008.
8. Donohoe M. Luxury primary care, academic medical centers, and the erosion of science and professional ethics. *J Gen Intern Med.* 2004;**19**(1):90–94.
9. Donohoe MT. Standard vs. luxury care. In: Buetow S, Kenealy T, eds. *Ideological Debatees in Family Medicine.* New York: Nova Science Publishers; 2007.
10. Brennan TA. Luxury primary care – market innovation or threat to access? *N Engl J Med.* 2002;**346**(15):1165–1168.

11. Donohoe M. Causes and health consequences of environmental degradation and social injustice. *Soc Sci Med.* 2003;**56**(3):573–587.

12. United States Government Accountability Office. Physician services: Concierge care characteristics and considerations for medicare. 2005.

13. Donohoe MT. Comparing generalist and specialty care: Discrepancies, deficiencies, and excesses. *Arch Intern Med.* 1998;**158**(15):1596–1608.

14. Donohoe MT. Unnecessary testing in obstetrics and gynecology and general medicine: Causes and consequences of the unwarranted use of costly and unscientific (yet profitable) screening modalities. http://www.medscape.com/viewarticle/552964_print.

15. Cunningham PJ, May JH. A growing hole in the safety net: Physician charity care declines again. http://www.hschange.org/CONTENTS/826/. Accessed May 17, 2006.

16. Pelliegrino T. *For the Patient's Good: The Restoration of Beneficence in Health Care.* New York: Oxford Press; 1988.

17. Whittmore C, ed. *Personalized Medicine: The Emerging Pharmacogenomics Revolution.* Price Waterhouse Coopers, Global Technology Centre; 2005.

18. Beauchamp TL, Childress JF. *Principles of Biomedical Ethics.* 5th ed. New York: Oxford University Press; 2001.

19. Ubel PA, Jepson C, Asch DA. Misperceptions about beta-blockers and diuretics: A national survey of primary care physicians. *J Gen Intern Med.* 2003;**18**(12): 977–983.

20. Wazana A. Physicians and the pharmaceutical industry: Is a gift ever just a gift? *JAMA.* 2000;**283**(3):373–380.

21. Dana J, Loewenstein G. A social science perspective on gifts to physicians from industry. *JAMA.* 2003;**290**(2):252–255.

22. Dunning D, Meyerowitz JA, Holzberg AD. Ambiguity and self-evaluation: The role of idiosyncratic trait definitions in self-serving assessments of ability. *J Pers Soc Psych.* 1989;**57**:1082–1090.

23. Svenson O. Are we all less risky and more skillful than our fellow drivers? *Acta Psych.* 1981;**47**:143–148.

24. Messick DM. Social interdependence and decision making. In: Wright G, ed. *Behavioral Secision Making.* New York: Plenum; 1985:87–109.

25. Loewenstein G, Issacharoff S, Camerer C, Babcock L. Self-serving assessments of fairness and pretrial bargaining. *J Leg Stud.* 1992;**12**:135–159.

26. Pronin E, Lin DY, Ross L. The bias blind spot: Perceptions of bias in self versus others. *Pers Soc Psych Bull.* 2002;**28**:369–381.

27. Katz D, Caplan AL, Merz JF. All gifts large and small: Toward an understanding of the ethics of pharmaceutical industry gift-giving. *Am J Bioeth.* 2003;**3**(3):39–46.

28. Avorn J, Chen M, Hartley R. Scientific versus commercial sources of influence on the prescribing behavior of physicians. *Am J Med.* 1982;**73**:4–8.

29. American Medical Association. Advertising and publicity. In: *Code of Medical Ethics of the American Medical Association: Current Opinions with Annotations.* Chicago, IL: AMA; 2006:127.

30. American College of Obstetrics and Gynecology. ACOG committee opinion. commercial enterprises in medical practice; 359.

31. AMA (Ethics) AMA Code of Medical Ethics. http://www.ama-assn.org/ama/pub/category/2498.html. Accessed July 11, 2008.

32. ABIM Foundation. American Board of Internal Medicine, ACP-ASIM Foundation. American College of Physicians-American Society of Internal Medicine, European Federation of Internal Medicine. Medical professionalism in the new millennium: A physician charter. *Ann Intern Med*. 2002;**136**(3):243–246.

33. Lader EW, Cannon CP, Ohman EM, et al. The clinician as investigator: Participating in clinical trials in the practice setting. *Circulation*. 2004;**109**(21):2672–2679.

34. American Academy of Pediatrics Subcommittee on Management of Acute Otitis Media. Diagnosis and management of acute otitis media. *Pediatrics*. 2004;**113**(5):1451–1465.

35. Morin K, Rakatansky H, Riddick FA, Jr, et al. Managing conflicts of interest in the conduct of clinical trials. *JAMA*. 2002;**287**(1):78–84.

36. Hampson LA, Agrawal M, Joffe S, Gross CP, Verter J, Emanuel EJ. Patients' views on financial conflicts of interest in cancer research trials. *N Engl J Med*. 2006;**355**(22):2330–2337.

37. Crowninshield R. The orthopaedic profession and industry: Conflict or convergence of interests. *Clin Orthop Relat Res*. 2003;(412):8–13.

38. Patent Act of 1790, HR and S 109–112(1790).

39. Brand RA, Buckwalter JA, Talman CL, Happe DG. Industrial support of orthopaedic research in the academic setting. *Clin Orthop Relat Res*. 2003;(412):45–53.

40. Feder BJ. Subpoenas seek data on orthopedics makers' ties to surgeons. *The New York Times*. 2005:12.

41. Bhandari M, Busse JW, Jackowski D, et al. Association between industry funding and statistically significant pro-industry findings in medical and surgical randomized trials. *CMAJ*. 2004;**170**(4):477–480.

42. Bahamonde R, Zimmer, DePuy. Inside Indiana Business. http://www.insideindianabusiness.com/newsitem.asp?id=25688&ts=true. Accessed September 28, 2007.

43. Bloche MG. Clinical loyalties and the social purposes of medicine. *JAMA*. 1999;**281**(3):268–274.

44. NIHCM. Changing Patterns of Pharmaceutical Innovation. www.nihcm.org. Accessed September 20, 2007.

45. Mirza SK. Accountability of the accused: Facing public perceptions about financial conflicts of interest in spine surgery. *Spine J*. 2004;**4**(5):491–494.

46. Wenger DR. Spine surgery at a crossroads: Does economic growth threaten our professionalism? *Spine*. 2007;**32**(20):2158–2165.

47. Jacobs JJ, Galante JO, Mirza SK, Zdeblick T. Relationships with industry: Critical for new technology or an unnecessary evil? *J Bone Joint Surg Am*. 2006;**88**(7):1650–1663.

48. Moses H, 3rd, Martin JB. Academic relationships with industry: A new model for biomedical research. *JAMA*. 2001;**285**(7):933–935.

49. Brennan TA, Rothman DJ, Blank L, et al. Health industry practices that create conflicts of interest: A policy proposal for academic medical centers. *JAMA*. 2006;**295**(4):429–433.

50. Brand RA, Buckwalter JA, Talman CL, Happe DG. Industrial support of orthopaedic research in the academic setting. *Clin Orthop Relat Res.* 2003;(412): 45–53.

51. Medical Professionalism Project. Medical professionalism in the new millennium: A physician's charter. *Lancet.* 2002;**359**(9305):520–522.

52. Reczek PR. Research and the Bayh-Dole Act. *Science.* 2004;**303**(5654):40.

53. Klanica K. Conflicts of interest in medical research: How much conflict should exceed legal boundaries? *J Biolaw Bus.* 2005;**8**(3):37–45.

54. Gelsinger P, Shamoo AE. Eight years after Jesse's death, are human research subjects any safer? *Hastings Cent Rep.* 2008;**38**(2):25–27.

55. Association of American Medical Colleges. Protecting Subjects, Preserving Trust, Promoting Progress. Principles and Recommendations for Oversight of an *Institution's* Financial Interests in Human Subjects Research. https://services.aamc. org/Publications/index.cfm?fuseaction=Product.displayForm&prd_id=106& cfid=1&cftoken=C82606B7–F8B6–41EE-99E6B7610BEB75CB. Updated 2002.

56. Association of American Medical Colleges, Association of American Universities. Protecting Patients, Preserving Integrity, Advancing Health: Accelerating the Implementation of COI Policies in Human Subjects Research. AAMC Web site. https://services.aamc.org/Publications/index.cfm?fuseaction=Product.display Form&prd_id=106&cfid=1&cftoken=C82606B7–F8B6–41EE-99E6B7610BEB75CB. Updated 2008. Accessed August 13, 2008.

57. Campbell EG, Weissman JS, Ehringhaus S, et al. Institutional academic industry relationships. *JAMA.* 2007;**298**(15):1779–1786.

58. Accreditation Council for Continuing Medical Education. ACCME Annual Report Data 2006. http://www.accme.org/dir_docs/doc_upload/f51ed7d8-e3b4–479a-a9d8–57b6efedc27a_uploaddocument.pdf. Accessed August 13, 2008.

59. Brennan TA, Rothman DJ, Blank L, et al. Health industry practices that create conflicts of interest: A policy proposal for academic medical centers. *JAMA.* 2006;**295**(4):429–433.

60. JosiahMacy, Jr. Foundation. Continuing Education in the Health Professions: Improving Healthcare Through Lifelong Learning, 2007. http://www.josiahmacy foundation.org/. Accessed August 13, 2008.

61. Association of American Medical Colleges. Task Force on Industry Funding of Medical Education. AAMC Web site. http://www.aamc.org/research/coi/ industryfunding.pdf. Accessed August 13, 2008.

62. AMSA Web site. http://www.amsa.org. Accessed August 13, 2008.

63. No Free Lunch Web site. http://www.nofreelunch.org/aboutus.htm. Accessed August 13, 2008.

64. Brand RA, Buckwalter JA, Wright TM, et al. Editorial from journal editors: Patient care, professionalism and relations with industry. *Clin Orthop Relat Res.* 2008;**466**(3):517–519.

65. Sierles FS, Brodkey AC, Cleary LM, et al. Medical students' exposure to and attitudes about drug company interactions: A national survey. *JAMA.* 2005;**294**(9): 1034–1042.

10 Commitment to Professional Responsibilities

Cases and Commentaries

COMMITMENT TO PROFESSIONAL RESPONSIBILITIES – ADULT PRIMARY CARE

A family physician has seen an unmarried female patient for many years. She is now fifty years old. He has been managing her preventive medical care as well as osteoarthritis and "white-coat hypertension." Following his divorce, he encounters this patient at a social event and they become romantically involved.

A Perspective from a Primary Care Physician

Clinical Background

"White coat hypertension" is a common clinical finding in which patients are found to have high blood pressure readings in the medical office, but normal readings when home or at rest. Blood pressure normally varies with different activities and times of day. However, some people have hypertensive readings while in stressful or anxiety-producing situations, but normal pressure at other times. White coat hypertension is an example of this phenomenon. Continuous ambulatory blood pressure testing permits determination of mean systolic and diastolic pressures over twenty-four hours. Many authorities believe patients with mean pressures of 135/85 or above should be treated.[1] However, the value of treating white coat hypertension with medication remains controversial.[2]

Professionalism Considerations

The ancient oath of Hippocrates includes several specific injunctions that contemporary oath-takers might find archaic or controversial. Among these are pledges to avoid performing surgery, abortion, and euthanasia. In addition, Hippocratic physicians affirmed that they would work "for the benefit of the sick, remaining free of all intentional injustice, of all mischief and in particular of sexual relations with both female and male persons, be they free or slaves."[3] In contemporary physicians' oaths, the last injunction is usually omitted or replaced with a more general statement about treating patients with respect.[4] Nevertheless, prohibition against sexual liaisons with patients remains a part of the professional ethos of medicine.

But why should it? The prima facie case against romantic relationships between doctor and patient is based on the principles of beneficence, non-maleficence, and respect for autonomy. The physician's primary duty is to help his or her patient, or at least not cause harm. To accomplish this, physicians must be responsive to patients' vulnerability, suffering, uncertainty, and emotional stress. This requires that they cultivate and maintain professional objectivity, as well as empathic understanding. Given these dynamics, the American Medical Association's Council on Ethical and Judicial Affairs summarizes the doctor's ethical responsibility in this way, "Sexual or romantic interactions between physicians and patients detract from the goals of the physician-patient relationship, may exploit the vulnerability of the patient, may obscure the physician's objective judgment concerning the patient's health care, and ultimately be detrimental to the patient's well-being."[5]

However, this analysis may fail to provide us with nuanced guidance in certain contemporary health care situations. First, what about termination? Does the prohibition of intimate relationships continue even after the physician–patient relationship has ceased? In today's medicine, therapeutic relationships are frequently short term rather than long term, or intermittent rather than continuous. Moreover, what role does therapeutic intensity play? Does the prohibition apply equally to psychiatrists conducting psychotherapy, surgeons performing a mastectomy, family doctors treating diabetes, and dermatologists removing a benign mole? It seems reasonable to assume that the higher the physical and emotional intensity of the therapeutic relationship, the more vulnerable the patient is, and the more likely he or she might be harmed by intimacy with the physician, even after active treatment has ceased. For example, given the nature of psychiatric treatment, the American Psychiatric Association absolutely prohibits sexual relationships with patients, even former patients.[6]

Opinion

If the physician develops a romantic relationship with this patient, he will not be able to treat her with non-judgmental empathy, openness, and clinical objectivity in his professional capacity. The patient would suffer as a result of her vulnerability and possible inhibition, and because of the doctor's lack of objectivity and possible manipulation. Thus, it is unethical for this physician to become romantically involved with this patient while remaining her doctor. He must refer her to another physician.

But would it be appropriate for him to date her when she becomes his former patient? This is a more complex issue. While the two have shared a long-term primary care relationship, given the nature of her medical problems, it is conceivable that self-disclosure has been minimal and the patient sees herself as an equal partner. Primary care relationships vary in intensity from close to psychiatric in nature (in which case intimacy even with a former patient would be unethical) to "care-lite" involving only the occasional sore throat or sinus infection (in which case there may be little or no ethical objection to future intimacy).

This case falls somewhere in between. However, we do have one additional bit of information: The physician has recently been divorced. This suggests that he may be on the rebound, seeking solace wherever he can. What could be easier than crying on the shoulder of one of his patients? Thus, his sudden romantic interest may be a case of (perhaps unconscious) self-serving manipulation. It would clearly be unethical for the doctor to "use" his patient – or former patient – in this way. Although there well may be situations in which it is ethical for a family doctor to date a former patient, I don't believe this is one of them.

Jack Coulehan, M.D., M.P.H.
Head, Division of Medicine in Society, Department of
Preventive Medicine
Institute for Medicine in Contemporary Society, SUNY at Stony Brook

A Perspective from an Attorney and Ethicist

Becoming "romantically involved" – leading to sexual involvement – with a current patient is a bad idea. Medical professional society ethics codes and state medical boards say such behavior is unethical. Hippocrates agreed, pronouncing the prohibition in the fourth century B.C., as Dr. Coulehan notes.

Caring for patients is a privilege that requires trust in the physician, and in the profession.[7,8] Patients need to know that their best interests are being served, and that boundaries in the patient–physician relationship protect those interests. Many state laws prohibit physician (especially psychiatrist) sexual relationships with patients. Physicians could end up facing not only state medical board and professional society review, but also criminal and/or civil proceedings.

Different terms and definitions are used, but the bottom line is protecting the patient, and the patient–physician relationship, from exploitation. The Federation of State Medical Boards defines sexual misconduct as "behavior that exploits the physician–patient relationship in a sexual way."[9] Further, sexual misconduct is sexual impropriety – including among other things "using the physician–patient relationship to solicit a date or a romantic relationship" – or a sexual violation, which is physical sexual contact, including sex or "kissing in a romantic or sexual manner."[9]

The American College of Physicians (ACP) has said in its *Ethics Manual* (fifth edition, 2005) that sexual involvement between the physician and a current patient is unethical even if the patient initiates or consents to the contact.[7] Is this paternalistic? Is it an affront to patient autonomy, especially when patients today are very knowledgeable and sophisticated about their rights? The answer is yes, as there is an inherent imbalance of power in the therapeutic relationship, and patients are often vulnerable.[10] Patients provide sensitive information to their physicians and allow themselves to be examined – intimate contacts that do not run both ways. They rely on the physician for his or her expertise and recommendations about care. This must not be exploited. The physician must be in a position to be objective about the patient's medical care, without his or her own competing interests (usually "his" interests, as physicians who have sexual contact with patients are usually male and older; patients are usually female and younger).[10]

Where is the physician practicing? What about the clinician in a rural area, who sees most of the community members as patients? The American Psychiatric Association has said in its ethics code that sexual activity with a current or former patient is unethical. Period. But others have said that a relationship with a former patient may be acceptable under certain circumstances.[11] Key for the AMA and ACP is that a sexual or romantic relationship with a former patient would be unethical if the physician "uses or exploits the trust, knowledge, emotions or influence derived from the previous professional relationship."[7,10] The United Kingdom's General Medical Council recently reiterated and refined its guidance prohibiting sexual relationships with patients,[10] echoing the same concerns and spelling out a process for evaluating whether a relationship with a former patient may be ethically acceptable:

> If circumstances arise in which social contact with a former patient leads to the possibility of a sexual relationship beginning, you must use your professional judgment and give careful consideration to the nature and circumstances of the relationship, taking account of the following:
> - when the professional relationship ended and how long it lasted
> - the nature of the previous professional relationship
> - whether the patient was particularly vulnerable at the time of the professional relationship, and whether they are still vulnerable
> - whether you will be caring for other members of the patient's family[11]

What about the vignette presented here? It seems so innocuous, as it is between consenting adults. The care has been for osteoarthritis, white-coat hypertension – did the doctor take that as a sign?! – and prevention, not mental health or other disorders, nor an acute condition, that could make a patient particularly vulnerable. The involvement does not appear unwanted by the patient. The patient–physician relationship, however, has been long-standing and may include a dependence on the doctor that neither the doctor nor the patient have identified. Is the physician being objective? In addition, they may each view the romantic relationship differently.

What if it all works out and they live happily ever after in the end? Irrespective of whether they do or not, a relationship outside of the therapeutic relationship is cause for concern. In this case, the obvious first step, before even considering the factors outlined, is to terminate the doctor–patient relationship. The physician should transfer her care, then evaluate the factors outlined. He might do so with the help of an impartial colleague, especially in determining a suitable post-termination period of time, since it may be difficult to judge the effects of the previous patient–physician relationship on current feelings.[7]

Physicians must individually and collectively fulfill the duties of the profession, put the best interests of the patient first, and engage in self-regulation and review of those who fail to meet the standards of ethics and professionalism.[7,8] Even in seemingly benign situations involving consenting adults, there are potential ethical and legal consequences.

Lois Snyder, J.D.
Director, Center for Ethics and Professionalism
American College of Physicians

COMMITMENT TO PROFESSIONAL RESPONSIBILITIES – PEDIATRICS

A semi-retired pediatric allergist gives expert testimony in court on a pediatric issue in which the pediatrician has no prior experience. The case involves a child who was not properly diagnosed as having a developmental dysplasia of the hip.

A Perspective from a Pediatrician

When a physician or scientist accepts the responsibility to testify in a court of law as an expert for either the plaintiff or the defendant, that individual should be aware of the criteria that determine whether he/she has the credentials to participate as an expert. As an expert, you should determine whether you have the qualifying credentials.

First, are you considered by your colleagues, locally and even nationally, to be an expert in the issues in this negligence lawsuit? Ask yourself the following questions:

- Do I have prior and present ongoing clinical experience in evaluating patients with this problem?
- Have I published medical or scientific articles in peer-reviewed journals dealing with the clinical problem being adjudicated in the lawsuit?
- Have I performed any research studies dealing with this particular problem? If you have not performed the studies, are you very familiar with medical literature dealing with the issues that will be adjudicated in this case?

Second, how were you contacted to participate in this particular lawsuit? If you are concerned about your qualifications you should ask a neutral attorney. Who are the other experts in this case and have any experts refused to participate? Attorneys will frequently review the literature in an attempt to obtain experts who have published in this area and have experience in evaluation of this particular clinical problem. It is the responsibility of the attorney to find a qualified expert in order to pursue the plaintiff's accusation or prepare a proper defense. Sometimes the plaintiff or defendant's case is so weak that the attorney has difficulty obtaining a qualified expert. So the attorney may seek professional experts who advertise their services or contact physicians who are convinced to participate, although they may lack the expertise necessary.[12–14] The courts are more lenient with regard to approving experts in comparison to the medical and scientific community.[13–15] So a non-qualified expert can be accepted by the court, which is frequently not to the benefit of the expert or the litigants.

Third, each expert has to decide whether the defense or plaintiff's case has medical or scientific merit. If the side on which the expert has been asked to participate is clearly non-meritorious, the expert should withdraw from the case, unless he/she may be of assistance in negotiating a settlement, which may be of benefit to both sides.

As physicians and scientists we must realize and recognize that the only area of litigation over which science and medicine could have legitimate control is in the performance of expert witnesses.[13,14,16–18] Most non-meritorious lawsuits would not proceed if the attorneys could not find a physician or scientist who was willing to say that a non-meritorious case had merit.[14] Therefore, while we may be displeased with some attorneys and blame them for the epidemic of litigation, the fact is that unscrupulous scientists and physicians have an important role in promoting non-meritorious actions. Since we are not able to modernize the legal system, our best initiative is to alter drastically the activities of the irresponsible expert, by raising the quality of expert-witness testimony.[14,17,19] We must strengthen the guidelines of universities and professional organizations in the United States to train and encourage scientists and physicians to perform as scholars and to monitor their contributions to the courts. We should expect them to behave as scholars in the courtroom, and if they do not provide competent and scholarly testimony, they should be criticized or expelled by their universities or their professional scientific and medical organizations.

While some aspects of this discussion are critical of the legal profession, it is important to place this criticism into perspective. Physicians, as a group, tend to be hypercritical of the legal profession because of the escalation of malpractice litigation and malpractice insurance premiums. Recommendations from the medical community to modify the law in order to reduce the frequency of non-meritorious litigation and the size of the awards have been minimally successful, primarily because lawyers dominate the legislatures. Furthermore, many of these attempts by physicians to change the law are naïve. My suggestions in the past have directed the medical community to focus their attention on junk scientists and their junk science, since these are problems that emanate from the medical and scientific community, over which physicians should have some authority.

More importantly, we should respect and admire the importance and accomplishments of the legal profession, because it is the foundation of any thriving democracy. Without the law, we could never have rid ourselves of a sitting president or protect all of the rights bestowed on individuals in our constitution. Because a very small percentage of attorneys exploit the power of the law to their own advantage, it does not mean that the legal system has to be drastically altered. It is to everyone's advantage to have a functioning legal system with its benefits and risks. Will the situation improve? I cannot predict the future of malpractice litigation but we are not doing our job by allowing the participation of irresponsible expert witnesses in matters of litigation without being censured by their university or professional organizations.[14,17,20]

Robert I. Brent M.D., Ph.D., D.Sc. (Hons.)
Distinguished Professor of Pediatrics, Radiology and Pathology
Louis and Bessie Stein Professor of Pediatrics
Jefferson Medical College
Alfred I. duPont Hospital for Children

A Perspective from a Legal Scholar

A 1988 report of the American Medical Association voiced a common complaint about the ability of jurors to decide medical negligence:

> Juries are not optimally suited to decide the complicated issues of causation and duty of care ... With respect to the major elements of liability – duty of care and

causation – the parties must present expert testimony, which the jurors cannot evaluate independently.[21]

Systematic research, however, is inconsistent with this assertion. Before giving some examples, jury trials need to be placed in context. Trial by jury occurs in only about 7 percent of malpractice claims. Of cases that do go to trial, doctors prevail in roughly three cases out of four. In Florida, between 1990 and the end of 2004 there were 801 cases involving payments of $1 million or more. Only 54 of the 801 payments were made after a jury trial. The rest were the result of pretrial settlements.

Critics of the jury system and the use of expert testimony to juries often fail to consider that at trial, experts are cross-examined and that the jury is usually exposed to experts from both sides, a process that educates them about not only potential weaknesses in an expert's testimony but often the basis of disagreement between experts. The jurors are also given instructions on the law by the trial judge, including how they are to evaluate expert testimony.

So what about the incompetence assertion? If the AMA is correct, jury verdicts should deviate from how medical professionals would decide cases. Tarragin et al. studied closed claim files of a major medical liability insurer that had medical doctors evaluate each case for negligence.[22] Tarragin et al. compared these ratings with verdicts in cases that went to trial and found substantial agreement with the juries' verdicts. In 2006 Studdert et al. reported a similar study. In this study, teams of medical doctors systematically rated the medical records from over 1,400 randomly chosen closed claims in four different regions of the United States.[23] Ratings were made as to whether the case involved a negligent error or not. Fifteen percent, or 208 claims, were decided at trial; plaintiffs prevailed only 21 percent of the time. The jury verdicts were generally consistent with the doctors' ratings of whether negligence had occurred.

These findings are consistent with a number of studies comparing jury verdicts with the opinions of the trial judges who heard the same evidence as the juries. The agreement rates between judges and juries are typically around 80 percent. When judges and juries differ, the disagreement cannot be ascribed to greater complexity or difficulty of the evidence; instead juries apply a slightly different set of values to the evidence.

The unique Arizona Jury Project studied fifty civil jury trials and included videotaped records of the actual jury deliberations.[24,25] Some of the trials involved claims of medical malpractice. Analysis of the deliberations showed jurors paying close attention to the judges' instructions on the standard of care.

We can get a flavor of juror attention to experts from the questions the Arizona juries submitted immediately after medical experts finished their testimony. In a personal injury trial the jurors asked these questions of a medical expert:

Why [are there] no medical records beyond the two years prior to the accident? What tests or determination besides subjective patient's say-so determined [your diagnosis of] a migraine? What exact symptoms did he have regarding a migraine? Why no other tests to rule out other neurological problems? Is there a measurement for the amount of serotonin in his brain? What causes serotonin not to work properly? Is surgery a last resort? What is indomethacin? Can it cause problems if you have prostate problems?

In still another accident case a radiologist testified about a knee injury. Here are the written questions that jurors wanted the witness to answer:

Did you see the tears in the meniscus? Do you see degeneration in young people and what about people of the plaintiff's age? Is a tear in the meniscus a loosening, lack or gash in the cartilage? Can you tell the age of a tear due to an injury? Can you see healed tissue in an MRI? Do cartilage tears heal by themselves? Can healed tears appear younger [more recent] than they really are?

These comments are typical of the way juries respond to expert evidence.[26,27] In a thorough review of the research literature bearing on juries and experts, Diamond and I concluded:

> There is a consistent convergence [in the various studies.] Jurors appear motivated to critically assess the content of the expert's testimony and weigh it in the context of other trial evidence, as they are instructed to do. They appear to understand the nature of the adversary process, at least in the context of their specific trial. Even though many jurors may not have had prior exposure to the trial process, it appears that they develop an understanding from the give and take of cross-examination and exposure to opposing experts. Indeed, rather than deferring to experts, as critics have claimed, the trial process appears to make them aware of the fallibility of expert testimony.[28]

Medical malpractice litigation is a contentious topic. However, careful research findings consistently reveal that most of the time juries do a good job in carrying out the task they are assigned.

In my opinion, if the defense lawyer does his or her job properly, the semi-retired pediatric allergist will have his credentials challenged before trial (in what is called a "Daubert hearing") and the judge may disqualify him as an expert. If the challenge fails, and assuming there are no other experts for the plaintiff, cross-examination of the pediatric allergist and contrary testimony from defense experts will likely result in another instance of jurors deciding in favor of the defendant doctor.

Neil Vidmar, Ph.D.
Russell M. Robinson II Professor of Law, Duke Law School
Professor of Psychology, Duke University

COMMITMENT TO PROFESSIONAL RESPONSIBILITIES – PULMONARY MEDICINE

An ICU (intensive care unit) physician manages the care of a patient who was transferred from a rehabilitation inpatient unit. The patient had a total hip replacement last week and now has a pulmonary embolism. Anticoagulation is discussed with the patient and family and is begun. The orthopedic surgeon does not agree with the decision to use anticoagulation, does not speak with the ICU physician, but tells the family that it should be stopped and an inferior vena cava filter should be placed.

A Perspective from a Pulmonologist-Critical Care Physician

Clinical Background

Pulmonary thromboembolism (DVT-PE) represents a potentially fatal post-surgical event and there is a high incidence after joint replacement or orthopedic surgery. Understandably, because of the high risk of pulmonary thromboembolism, most patients undergoing hip or knee replacement are treated with preventive anticoagulation to avoid symptomatic DVT-PE. The exact protocols vary despite well-established guidelines.[29] Despite such preventive therapies DVT-PE can still occur, although such events are uncommon in patients who receive adequate prophylaxis. A PE which the patient survives should be viewed as a marker of a potential recurrent event, which conceivably could be fatal. Treatment is aimed primarily at preventing any further occurrence.

There are two primary modalities of therapy.[30] First, in patients without contraindication, full anticoagulation would be considered standard treatment. Acceptable agents would include unfractionated heparin or low molecular weight heparin dosed at therapeutic levels (such as enoxaparin at 1 mg/kg SC q 12 hours).[31] Second, patients with contraindication or who fail anticoagulation should undergo vena cava filter placement. Thrombolytics cannot be utilized so soon after a surgical procedure. In the presented case, we will assume that prophylactic therapies did not lead to full anticoagulation or that prophylactic therapies were stopped too soon, otherwise, this would be considered a case of failed anticoagulation and a filter would indeed be appropriate from the perspective of the ICU physician as well as the orthopedic surgeon. Assuming preventive anticoagulation was sub-therapeutic or had been stopped at the time of the event, the medical literature would support full anticoagulation as the preferred treatment plan. The arguments for this approach include the demonstrated effectiveness in preventing recurrent events, the low rate of bleeding complications, and the ability to avoid placing a device that could lead to long-term complications such as recurrent deep vein thrombosis (DVT), post-phlebitic syndrome, or, rarely, phlegmasia cerulea dolens.[32] In a major scientific article comparing filter placement with anticoagulation, DeCousis et al. showed that filters are indeed effective in preventing pulmonary embolization in the short run.[33] However, DeCousis also showed a much higher rate of recurrent DVT by twenty-four months post-placement (20.8 percent vs. 11.6 percent). Two-year survival was comparable between the two groups.

Professionalism Considerations

The case in point represents an important therapeutic dilemma and professionalism challenge: Two physicians can approach the care of an individual patient from separate perspectives depending on their background, primary concerns, and view of the medical literature. In this particular case the orthopedic surgeon, concerned about bleeding into the joint which was just replaced, would prefer to avoid anticoagulation as a primary treatment for pulmonary thromboembolism. By contrast, the medical intensivist, concerned primarily about the overall outcome of the patient with regard to the pulmonary embolism, a potentially life-threatening event, recommends anticoagulation as the treatment which would lead to the best general outcome (perhaps less concerned with the joint itself). Both physicians are right to be involved in the care of the patient. However, managing their differences is key to ideal patient care.

The motivation for an orthopedic surgeon to suggest filter placement could be two-fold. It could mean that the orthopedic surgeon is still primarily concerned about the hip replacement and the risk of bleeding into the joint space, which could compromise the overall outcome of the joint surgery. Alternatively, it could reflect a lack of complete understanding on the part of the orthopedic surgeon regarding the literature on outcomes after filter placement.

Understanding the nuances of the professionalism dilemma posed by this case requires a discussion of the standards with regard to the admitting physician in contrast to the role of a prior treating physician. Technically, when the ICU physician serves as the attending of record, he/she is in charge and has the final authority over the treatment plan. Having stated that, it is important to include the previous treating physician in the dialogue of patient care for several reasons. These include identifying important technical details of the recent surgery, respecting the surgeon's role as an involved physician, and notifying him/her of the patient's course and complication. Assuming the medical intensivist disagrees with the suggestion of the orthopedic surgeon to place the filter, the best course of action would be to contact this physician directly, state the rationale for the proposed care plan, invite questions and comments, but then inform the orthopedic surgeon of the final plan. It would be important to inform the family that such a discussion has taken place and the outcome. As Merli and Weitz have noted in their text on medical consultation, "talk is cheap . . . and effective".[34] This conversation could help the family understand the care plan and reassure the family and patient that all opinions had been registered. In its Physician Charter, the American Board of Internal Medicine has emphasized the necessity of open and honest communication with patients and peer physicians.[8] In dealing with the divergent views of patient management head-on, the intensivist can help the family understand the management plan, avoid confusion, and establish proper authority regarding the care of the patient.

Opinion

One could argue that the "captain of the ship" mentality would be applicable in this scenario. While the orthopedic surgeon was at the helm during the hip replacement surgery, the patient has now encountered postoperative complications and it is time for the medical intensivist to set the course and provide direction. Although the input of the orthopedic surgeon should be sought and considered, this patient is at significant risk and aggressive care is warranted. As a courtesy, the orthopedic surgeon should be contacted. The surgeon's advice however, should be provided directly to the intensivist without creating conflict with the family. I would also point out the importance of clear communication and the need for one attending of record. With rare exceptions, such conflicts can be resolved before they escalate into a diversion from the care of the patient.

Gregory C. Kane, M.D.
Professor of Medicine, Vice Chair for Education
Jefferson Medical College

A Perspective from an Expert in Organization Development

This particular clinical scenario highlights the all too common realities that complicate a physician's work life:

- Optimal, effective quality patient care is dependent on all members of a patient care team establishing and maintaining, collaborative work relationships.
- Conflict between individuals and groups in the workplace is inevitable.[34]

The good news is that these two realities are not mutually exclusive. The fact is that when conflict is managed well, team functioning can actually improve rather than descend into dysfunction. The assumption usually is that in high-performing teams, conditions of conflict, disagreement, and discomfort are rarely experienced. This is a myth and nothing could be further from the truth. High-performing teams are filled with conflict and disagreement. The difference between low- and high-functioning teams is that in the latter, conflict is managed well and the conflict centers on the task and not on the interpersonal dynamics between individuals or between disciplines, specialties, or work groups.[35] In low-performing teams where conflict is handled poorly and/or the conflict centers on the other and not on the task, dysfunctional outcomes are guaranteed.

In the particular scenario before us, the ICU physician is faced with a difficult situation: A colleague involved in caring for the patient disagrees with the ICU physician's treatment plan and has communicated those concerns with the patient's family. What should the ICU physician do in this situation? How does he/she handle him/herself professionally to manage the conflict and benefit the patient? The first thing the ICU physician should do is to step back and remind him/herself of three core truths:

- Conflict is a normal and inevitable aspect of human interaction.
- Conflict can result in positive consequences for those involved.
- Complete lack of conflict in work interactions is a sign of an unhealthy work environment.

Adopting these attitudes encourages the ICU physician to focus on and address the behavior of a colleague, not to evaluate the personhood of the orthopedic surgeon. With these attitudes in mind the ICU physician is now at a decision point. How does he/she manage this conflict? Thomas and Killman postulate five conflict management modes to handle situations where two people's concerns, wishes and/or needs appear to be incompatible.[36] According to Thomas and Killman, an individual's behavioral response to this situation is dependent on two dimensions: (1) *assertiveness* – the extent to which an individual attempts to satisfy his/her own concerns; and (2) *cooperativeness* – the extent to which the individual attempts to satisfy the other person's concerns.[36]

A person's position on these two dimensions determines his/her response. Listed here are the five basic conflict management modes resulting from the intersection of assertiveness and cooperativeness. Each of these five modes has its costs and benefits. Ideally physicians should have the ability and skill to use any one or combination of these modes as the situation dictates.

1. A *competing* approach is assertive and minimally cooperative. It is important to understand here that assertive does not mean aggressive.

Aggressive behavior is behavior that an individual uses to get his/her needs/wants/desires met at the expense of another; assertive behavior is that type of behavior that an individual uses to stand up for his/her position while respecting the rights and personhood of the other. A competing approach is a good choice when: quick, decisive action is required; important issues are at stake and the right course of action may not be popular; the relationship is short-term and relatively unimportant; there is a need to protect oneself from people who may take advantage of non-competitive behavior.[36] A physician overusing this style risks negative consequences, including threatening important relationships, winning a battle but losing the war, and engendering feeling of revenge in colleagues.[36]

2. *Accommodating* is minimally assertive and highly cooperative. It is a useful choice when: you realize you are wrong; when the issue is more important to the other person; a goodwill gesture may act to maintain an important relationship; the other person is insistent and has ultimate power over the decision; preserving harmony and avoiding disruption are especially important.[36] When accommodating is overused, a physician can find him/her self in a lose-win situation where important and vital goals are constantly being sacrificed.

3. *Avoiding* is both unassertive and uncooperative. It is a good choice when: an issue is trivial; time is needed to cool down, and gather more information; the potential damage of confronting a conflict outweighs the benefits of a resolution; others can resolve the conflict more effectively.[36] If overused, the style has the consequence of leaving important conflicts unresolved and/or allowing a conflict to fester and grow to virtually irresolvable proportions.

4. *Compromising* is part assertive and part cooperative. Both parties give up something and gain something. This is a useful style when: the goals are somewhat important but not worth the potential disruption of competing; when two equal opponents are committed to mutually exclusive goals; a temporary solution to a complex issue is needed; expediency is needed due to a time pressure; competing or collaboration have failed to lead to successful resolution.[36] When overused, a compromising approach may cause a physician to lose sight of important principles, values, and long-term objectives in pursuit of a solution.[36]

5. *Collaboration* is both assertive and cooperative. It is a useful approach when: the interests of both parties are interdependent; it is important for the relationship to have a good future; values or principles are involved and compromise is unacceptable; innovative solutions are valued or needed.[36] The downside of collaboration is that it takes

enormous time and energy (both scarce and important resources for a physician) and it requires and assumes a level of trust that may not be present with the individual with whom the physician is in conflict.[36]

The ICU physician in our case has all of these modes available. It is important that an approach is chosen that matches the dynamics of the situation and that an approach is not taken because of habit, temperament or just because it worked before. Most people overuse a style or two repeatedly and consequently underuse certain modes – both to the detriment of good resolution of conflict.

Once the ICU physician is engaged with the orthopedic surgeon, the former should try to match the conflict mode with goals of the interaction and the emerging dynamics and new understandings that could arise during the conversation. It is important for our ICU attending to realize that he/she is never stuck with an outcome. He/she can always clarify a situation, gather more information, or change conflict management modes.

At the beginning of and throughout the conversation, the physician should remind him/herself that people hear best when they are not feeling threatened. For instance, when empathy and an awareness of the other's concerns and feelings are evident, the sense of threat abates. The physician should demonstrate through active listening skills and nonthreatening nonverbal and verbal responses that the focus is on the task of resolving the conflict amicably.

Conflict managed well can have important beneficial outcomes for a relationship, a team, and optimal patient care. While nothing is guaranteed, understanding the principles and utilizing the techniques outlined here will help physicians and health care teams move forward by using effective conflict management skills to create environments characterized by professional values and dedicated to high quality patient care.

Timothy Brigham, M.Div., Ph.D.
Senior Vice President, Department of Education
Accreditation Council for Graduate Medical Education

COMMITMENT TO PROFESSIONAL RESPONSIBILITIES – PSYCHIATRY

A psychiatrist, concerned that his forty-eight-year-old wife has been frequently anxious over the past several months, recommends and then prescribes the anxiolytic, lorazepam for her to take every six hours as needed. She has a gynecologist whom she sees annually, but does not regularly see another physician. Other than her anxiety, she feels well and has been in good health. They have had no marital difficulties.

A Perspective from a Psychiatrist

Clinical Background

Panic disorder occurs in about 2 percent of the populations studied in Europe and North America. An even higher percent of the populations report panic attacks, but do not meet the full criteria for panic disorder.[37] The symptoms of panic attacks involve intense fear for a discrete period (usually around ten minutes), during which the patient may experience a variety of physical and emotional symptoms such as palpitations, sweating, trembling, shortness of breath, choking, chest pain, nausea, dizziness, feeling unreal, fear of losing control, fear of dying, numbness, or chills.

An anxiety disorder can be treated with benzodiazepines with great efficacy. Panic disorder is also very responsive to selective serotonin reuptake inhibitors (SSRIs). A common treatment practice is to use benzodiazepines for the short term, while waiting for the SSRI to begin to take effect (which can take up to six weeks in some cases).

Professionalism Considerations

Treating "non-patients" is a common practice among physicians. One study of 465 physicians reported that 99 percent of those surveyed delivered some sort of medical care to family members, care which ranged from medical advice to performing surgery. In this study, 83 percent of the physician respondents had prescribed medication for family members, although the type of medication was not listed.[38] Another study of 92 resident physicians reported that 85 percent of those surveyed had written prescriptions for "non-patients."[39] This would suggest that the practice of treating non-patients starts during the training years, when physicians begin to establish their own practice habits and rules.

There are two areas of discussion here: one ethical and one legal. The AMA *Code of Medical Ethics* states "Physicians should not treat themselves or immediate family members," and the Code goes on to list several reasons why. For example, a physician may not be comfortable discussing very personal issues with a family member. In addition, that family member may not feel comfortable expressing disagreement with the physician if the physician is a family member. Further, the AMA Code states "Except for emergencies, it is not appropriate for physicians to write prescriptions for controlled substances for themselves or immediate family members."[40] The American College of Physicians' *Ethics Manual* echoes these ideas.[7]

There is scant literature about this dilemma, and when this author consulted legal advice about this issue, there was considerable disagreement about where the line should be drawn. For example, is it okay to prescribe antibiotics, but not narcotics? What constitutes a family member? A wife? A cousin? What constitutes an emergency?

Federal law identifies "non-patients" as individuals who seek medical care from someone who is not their regular physician. The law also states that a patient–physician relationship begins as soon as the physician begins treatment (e.g., writes a prescription). The law goes on to state that any time a controlled substance is prescribed, there must be a bona fide patient–physician relationship, and that includes the maintenance of a written medical record.[7]

This physician is at risk for several errors in judgment. First, the psychiatrist's objectivity would almost certainly be compromised due to the close relationship that already exists between him and his wife.[40] Second, performing an examination on a relative can be disturbing to patient and physician alike, and performing a mental status exam is even more troubling.[7] If this physician makes an error, either in diagnosis or treatment, tensions may develop, and those tensions may spill over into the personal relationship.[40] In addition, how can this physician guarantee that his wife's autonomy has been preserved? She may be reluctant to state her preference for treatment to her husband. Lastly, according to federal statutes, this physician may be breaking the law by prescribing a controlled substance for a family member. There is no mention here about a medical record, but one would assume that there is none, and, if so, this physician's action violates federal law as well.

Opinion

It is understandable that this physician would be concerned about his wife's symptoms. Panic disorder can be disabling, and may even prevent the patient from leaving the house. In such a scenario, if the patient could not function, it might be conceivable for the physician to prescribe a very limited amount of alprazolam. Even that seems risky to this author, and presenting to the ER seems a better route to procure treatment. That way, the burden of and responsibility for diagnosis, workup, and treatment would be transferred to another physician.

If the psychiatrist elected to write a prescription for his wife, it would definitely be appropriate to refer his wife to another physician as soon as possible.[7,40,41] In the meantime, it would be necessary for the psychiatrist to keep a record of the medical history, examination, and treatment, which can then be communicated with the subsequent treating physician when care is transferred.[7,40,41]

Josephine Albritton, M.D.
Assistant Professor, Department of Psychiatry and Health Behavior
Medical College of Georgia

A PERSPECTIVE FROM AN EXPERT ON PHARMACY ETHICS

The practice of prescribing medications for non-patients, that is, individuals such as friends and family members, is probably a common occurrence, although there are few studies that have explored the prevalence.[38,39,42] There is considerably more data on physician self-prescribing and the potential problems that can result.[43] The practices of self-prescribing and prescribing for non-patients usually begin in medical school, where the habit of not seeking professional help from a qualified colleague is established.

Physicians say they prescribe for non-patients because it saves the non-patient time and, if they possess the appropriate clinical expertise, they could help the non-patient. Physicians are more likely to write prescriptions for non-patients with whom they have a close relationship, such as a family member. Furthermore, physicians are more willing to write a prescription when the case involves what appears to be a simple health problem such as a urinary tract infection or a drug that is not addictive or has limited side effects. Finally, physicians prescribe for non-patients because they are often motivated by genuine concern and a desire to help.

There are some ethical and legal guidelines regarding treatment of family and friends. As noted, the American Medical Association *Code of Medical Ethics* states that physicians generally should not treat themselves or members of their family.[44] The exceptions are for a short-term, minor problem or an emergency. However, there is considerable room for interpretation by individual physicians as to whether treatment is appropriate. I would argue that prescribing for a non-patient is generally wrong for clinical and ethical reasons.

Possible Clinical Harms

The case in question involves a psychiatrist prescribing for a non-patient, his wife. The health problem in question, anxiety, does fall within the psychiatrist's area of expertise as does the drug he prescribes for his wife. However, the fact that he is qualified to diagnose and treat patients who are suffering from anxiety does not mean that it is appropriate for him to do so for his wife.

Inappropriate treatment is the greatest possible physical harm evident in the case. We do not know if the psychiatrist conducted as thorough an examination as he would with any other patient. Even if he did, he would not be able to approach his wife's symptoms with the same objectivity as with patients who are not his spouse. Nor would she be able to present her symptoms as honestly as she would with a more objective physician. The vague symptom of anxiety can have many causes, including organic problems that might be overlooked by a psychiatrist, who is primarily trained to look for mental and emotional sources of health problems. The wife could have hyper-thyroidism or consume too much caffeine, to name a few organic reasons for her anxiety. By prescribing for his wife, he could misdiagnose the problem and delay appropriate treatment. The degree of harm from delaying treatment could vary depending on the seriousness of the actual diagnosis.

Ethical Harms

The ethical harms arise from several sources. Any discussion of harms and benefits in the physician–patient relationship necessarily draws on the basic ethical principles of nonmaleficence (avoiding harm) and beneficence (doing good). According to these principles, physicians and other health professionals are to refrain from harming patients and to further the interests of others. Thus, there is a fundamental professional obligation to keep patients' best interests as the goal of the interaction. Because of the proximity of the psychiatrist to his wife, it is difficult for him to be objective, thus increasing the possibility of harm.

Another factor that compromises the psychiatrist's perspective is the existence of a dual relationship in the case, wherein "dual relationship" is defined as those in which a professional assumes or has a second role with a patient.[45] The psychiatrist may rationalize his behavior, arguing that the situation is unique. "However, dual relationships are potentially exploitive; crossing the boundaries of ethical practice, satisfying the practitioner's needs and impairing his or her judgment."[45] The psychiatrist cannot treat his wife like other patients because she isn't like other patients. The patient–physician relationship is founded on trust and confidence that offsets inequities in power and protects the vulnerability of the patient. The spousal relationship is also founded on important principles such as fidelity or faithfulness to promises. A dual relationship sets the stage for competing moral obligations that may not be apparent to those involved in the situation.

Finally, it is not clear if the wife exercised her autonomy in choosing who would treat her. If the husband unilaterally decided he was in the best position to treat his wife, he would be guilty of paternalism. The wife may not wish to share sensitive, personal information with her husband but rather seek help from a neutral medical advisor. It is not out of the realm of possibility that the source of the wife's anxiety lies within her relationship with her husband.

Amy M. Haddad, Ph.D.
Director, Center for Health Policy and Ethics, and the Dr. C.C.
and Mabel L. Criss Endowed Chair in the Health Sciences
Creighton University Medical Center

COMMITMENT TO PROFESSIONAL RESPONSIBILITIES – SURGERY

The head of nursing at a community hospital complains to the chairman of surgery about a general surgeon who has had difficulty collaborating with many of the nurses. This surgeon has thrown surgical instruments in the operating room, used abusive language, and berated nurses. Most recently, he loudly, and in the presence of the patient, criticized a nurse after noting that the patient's pneumatic compression boots were not applied as ordered.

A Perspective from a Current and Former Chair of Surgery and a Surgery Administrator

Professionalism Considerations

The scenario described in this vignette is believable, and describes activities that, at least in the past, were not unheard of in the hospital setting. Four aspects of this vignette are important to note.

First, the head of nursing has followed the typical chain of command, having been presented with evidence of a surgeon's unprofessional behavior, likely from the primary sources (the nurses involved). It would not be uncommon that most of the nursing staff at this community hospital recognize this particular surgeon as a "difficult," "problematic," or simply "nasty" surgeon. The head of nursing has taken these issues to the chairman of the Department of Surgery, with the expectation that the chairman will assess the situation, interact with the surgeon in question, and "fix" the problem. It is possible, even likely that the chairman of surgery has had previous complaints about this surgeon, and that the chairman has even dealt with these issues before, since behaviors such as these are difficult to eradicate.

Second, on a historical note, behaviors such as the throwing of surgical instruments, abusive language, berating nurses and other personnel, and criticisms of nursing care were not uncommon many years ago in a very hierarchical system where the surgeon was considered the "captain of the ship." In that bygone era, it was expected that the staff be very much subservient to the surgeon's leadership. Fortunately, this is no longer the case. All health care providers have come to the recognition that delivery of care to patients is best performed via a cohesive team, on which all types of health care professionals interact collegially, amiably, and with the patients' best interests in mind.

Third, the unacceptable behaviors manifested by this surgeon may not occur solely in the hospital setting, but may have deeper roots in the surgeon's personality, family situation, financial difficulties, medical-legal status, or personal health status. While not an excuse for this surgeon's unacceptable behaviors, this surgeon's private life, family life, practice partners, and many other stresses may be contributing factors.

Fourth, it is important to recognize that the health care setting can be a stress-filled environment, and that the operating room, and the treatment of postoperative patients, can be one of the most challenging environments in which to work. The stakes are high in the operating room and on the post-op surgical wards. The level of acuity of hospitalized patients has risen dramatically over the last decades, and the expectations of the patient, public, and legal profession, are clearly at all-time high levels. Errors in judgment, errors in technique, anesthetic errors, poor patient outcomes, deviations from critical pathways – all of these events can add to a surgeon's stress level and sense of urgency in providing optimal care twenty-four hours a day, seven days a week to all patients under his/her care.

Recent work at our institution has generated a document entitled "The Statement of Professional Conduct," which provides important and relevant information for this topic.[46] As part of this document, the general principles of medical professionalism include the concept that the medical profession places the welfare of the patient above self-interest, and notes that the practitioners accept their responsibility to educate future physicians in the values and ethical standards of medical professionalism. The faculty acknowledges that this can best be achieved by serving as strong role models and advocates, while maintaining professional relationships based on mutual respect and concern. Overall, it is critical that we promote an atmosphere of cooperation and learning, of intellectual openness, honesty, and sincerity, in order to constantly protect, redefine and make meaningful our core values and covenant of trust with society.[46]

An important aspect of medical professionalism involves the core values of the institution. These core values of professionalism should guide the actions of the medical practitioners on a daily basis. At Jefferson the core values include:

- *Integrity* – our word is our bond.
- *Respect* – we respect each other and all with whom we come in contact.
- *Compassion* – we care about and attempt to ameliorate the suffering and pain of illness.
- *Excellence* – we are committed to excellence and lifelong pursuit of new knowledge and personal and professional growth.
- *Altruism* – we aspire to do the right thing, for the right reason, even if it involves pain or sacrifice.
- *Collaboration* – we are committed to each other and to those we serve. We work together to achieve our mission and goals.
- *Stewardship* – we are committed to the prudent use of resources.

In the particular vignette discussed here, the general surgeon with unprofessional behavior appears to have violated, at minimum, the three core values of respect, compassion, and collaboration. The violations of these core values can be seen as creating a dysfunctional interpersonal interplay between this surgeon and the staff in the operating room, and the staff taking care of his patients on the hospital wards. While striving for high levels of performance and patient results are lofty goals, there can be no doubt that each of us as physicians ultimately wishes the absolute best for all of our patients at any time. The shortfalls and inappropriate behaviors exhibited by this surgeon in the areas of respect, compassion, and collaboration must be seen as contributing very negatively to the work of the entire professional health care team. Additionally, the loud criticisms of a nurse in the presence of a patient serve to erode the physician–patient relationship, and may lead to the patient calling into question the surgeon's commitment to those same core values (respect, compassion, collaboration).

As a result of the eighty-hour resident work rule on academic institutions sanctioned by the ACGME (Accreditation Council for Graduate Medical Education), we have observed attending physicians spending more time on hospital grounds than they did just five years ago. Increased surgeon work hours present the potential for increased surgeon stress and decreased professionalism.

Currently, clinical department chairs conduct annual physician performance reviews. In addition to addressing clinical, financial, academic, and research accomplishments, these reviews now include interpersonal skills, teaching abilities and "good citizenship." Deficiency in these areas may result in decreased compensation or the requirement to attend one of several educational programs offered by the institution.

Opinion

The relevant steps for addressing the surgeon's professionalism issues are to:

1. collect information about the extent of the surgeon's inappropriate behavior (be a detective and see if these are isolated events);
2. speak to the surgeon about these behaviors in the broader context of personal and professional life;
3. initiate a formal counseling process, using the resources of the medical center or an independent counselor, to address these inappropriate behaviors;
4. put in place a clear expectation that such behaviors will not be tolerated;
5. define the sequelae, should the behaviors recur.

Fortunately, the behaviors of the surgeon in this vignette are becoming less common. They are clearly not acceptable. In fact, the pendulum is swinging toward a zero tolerance policy. In the past, surgical residents in training were exposed to attending surgeons who practiced such unacceptable, demeaning, even misogynistic behavior, and the residents may have concluded that this behavior was acceptable – but such is no longer the case.

Upon completion of their formal medical school education, one of the rites of passage for medical students is the recitation of the Oath of Hippocrates or one of many variations thereof. In it one states *primum non nocere*, first do not harm. While the ancient intent may have referred to the physician–patient relationship, in today's world of high acuity medical practice, where teamwork is so critical, the intent goes well beyond that, to include our interactions with other members of the health care team. It is one of the key elements of professionalism that we must adhere to at all times. Included in the "core values" of both undergraduate and graduate medical education are professionalism and interpersonal skills and communication. They are essential components upon which successful medical and surgical practices are built.

Charles Yeo, M.D.
Samuel D. Gross Professor and Chair of Surgery,
Jefferson Medical College

Herbert Cohn, M.D.
Professor of Surgery, Jefferson Medical College

Dianne MacRae
Department of Surgery, Jefferson Medical College

A Perspective from a Nurse Educator

The most challenging areas for physicians and nurses when working in the operating room are communication, conflict resolution, and collaboration. These three Cs are key ingredients to providing safe and quality care.[47,48] When physicians and nurses do not communicate, collaborate, or resolve conflict responsibly, in a civilized manner with each other, the consequences may be great indeed. In this case, the issue was addressed at the chief nursing officer (CNO) and chairman level. How might it have been resolved in an equitable fashion between the nurse and the general surgeon? Two questions to consider are:

1. What are the obligations of the general surgeon, the nurse, the head of nursing, and the chairman of surgery?

2. In analyzing and evaluating the patient's risks related to this case, how should risk to patient safety be taken into account in this context?

Effective nurse–physician communication is a responsibility of all members of the health care team. This is critical in the operating room because the more specialized the work of nurses, the more complex the communication lines. The multiple communication lines are compounded by specialization across surgeons with whom nurses must communicate when caring for heterogeneous groups of patients.[49] This case study is shaped by the fact that the general surgeon did not exhibit professional behavior, he did not communicate directly with the nurse affected by his disruptive behavior and the exchange occurred in the presence of the patient. Events such as this are known to increase the likelihood of adverse events.[48] Rather than the CNO discussing the situation with the chairman, direct peer communication at the time of the incident between the general surgeon and nurse would have been a more appropriate strategy. Also, the preferred exchange would be a calm, private conversation unbeknownst to the patient.

Given the importance of the working relationship between physicians and nurses and the frequency of conflict between them, more effort should be devoted to constructive ways to resolve conflict.[50,51] In this case study, addressing and resolving the conflict in a positive manner at the time of the occurrence would have demonstrated responsibility and accountability on behalf of the nurse and the general surgeon. Since it was addressed at the CNO and chairman level, these two leaders were obligated to use this as a teaching moment for both the nurse and physician. For example, the nurse and the general surgeon should have been made aware of the importance of cooperation and be encouraged to learn the most constructive ways to settle conflicts. If the conflict was addressed at the peer level, a dialogue could have identified that rather than an error, there was evidence for not applying the sequential compression device (SCD). There may have been a contraindication to the use of an SCD and this is why the nurse did not apply them. Resolving conflict and building relations at the peer level prevents potential patient consequences.

It is fundamental to acknowledge that relationships between physicians and nurses can be improved and that there is a responsibility of each professional to change behaviors toward that improvement.[52] Working toward more collaboration requires willing participants in change and growth opportunities. Collaboration within peer groups and daily working teams leads to smoother functioning and improved patient outcomes.[47]

In this case study, all the health care providers involved owe it to the patient and their colleagues to work, act, and look like a team. The delivery of safe and quality care is enhanced when teams are functioning and striving together for excellence. Professional demeanor should include visible respect for each other. At the very least, the nurse and general surgeon should be able to conceal their displeasure and aggravation, and exhibit behavior that indicates teamwork in front of the patient.

Beth Ann Swan, Ph.D., CRNP, FAAN
Associate Professor and Associate Dean of the Graduate Program
Jefferson School of Nursing

COMMITMENT TO PROFESSIONAL RESPONSIBILITIES – NEUROLOGY

An eighty-two-year-old man with a history of chronic atrial fibrillation comes into the emergency room on a Sunday morning with sudden onset of hemiparesis. A non-hemorrhagic stroke is diagnosed and TPA (tissue plasminogen activator) is administered by the emergency room staff. The hemiparesis begins to resolve. The covering neurologist is called but is unable to be reached. After several hours of unsuccessful calls, the neurologist's partner is reached and comes in to continue care for the patient. The following day, the neurologist who was reached discusses the inaccessibility with her partner and the fact that there have been other behavior problems such as patient and staff complaints about his conduct. She also is aware that her partner has had a past history of alcohol abuse and is concerned that her partner is impaired.

A Perspective from a Neurologist

Clinical Background

Acute stroke is a neurological emergency that requires emergent care and ready consultation to a neurologist. Tissue plasminogen activator (TPA) administered within three hours of the onset of stroke improves clinical outcomes at three months compared to placebo.[53] However, TPA carries risks, including a 6 per cent risk of symptomatic intracerebral hemorrhage within thirty-six hours,[53] that require urgent neurological and neurosurgical evaluation.

The partner of the neurologist on call in this vignette is confronted with a possible impaired physician. Several causes for physician impairment exist, and in this case, alcohol abuse appears to be possible. Among the criteria for substance abuse, according to the *Diagnostic and Statisitical Manual of Mental Disorders*, fourth edition, is repeated failure to fulfill work, school, or home obligations,[54] which may be the case here. Substance abuse among physicians is common: approximately 10–15 percent of physicians will misuse drugs or alcohol at some point during their career,[54] a statistic that mirrors that of the general population.[54,55]

Professionalism Considerations

The neurologist who was finally reached has many duties to address with the possible impairment of her partner. In this case, she has moral obligations to at least four parties. The first is an obligation to the health of current and future patients. The physician has a duty to protect patients from harm that may occur from acts of omission (e.g., failing to provide TPA) or commission. From this standpoint alone, the neurologist should confront her partner and seek ways to help him address his impairment.

The second obligation is to her partner. More than likely, the neurologist who was reached has at least a cordial relationship with her errant partner and has a genuine interest in his well-being. The neurologist should thus avail herself to help her partner, and likely friend, in need.

The next obligation is to her profession. One of the hallmarks of a profession is the ability and willingness to self-regulate. In this case, having a physician with a substance abuse disorder who is not receiving appropriate treatment could lead to harmful results and erode the overall trust of the profession. Failure of a profession to self-regulate inevitably leads to regulation from parties outside the profession (e.g., the government).

Finally, the neurologist has an obligation to her partnership. The partnership and its assets, including those of the physicians, may be exposed legally to any misconduct on the part of the impaired physician. Thus, the financial livelihood of the neurologist, other partners, employees, and their families may all be threatened by the potential misconduct of an impaired physician.

Some of these duties are codified into law. Some states, for example, have mandatory reporting requirements to the state board of medical examiners, physician health programs,[55] or other entities of any physician that "may be mentally or physically unable to engage in the practice of medicine."[56] In most states, physicians reporting such physicians are legally protected for their actions,[54] unless they commit perjury.[56]

Confronting and overcoming substance abuse is challenging. Fortunately, the prognosis for an impaired physician recovering from substance abuse is generally good. Reported recovery rates are variable and range from 27 percent to 92 percent.[54] However, most studies show that physicians have better outcomes than the general population, and recent reports demonstrate that comprehensive programs, which include rehabilitation, close monitoring (e.g., random drug screening), and follow-up, can lead to 75 percent to 85 percent of physicians returning to work.[54]

Opinion

Confronted with this case, I would (1) do my homework, (2) confront my partner, and (3) follow through. Given my lack of familiarity with my hospital and state's requirements, I would consult (without revealing the identity of my partner) with colleagues and an attorney who works in our department about these requirements. Absent ready access to an attorney, one could consult with respected colleagues, the physician health program for one's state (www.fsphp.org),[55] or with the ombudsman for the hospital. Appropriately informed, I would then confront my partner about my concern for his possible alcohol abuse (ideally I would have approached this subject previously) and his lack of availability the preceding day. Absent a clear and compelling explanation, I would ask him to refer himself to a physician's health program (either through the state or hospital)[54] and indicate that if he did not, that I would. I would support him (and his family) in this process. I would also ask for evidence that he reported himself, and absent that evidence, would indicate that I would contact the health program independently.

E. Ray Dorsey, M.D., M.B.A.
Assistant Professor of Neurology, University of
Rochester Medical Center

A Perspective from a Substance Abuse Psychologist

When a problem with a colleague is identified, it is the ethical obligation of the observer to intervene. Ignoring a concern could harm other patients and lead to an exacerbation of problematic behaviors. Despite this probability, research has shown that many physicians are reticent, if not unwilling, to report problematic behaviors of professional colleagues, even if serious concerns exist such as impairment from substance abuse and/or mental health issues.[57]

Substance abusers have a well-earned reputation for lying and unreliability. In the vignette provided, what we know is that the physician of concern did not attend to his on-call responsibilities, received "complaints about his conduct," and has a history of alcohol abuse. The colleague is appropriately "concerned that her partner is impaired" and has an ethical obligation to safeguard all patients in the practice. The partner might also worry about the impact of the presenting circumstances on her livelihood and professional reputation. Despite some very incriminating circumstances that alcohol is the cause, indisputable evidence is lacking. There is no slurred speech, no odor, and no ataxic gate. Other problems not directly evident (or without adequate information to determine) include familiar patterns, relationships, and habits associated with previous drinking episodes; shame; guilt; increased personal/professional difficulties; changes in mood; driving infractions; changes in appearance; and weight changes.

Emphasizing substance abuse prematurely or in error could lead the physician of concern to be defensive, to perceive the intervention as punitive thereby contributing to alienation and deterrence from seeking help, and to exacerbate the problematic behavioral patterns[58] while the true underlying issue is missed. In addition, accusing a colleague of poor patient management without "substantial evidence"[59] is also unethical.

Ethical guidelines exist about how to respond to the challenging scenario described in the vignette. There is an ethical obligation to utilize resources at one's disposal to try to get a handle on this situation so that the welfare of the colleague and the public is preserved. Depending upon the context and index of suspicion of alcohol abuse, any or all of the following responses are appropriate and ethical: speaking directly with the physician of suspected impairment (done in this case); speaking with the physician's family or close friends about the behavior of the colleague; consulting with other colleagues and/or supervisors about what is observed and what is appropriate; consulting with a member of the Professional Assistance Committee about observations and the appropriate next step; consulting with a faculty/staff assistance program; and reporting concerns to the Board of Physician Quality Assurance.[57] These interventions are also consistent with the standards of conduct and the "essentials of honorable behavior for the physician" as outlined by the American Medical Association[60] and state medical societies.[61]

In this vignette, the colleague took the proper first step by identifying concerns about the partner's unresponsiveness when on-call and informing him of patient complaints. Sometimes this is enough to motivate someone to initiate positive changes on his/her own (e.g., seek professional help), but if problems continue or if alcohol abuse is strongly suspected, it becomes necessary to gather information from family members and colleagues to identify patterns and corroborate suspicion. This should be done in a discreet, caring, and confidential manner. The degree of concern for the colleague and risk to others should match the urgency applied to this quest.

Once it is clear that the partner is drinking excessively, it is time to build an intervention plan. At this point the concerned colleague should contact the appropriate authorities in the institution for an intervention strategy. A thoughtful intervention would ideally involve family members and a faculty assistance program. If the colleagues are in private practice together and are not affiliated with an institution, it will be critical for the colleague to work with the family members and the local medical society, and possibly a professional with expertise in addiction treatment to help outline an intervention strategy. The state medical society and/or the employing institution will work with the state licensing board.[62] The intervention itself should identify specific behaviors that have been problematic, presented with firm support and tone of concern in order to get the person to agree that treatment is necessary. Treatment could include detoxification, psychiatric services, medication and rehabilitation/aftercare, including self-help meetings such as Alcoholics Anonymous.

To increase the likelihood of this working effectively, it may be necessary to plan for and provide professional coverage for the impaired colleague so that the reasons (i.e., excuses) to delay the onset of treatment are eliminated. This could include covering for on-call responsibilities, arranging for patients of the colleague to be seen, providing lectures, and attending meetings for the colleague. It might also require a commitment and availability to handle matters that the impaired colleague becomes concerned about after entering treatment.

Once the impaired colleague is in treatment, the role of the colleague can range from no direct contact while managing the professional obligations of the partner to support or even involvement in treatment sessions and planning. Once the patient is discharged from treatment, it is important for the partner with concerns to know what is expected of her colleague from the institution and licensing board because deviations from an identified plan serve as early warning signs of problems that the observing partner is ethically obligated to respond. It is also recommended that individuals be aware of their own reactions. Emotions such as anger and mistrust, as warranted as they may be, if left to fester, will contribute to a dissatisfying work environment with additional problems. When these feelings do not wane over time, there is reason to question the long-term viability of the professional arrangement. This process parallels what usually occurs within the family of the impaired professional.

The reader should be aware that 75–85 percent of physicians recover when coaxed into treatment in the manner described, particularly when appropriate aftercare, follow-up and monitoring is provided.[62–64] Thus, there is much to motivate the person to enter treatment. And such high success should also serve as strong motivation for the concerned colleague to intervene.

Brad Meier, Ph.D.
Delaware Health and Social Services
Division of Substance Abuse and Mental Health,
Delaware Psychiatric Center

COMMITMENT TO PROFESSIONAL RESPONSIBILITIES – EMERGENCY MEDICINE

A twenty-four-year-old man presented to the emergency department with a red, warm, tender, and swollen knee over the past three days. The attending emergency physician interviewed and examined the patient, reviewed the need for arthrocentesis with the patient, obtained consent, watched as the patient was prepped and draped, but left the patient's room for another emergency prior to the actual procedure. The senior emergency medicine resident along with the medical student successfully performed the knee arthrocentesis. The attending then returned to the patient's room to assess the patient after the procedure was complete. Thereafter, the attending emergency physician documented that she was present for the key portion of the exam and arthrocentesis and was aware that such documentation was required in order to submit a bill for the arthrocentesis.

A Perspective from an Emergency Medicine Physician

Clinical Background

Acute, monoarticular arthritis is a common problem encountered in the emergency department (ED).[65] Patients typically present with joint pain, immobility, swelling, erythema, increased warmth, and tenderness. Non-traumatic causes such as osteoarthritis, rheumatoid arthritis, and crystal-induced arthritis such as gout and pseudogout represent the majority of cases that present to the ED. Trauma may result in intra-articular blood (hemarthrosis) and may signify ligamentous disruption or a fracture. In the ED, the undifferentiated cause requiring the most urgent diagnosis and treatment is septic arthritis. Patients who present to the ED with joint swelling, tenderness, and erythema should be considered to have septic arthritis until proven otherwise.

Direct aspiration of a joint (arthrocentesis) is the procedure of choice.[66] It can be both therapeutic (removal of excess articular fluid lowers intra-articular pressure and relieves pain) and diagnostic. It is indicated for diagnosis of non-traumatic joint disease, diagnosis of ligamentous or bony injury, relief of pain, instillation of medications, and the need for joint fluid analysis.

Professionalism Considerations

The two main purposes of a teaching hospital are patient care and medical education. Teaching hospitals typically combine the two by having resident physicians participate directly in the care of patients under the supervision of the attending physician. The common scenario in the teaching hospital ED is that a resident evaluates a patient (typically alone, but possibly under the watchful eye of the attending physician) and then presents his/her findings to the attending. The evaluation and management is then discussed and a treatment plan is implemented. The attending evaluates the patient directly to confirm findings and/or obtain further information. Continued evaluation and treatment progresses under the supervision of the attending physician but the direct care is typically performed by the resident.

As the attending is ultimately responsible for the care of the patient, he/she must physically see and examine the patient and document the care that was provided. The time that the resident spends with the patient, the discussions between the attending and the residents related to the care of the patient, and the time spent by the attending physician in direct care are all part of the overall care and services provided by the attending. The attending will bill a patient for providing these services. The amount of the bill is dependent upon the level of service provided and is typically related to the severity of illness. It is also directly related to the procedures that may have been performed on the patient while under the care of the attending physician.

In this case, the patient appears to have received comprehensive care. A history was taken, a physical examination was performed and the required procedure was performed. The attending saw and examined the patient and supervised the overall care. The resident's and attending's time devoted to the overall care is primarily spent counseling the patient and obtaining consent. The majority of the time spent on the overall care by the resident and attending is spent on talking with and counseling the patient and obtaining consent for procedures. Further, the attending spends additional time on the case by discussing the care of the patient with the resident and providing teaching. The arthrocentesis represents a very small percentage of the patient care time: the procedure itself takes only a few minutes. The key portion of the procedure is the least time consuming of the patient's stay and may actually represent seconds of time. As a procedure, arthrocentesis is relatively minor, such that a resident or student could perform it safely without direct supervision by the attending physician. Residents, by virtue of the fact that they work under that attending's supervision, cannot directly bill patients for their services. The arthrocentesis was performed, and not billing for the procedure would represent a lost opportunity for income. Because much time and effort was spent on the overall care, the attending should be compensated to the fullest. It seems reasonable to include the arthrocentesis in the bill to optimize compensation for the good patient care. But what seems reasonable in this case is not what is legal.

The Center for Medicare and Medicaid Services states that, in order to bill for a procedure, the attending physician, "must be present during all critical and key portions of the procedure and be immediately available to furnish services during the entire procedure."[67] If the physician is not, then he/she is not able to submit a bill for it. In this case, the "key portion" of the procedure would have been the insertion of the needle into the joint space and the withdrawal of joint fluid. The attending physician clearly was not present for the key portion of the arthrocentesis. While it appears that there was a valid excuse (being called away to another emergency) for the attending's absence, the rules are clear that the attending was not present for the key portion of the procedure. Thus, a bill by the attending should not have been submitted and if it was, the attending physician is guilty of fraud.

Opinion

It may be tempting for physicians to bill for procedures done on patients by residents even if the key portion was not directly supervised. Reasoning such as "I discussed and directed the care, including the procedure, with the resident; I was physically present in the ED and could have been immediately present if needed; I felt comfortable with the skill of the particular resident and did not need to be there to supervise" are all legitimate reasonings. However, they do not allow one to circumvent the moral and legal rules. While the overall care provided to the patient was proper, the emergency physician, in this scenario, should not have submitted a bill for the arthrocentesis. She can submit a bill for other services provided (history and physical examination, decision making, time spent on the case), as long as those services were truly provided.

> *Bernard Lopez, M.D.*
> *Professor of Emergency Medicine*
> *Assistant Dean, Student Affairs*
> *Jefferson Medical College*

A Perspective from an Attorney Specializing in Health Care Services

The issue relating to the appropriate level of supervision of medical residents and the ability to seek payment by the attending physician was decided in a number of very costly settlements by academic medical centers and teaching hospitals commencing in 1995 through the early 2000s.[68] At that time, there was confusion relating to the instructions provided by Medicare and their fiscal intermediaries concerning services provided by residents which could be billed and those services which could not be billed by attending physicians. This became known as the Physicians at Teaching Hospitals Audit Program (PATH). Audits were conducted unannounced by Medicare's Office of Inspector General (OIG). Once the PATH Program audits became more commonplace, a general consensus was reached that physician services provided solely by a medical resident could not be billed by the attending physician. The theory behind the government's approach was a view that academic medical centers and teaching hospitals were double-dipping. The cost of medical residents was paid through medical education adjustments made to the hospital's reimbursement from Medicare and the attending physicians could not then bill for the service if the resident had actually performed the medical services.[69]

Many academic institutions signed Corporate Integrity Agreements (CIAs) with the OIG in which they agreed to pay large amounts to the government; follow appropriate billing guidelines in the future; have third parties review their billing practices periodically; institute comprehensive billing compliance plans; and conduct training of all personnel (including attending and consulting physicians, students, and residents) with respect to compliance issues.[70] While the fact pattern described in the vignette does not indicate whether a CIA is currently in place at this institution, all hospitals are required to maintain a billing compliance plan.[71] One must assume that if this is an academic training facility then both the medical residents and the attending physicians have received training on appropriate billing practices. Billing compliance plans are intended to prevent fraudulent billing practices. In this example, the physician knowingly bills for services that she did not render (the arthrocentesis). This is a clear violation of the Medicare statute and the False Claims Act,[72] and can result in disciplinary action. In order to bill for a service, there must be medical documentation in the patient's medical record showing which physician performed the service and what was performed. In this case, the attending physician is either falsifying the medical record to show that she was in attendance or, if not, the medical record will actually show that she did not perform the procedure. Both could lead to a violation of the institution's compliance plan, resulting in possible fines and other penalties if this is part of a pattern of conduct. All compliance plans contain a disciplinary process for those individuals found to have violated the plan. The compliance officer who administers the plan has the right to recommend that disciplinary action be taken against the attending physician whether or not the physician is an employee of the hospital.

In addition to the violations noted, an intentional violation of the billing methodologies of the hospital could be considered a violation of the code of ethics and code of conduct of the institution. Many organizations, in the wake of the passage of Sarbanes Oxley (a U.S. law passed in 2002 that introduced new regulations to financial accounting),[73] have adopted comprehensive codes of conduct.[74] These codes of conduct contain provisions that prohibit any contractor or employee from breaking any laws. Further, as the patient did not receive the medical service from the attending physician, this may also have been a violation of the hospital's patient bill of rights, which is required to be maintained by Medicare and the hospital accrediting organization.[75] Most patient bill of rights requires the institution to have honest dealings in the provision of medical treatment and billing practices.

It is my view that the attending physician may also have violated the written consent to treatment that the physician had obtained from the patient.[76] The fact pattern indicates that the attending had interviewed the patient, evaluated the patient's condition and prescribed treatment for the inflamed knee. The attending physician obtained the consent to treatment without advising the patient that she would not be conducting the arthrocentesis. This is a basic failure of medical ethics and a potential violation of state medical licensing laws. Even though the physician was called out of the room as a result of another emergency in the ED, she should have advised the patient that the medical resident and medical student were going to conduct the procedure without her supervision. The physician should have provided the patient with a choice as to whether to put off the timing of the arthrocentesis (as it was not life threatening) or obtain appropriate new consent. The medical boards of most states, hospital licensing, and accreditation authorities as well as accepted medical practice require the obtaining of prior written consent before performing a procedure which invades the patient's body. Failure to abide by such standards could lead to a report to the quality assurance staff at the hospital and discipline before the medical staff; discipline through suspension or loss of license through the state medical board; and, if this is a widespread practice in the hospital, possible suspension from the Medicare and Medicaid programs. Loss of the ability to bill Medicare and Medicaid could result both from the failure to follow appropriate medical consent guidelines with the patient and also the billing irregularities described.[77]

In conclusion, the attending physician should be required to participate in additional training in both medical ethics and billing compliance. Hopefully, if this is an isolated incident, this additional training will result in future appropriate behavior. If this is a widespread practice of this attending physician and the institution, the organization is at risk for a major fraud investigation and the payment of substantial fines and penalties.

Henry C. Fader, Esq.
Health Care Services Group of Pepper Hamilton LLP, Philadelphia, PA

SUMMARY – COMMITMENT TO PROFESSIONAL RESPONSIBILITIES

Background

The preamble to the document entitled *A Physican Charter* states that "professionalism is the basis of medicine's contract with society."[8] This statement was made because of a growing awareness that the complex relationship between medicine and the society which it serves is being reexamined. The Charter was created in response to changes to the practice of medicine brought about by science, perceived threats to the professionalism of physicians arising from contemporary health care systems, and the belief that physicians individually and collectively are failing to meet some of their professional responsibilities. Those who created the Charter identified a series of principles which they hoped could guide physicians as they attempt to practice medicine in an environment which often appears to subvert the values traditionally associated with the professional.[78]

The social contract provides a contextual framework within which the section entitled "Commitment to Professional Responsibilities," can be examined.[79,80] While the concept of the social contract was developed in the eighteenth century, it has only been invoked recently to describe the relationship between medicine and society. The contract is relatively simple. Society grants medicine substantial autonomy in practice, a monopoly over the practice of medicine through licensing laws, the privilege of self-regulation, prestige, and financial rewards. In return, both individual physicians and the medical profession are expected to be altruistic, to assure the competence of the practicing physician, to demonstrate morality and integrity in their daily lives, and to address issues within their domain of concern to society. This "bargain," as it has been called, has not changed appreciably since it was established in the middle of the nineteenth century, when licensing laws were enacted that established the modern professions in the developed world.[81–83] The contract is based upon the presence of mutual rights and obligations, with the obligations being linked to the expectations of both parties to the contract. Society has a right to receive competent medical care and it has obligations to meet in order that physicians may provide that care. If society fails to meet what physicians believe to be their legitimate expectations, there will be consequences in terms of changes in both physician attitudes and behaviors. Physicians also have rights under the contract and they must meet their obligations. When the obligations of the individual physician or of the profession are not met, society can change the social contract and hence the professional status of medicine.

A primary objective of the Charter is outlining these obligations. The section outlining the "Commitment to Professional Responsibilities"[7] is extremely important as it addresses many of the perceived failures of the medical profession. We will outline the nature of these professional responsibilities, indicate how they have changed through the years, and attempt to show how the vignettes in this chapter can illuminate these fundamental issues.

The Charter outlines medicine's commitment to professional responsibilities as follows:

As members of a profession, physicians are expected to work collaboratively to maximize patient care, be respectful of one another, and participate in the processes of self regulation, including remediation and discipline of members who have failed to meet professional standards. The profession should also define and organize the educational and standard setting process for current and future members. Physicians have both individual and collective obligations to participate in these processes. These obligations include engaging in internal assessment and accepting external scrutiny of all aspects of their professional performance.[8]

The majority of the responsibilities in this section of the Charter relate to the process of self-regulation of the profession, including the setting and maintenance of standards and the identification and subsequent remediation or discipline of incompetent or unethical physicians. The object is to assure society of the competence of each practicing physician. As Irvine has stated, "every patient deserves a good physician."[84] Also included are the necessity to be respectful of other members of the profession and to collaborate with other physicians and health professionals.

The Regulatory Process Requiring Physician Involvement

Guaranteeing quality in medicine occurs through a process of regulation which can be carried out internally through self-regulation via professional bodies, or externally, by governments, the legal system, or commercial organizations.[85,86] While regulation of the medical profession in different countries varies in how standards are set and performance is monitored, credentialing is universally regarded as fundamental to the process. Public trust in both the individual physician and in the profession as a whole is heavily dependant on the integrity, validity, and trustworthiness of the credentialing system. When patients use the services of a licensed physician who is certified as competent in family medicine or a specialty, they believe that those credentials constitute an assurance that the care will be consistent with contemporary standards.[84]

Randall Collins, in an influential book entitled *The Credential Society*, traced the origin and evolution of credentialing systems in Western society and emphasized their increasing importance as society came to require more complex services essential to the well-being of individuals.[87] In discussing medicine he linked the development of credentialing systems with the emergence of the concept of the profession. Thus, the evolution of credentials, including educational qualifications, licensing, and specialty certification and their maintenance, are inextricably linked to the evolution of professionalism.

Credentialing and Professionalism
The professions had their origins in the guilds and universities of medieval Europe and England.[81,82] From the beginning, criteria for admission to the

professions were established and reputed to represent an assurance of a certain level of knowledge and skill. Subsequent interpretations of the early professions indicated that they were exclusionary and attempted to establish monopolies,[87–90] but in their approach to the public an explicit guarantee of quality was always both intended by the profession and expected by society. In the middle of the nineteenth century the quality of modern scientific medicine and health care began to make it more important to the average citizen. At the urging of the recently established professional associations, governments throughout the Western world turned to the concept of the profession as a means of organizing the delivery of the complex services which were required.[79,81,82] Society delegated some of its authority to the medical profession on the understanding that it would assure the competence of its members through internally instituted and managed processes of self-regulation. The major reason for this approach was and remains the complexity of medicine's knowledge base,[79,81,82,86] which has two consequences. First, there is a substantial discrepancy in knowledge between the individual patient and the trained and credentialed physician. This discrepancy is accentuated because patients are often sick and in distress. It persists in spite of the wide availability of information about disease and treatment on the Internet as individual patients are not trained in the use of this information. For this reason an assurance of competence increases trust in the practitioner, and contributes to the process of healing.[91] Second, the complexity of the knowledge base makes it difficult for non-professionals to evaluate the performance of professionals. Therefore society, acting through its governments, enacted legislation which delegated responsibility for setting and maintaining standards in the health care field to the profession, acting through licensing, certifying, and accrediting bodies and professional associations.[86,92,93]

It is widely acknowledged that public trust in individual physicians and in the medical profession is essential if medicine's professional status is to be maintained.[79,82,87,94] During the first half of the twentieth century, public trust in the medical profession remained extraordinarily high.[95,96] The early social scientists studying professionalism described the rights and privileges granted to the profession and the obligations expected of physicians.[97–99] They noted the potential conflict between altruism and self-interest, but believed that the commitment to service of the medical profession would ensure altruistic behavior. They reflected public opinion in depicting a trustworthy medical profession. In the 1960s and 1970s throughout the world, a "questioning society" developed in which all forms of authority were greeted with skepticism.[81,82,89,90] Medicine's claims to altruism were not believed to be credible and the processes of self-regulation were found wanting. The profession was accused of abusing the collegiality inherent in professionalism[100] to protect incompetent or unethical colleagues. The public lost trust in the profession.[95,96]

It is interesting to observe the more recent opinions of the social scientists who have examined the state of professionalism during the past two decades.[79,82,101] During medicine's "dominant phase" it had great influence over public policy and carried out its regulatory duties with very little outside supervision.[81,82] As the state or the market place became dominant, the profession lost much of its influence over public policy.[82,101,102] Some felt that an autonomous and self-regulating profession did not benefit society. Recently as the results of state and market dominance of health care have become apparent, many sociologists have called for a return to professionalism in health care and virtually all have indicated that better self-regulation is an absolute requirement for this to take place.[79,81,82,101,103] This has been a major factor in the increased emphasis on self-regulation during the education of future physicians.

Self-Regulation of Medicine in the Western World

A fundamental aspect of self-regulation by the medical profession is the setting and maintenance of standards including discipline. This is carried out using two separate and distinct processes: accreditation of educational and training institutions and programs for licensing and certification of individual practitioners.[92,93] Licensure assesses knowledge and awards a license to practice medicine.[93,103,104] Certification is granted by specialty boards or societies and gives credentials of competence in a given specialty or subspecialty of medicine.

Fundamental to the success of both processes is the involvement of knowledgeable practitioners. In order to meet their commitment to professional responsibilities, physicians are responsible for maintaining their own competence and for ensuring that licensure and certification standards meet societal expectations.

Credentialing of Institutions and Programs

Accreditation is usually an ongoing process with recognition of conforming to standards being awarded for a set period of time.

Accreditation of Medical Schools. In 1904, the American Medical Association (AMA) established its Council on Medical Education and began establishing criteria for accrediting medical schools.[81,105] It was instrumental in initiating the Flexner Report, which assessed the adequacy of medical education in every medical school in North America and later in the United

Kingdom.[106] Since then medical schools have been assessed at regular intervals on their admissions criteria, the adequacy of their curriculum, the resources available for teaching and training, and the performance of their graduates. If inadequacies are identified, schools can be placed on probation until these are remedied, or the school may be forced to close. The process depends heavily upon a self-study document used by institutions to measure themselves against agreed-upon standards.[107] The certifying body includes representatives of various medical organizations and of the public.

Sanctions must be available for accreditation to be effective. Graduates of non-accredited schools are not eligible for postgraduate training in North American programs and have difficulty in being accepted to sit for licensing exams.

Those physicians associated with faculties of medicine must participate in the accreditation process, but every physician should be aware of the fact that the quality of the education which they have received is heavily dependent upon accreditation. In the United States and Canada this is granted by the Liaison Committee on Medical Education (LCME) and in the United Kingdom by the General Medical Council (GMC).

Accreditation of Postgraduate Training Programs. Individual physicians have for centuries traveled widely to study in renowned institutions or with recognized experts, often as apprentices. The growth of formal postgraduate training was essentially a twentieth-century phenomenon, having begun with a single year's internship offered by a small number of hospitals prior to the 1914 war.[81,105,108] As early as 1916 the AMA Council on Medical Education visited the sites of postgraduate training and by the early 1920s was setting standards for the content and minimum length of these programs.[81,108] In 1923 it began publishing a list of approved sites – essentially accrediting the training programs.

The growth of specialization in medicine greatly increased the need for credentialing, and throughout the world different bodies became responsible for the process. In the United States, specialty boards assumed primary responsibility with coordination being ensured by the Accreditation Council on Graduate Medical Education (ACGME) and the American Board of Medical Specialties (ABMS).[81,105,108] From the inception of postgraduate training in the United States, hospital-based programs were accredited. In Canada, the Royal College of Physicians and Surgeons was established as the single accrediting body for all postgraduate specialty training, to which was added the Canadian College of Family Practice in 1955 for family medicine.[109,110] These organizations originally accredited hospital-based programs, but in 1970 they made a policy decision that all postgraduate education would be university-based and accreditation was only given to integrated university programs. In the United Kingdom, programs are accredited by the various Royal Colleges, many of which have long and rich histories.[82,108]

Again, the accreditation process depends heavily upon self-study documents and peer review. The sanction applicable to those programs not meeting acceptable standards is a ban on their ability to issue certificates of competence, which are essential if an individual is to obtain a position in today's medical marketplace.

Once again, physicians involved in postgraduate education have a responsibility to participate in the setting and maintenance of standards and in assuring compliance with them. However, because postgraduate training is a requirement to practice, it directly affects every practitioner.

Accreditation of Hospitals. While not directly involved in credentialing individuals practicing medicine, accreditation of hospitals must be mentioned when discussing participation in the credentialing process as a professional responsibility. Because much medical education takes place in a hospital setting, the standards of the hospital can have a profound impact on the outcome of the educational process. This was not the original intent of hospital accreditation, which was started in 1916 by the American College of Surgeons in order to improve the quality of surgical care.[111] However, as the accreditation process in North America developed, it became apparent that postgraduate education should only take place in institutions that not only met minimal standards, but hopefully would exceed them.[81,108] Consequently, when teaching hospitals are accredited, the quality of patient care, the adequacy of the facilities and the resources devoted to teaching constitute an important aspect of the process. As is true in other forms of accreditation, extensive self-study documents and peer review, including physicians, remain the basis of the process. Accreditation occurs at regular intervals and the sanctions are important, as postgraduate training may not take place in a hospital which is not credentialed as meeting established standards.

Credentialing of Individuals
Licensure. The history of medical licensure varies from country to country, but the necessity for some form of license became apparent in the middle of the nineteenth century in most.[81,82,108,112] There were a variety of health care providers and the public required some assurance of quality as science made modern health care more complex and therefore more difficult to regulate. The recently constituted national professional associations lobbied their respective governments to be given the privilege of setting and maintaining the

standards for entry into practice and monitoring its quality. In addition, they petitioned for and were granted a monopoly over the practice of medicine. In the United Kingdom, the centralized system of registration of qualified practitioners was established by the General Medical Council.[113] In the United States and Canada, both of whom enjoy federal systems, the various states and provinces legislated the establishment of physician-run licensing bodies.[81,109] These organizations established the criteria for eligibility for licensure, which generally include graduation from a recognized medical school, a minimum amount of postgraduate training, and passage of an examination testing skills and knowledge using validated methods.

There is an impression amongst physicians that licensing bodies are a part of an ever expanding bureaucracy intruding into their daily lives. This is not true. Their mandate is to protect the public and they are a fundamental part of the process by which the profession regulates itself. They are "us" and individual physicians must be aware of their role and, when required, must participate in their activities.

Relicensure and Revalidation. Until recently, in the absence of documented incompetent or unethical behavior, licensure was for life. During the past few decades, it has become apparent that a credential given to a young physician is no guarantee of continued competence[112,114,115] and pressure has grown for a reassessment of competence on a regular basis. There has been great resistance on the part of the medical profession to this concept[94] and as has been pointed out by Irvine, "performance based relicensure does not exist despite there being much talk about it."[104] The emphasis has been on a revalidation of the continuing ability of an individual to meet contemporary standards through documented participation in a wide variety of accredited educational programs or activities, an examination of knowledge and practices, and an assessment of the opinions of patients and colleagues as to the individual's professional competence and behavior.[104,114,115] Extensive processes have been developed in order to gather and act upon this information and validate the processes. There is a strong emphasis on identifying marginal practitioners and establishing remedial educational or counseling programs. The ultimate sanction available is the temporary or permanent loss of the license to practice.

Again, participation in these activities is an essential individual professional responsibility which will undoubtedly become even more important in the future as the processes become more universal, reliable, and sophisticated.

Certification. A medical license is essential to practice. Certification as it was originally conceived was voluntary and represented a credential indicating that the individual concerned had demonstrated a pre-established and verified level of competence in a specialized field of medicine.[81]

The development of specialty boards was contemplated in the United States before the First World War and the first (ophthalmology) was established in 1913.[116] Other disciplines followed, and in 1933 the American Board of Medical Specialties was established to ensure uniform standards, a function which it still carries out.[117] Specialty certification arrived in Canada in 1929, when the Royal College of Physicians and Surgeons was chartered and given the mandate to establish and maintain standards for all specialties.[109] Certification in family medicine became a reality during the second half of the twentieth century in both countries.[81,109,118] In the United Kingdom, for over two hundred years specialists have become credentialed when they joined one of the Royal Colleges. Credentialing in general practice developed during the latter half of the twentieth century.[82,94,108]

In general in North America, credentialing of competence in a specialty has been documented by requiring candidates to pass an exit examination after they have completed training in accredited programs. In the United Kingdom, exit exams are still not the norm, the emphasis being on satisfactory completion of training within an approved program.

The growth of subspecialization has greatly expanded the number of certifying bodies and increased the variety of the credentials being presented to the general public. Although this has added to the complexity of health care systems, it is a reality of contemporary medicine and the trend will undoubtedly continue.

Recertification. As is true of licensure, the idea that certification of competence at one stage of a practitioner's career will guarantee that competence for the rest of that practitioner's professional lifetime is no longer tenable.[112,119] The rapid growth of knowledge and of technology require that practitioners constantly renew their knowledge and skills. There has been sufficient evidence of incompetent and unethical practice that the public now demands assurance of continued competence.[120,121] This has led to demands for recertification of practitioners (see the discussions by Cassell and Nash in Chapter 8).[121] It is now a requirement of the American Board of Medical Specialties and has been instituted by several of the examining boards.[122] There is a time limit on the credentials granted and some form of scrutiny of practice is required for their maintenance. A variety of means is used to accomplish this, including assessment of knowledge by examination, documentation of practice patterns, peer review, and the solicitation of information from other health professionals and patients.[116] Because practices vary greatly, fairness dictates that the process be tailored to the individual, taking into account what he or she actually does. The aim is to document the "maintenance of competence" and to issue a credential attesting to this. It can be anticipated that these methods will grow more rigorous and sophisticated in time and that the information will be made public in order to offer assurance of competence.

As is true with relicensure, recertification is a professional responsibility.

Discipline

The role of the regulatory bodies in licensing and certifying the competence of physicians and requiring evidence of continuing competence is reasonably straightforward. It is clear that individual physicians have an obligation to meet the standards set by these physician-led organizations and that some practitioners must be actively involved in setting the policies of the regulatory bodies if medicine is to meet its obligations to society. In fact, the process of credentialing works reasonably well, although revalidation and recertification at the present time must be regarded as works in progress since the tools required to carry out this difficult task are only now being developed.[122]

Every physician faces two challenges in meeting his or her commitments in the area of professional responsibilities. The first is of course in maintaining his or her own competence. The second, and in many ways the more difficult one, is in the identification of incompetent, unethical, or immoral colleagues. As George Bernard Shaw said almost a hundred years ago, "every doctor will allow a colleague to decimate a whole countryside sooner than violate the bond of professional etiquette by giving him away."[123] The profession encourages a sense of collegiality in students, residents, and practitioners. Sullivan said that "a profession is a means of livelihood that is also a way of life"[79] and collegiality is used in order to gain agreement on the common goals involved in this way of life and to ensure voluntary compliance with these goals.[100] There is a strong sense of commitment to fellow physicians who share the satisfactions and the stresses inherent in the practice of medicine. There is a reluctance to report them, even if their conduct carries potential harm to patients and the public (see commentaries by Dorsey and Meier).[124] While this attitude has never been acceptable, current circumstances make it imperative that every physician realize that as professionals they are responsible for the actions of their colleagues. They are "their brother's and sister's keepers."[125] The reasons why this responsibility must be stressed at the present time is that the public has become aware of the deficiencies of self-regulation. In all countries surveyed, the number of medical errors causing harm or death to patients has been documented and is unacceptably high.[126] While there are certainly systems errors involved, many errors are caused by incompetent practitioners and the public is aware of this. In the United Kingdom several well-documented failures of both individual physicians and of the regulatory processes have caused the public and the government to doubt the ability of the medical profession to police itself.[94,127,128] The U.K. government has recently introduced legislation withdrawing many of the regulatory powers of the medical profession.[129] In this globalized world, no country can insulate itself from happenings elsewhere. If we are incapable of regulating ourselves, external regulation will be imposed upon us. This is why each individual physician must not tolerate anything less than competence in their colleagues and must take appropriate action when necessary. It is a primary professional responsibility.

The actions taken will depend upon the circumstances. Responsibility for the protection of patients is shared. There is general agreement that the first step is to deal directly with the colleague involved if there are not serious personal contra-indications. Each chief of service is responsible for the activities on that service and reporting the colleague at this level is the next logical step. Every accredited hospital will have a medical director or its equivalent and there will be both quality control and disciplinary committees operating under publicly understood bylaws. If none of these routes are available, or if the colleague's conduct is deemed to be egregious, reporting directly to the licensing authority is the proper course of action. It goes without saying that every physician whose conduct is being questioned has the right to be treated fairly, taking note of the principles of natural justice and due process. However, the primary concern must be the welfare of patients and the public.

The responsibility of every practitioner is to know the code of ethics which should guide the behavior of all physicians, to understand what constitutes a breach of this code, and to be knowledgeable about the most appropriate actions which he or she should take when they become aware of a breach. In addition, many individuals will be asked to serve on disciplinary committees or will choose to become involved with the regulatory bodies. They then must recognize that their primary obligation is to patients and the public.

Collegiality

The Charter states that it is a professional responsibility of physicians to "be respectful of one another." This involves a principle which was included in the first versions of the Hippocratic Oath and which has been deemed to be important ever since.[130] It invokes the concept of collegiality, which is fundamental to the structure and organization of all professions and to the identity of professionals.[79,81,100] Collegiality gives a sense of "connectedness," the awareness of sharing with others a feeling of being part of a larger and interdependent whole, with a set of values and beliefs that give meaning to the practice of medicine. Other physicians are viewed as colleagues who enjoy mutual respect and who can rely on each other to perform as they should.

While collegiality is important to individual physicians, it also has implications for society, which relies upon the profession to utilize collegiality as a means of agreeing upon the common goals of the profession and ensuring compliance with them. In this way, the value system of the healer, which is so essential to patients, becomes internalized and is manifested by professional behavior.[131] It is not possible to legislate commitment or altruism. They must come from within the individual practitioner and collegiality is a powerful force in bringing this about. It also creates the sense of obligation necessary for physicians to be aware of the very real nature of their public roles and the necessity of filling them.[132,133]

Team Medicine

Finally, this section of the Charter states that physicians must "work collaboratively to maximize patient care." In contemporary terms, this means that practitioners must function as members of a health care team which may consist of physicians from their own or other medical disciplines and/or other health care professionals. The days of the solo practitioner are over.[81,82,101] The complexity of contemporary medicine resulting from technology and subspecialization has meant that optimum patient care requires the services of individuals from many disciplines. Physicians have a professional responsibility to be able to function in teams, to communicate with other team members in a respectful fashion, and to understand the dynamics of teamwork.[134] All evidence indicates that this is what patients wish.[135]

Review of the Cases and Commentaries

The vignettes which have been chosen by the editors for this chapter highlight many of the professional responsibilities included in the Charter and can serve as essential aids in ensuring that students and residents understand their professional responsibilities and are prepared to meet them. There is general agreement that teaching professionalism at all levels includes two essential steps which are separate but linked.[136,137] In the first place, students must understand professionalism, the nature of the obligations necessary to sustain professional status, and the reasons for their existence. This could be called the cognitive base and it must be communicated to students. The Charter serves this purpose very well. However, if the teaching program is limited to reading a section or listening to a lecture, the material will remain largely theoretical and will not be incorporated into the professional identity of the future physician.[138] It is necessary to provide opportunities for the learner to reflect upon the issues in a safe environment, preferably before he or she must address them in real life. There are several educational methods to ensure that this will take place and the use of vignettes is one of the most powerful.[139] It is particularly important that this occur during the teaching of professional responsibilities because it is an area where the profession is widely regarded as failing to meet its responsibilities[78,81,82,88,94,97,127] and because meeting these responsibilities often entails difficult personal decisions or sacrifices.

The vignettes provided describe a variety of situations, but all include the presence of common situations in which individual physicians are seen to breach their professional responsibilities. This breach, when observed or known, imposes often unpleasant responsibilities upon their colleagues who have either observed the unprofessional conduct or are in positions of responsibility for enforcing the standards of the profession. In using the vignettes to promote reflection on the professional responsibilities of physicians it is most important to identify the positive or negative characteristics of professionalism illustrated in the situations described and to encourage reflection upon them. Only when this has occurred should the individual or groups engaged in the exercise be encouraged to outline what actions might be taken. There is always a tendency to solve the problem first, which can actually discourage discussion of the issues.

The contributors to this work who have discussed the individual vignettes have covered the actions to be taken and this will not be repeated. The vignettes will be discussed in terms of how they can be used to promote reflection on the issues by students. The common threads are quite straightforward. A student or health care professional fails to meet his or her professional responsibilities. Most often patient care and the reputation and collegial nature of the profession are threatened and individual physicians must respond by participating in medicine's self regulatory processes. If no actions are taken, present and future patient care can be compromised. This is unacceptable since the unprofessional behavior may continue, the integrity of medicine's regulatory processes can be called into question, and public trust in the profession will diminish. Furthermore, other physicians may come to believe that they are entitled to behave in a similar fashion. The reflective process should center on these common themes.

The case commented on by Kavan and Potter (Chapter 2) involves a student arrested for drunk driving and a classmate who becomes aware of it, and ultimately it will involve physicians in an administrative capacity in the medical school should the school be made aware of the incident. The student who was arrested has clearly failed to uphold the standards of the profession. The classmate who is aware of the incident and those directing the medical school have an obligation to participate in the process of self-regulation. The classmate must report the incident and those physicians in the school must take actions to ensure that the public will not be harmed in the future.

The case commented on by Kairys and Yingling (Chapter 2) involves a resident who performs a cursory physical examination and then lies in communicating its results. Patient welfare is endangered, professional competence is questioned, and the resident is dishonest. Again, the student must take action and the chief of the department of surgery must react.

Another case in this chapter involves a physician who fails to maintain appropriate relations with a patient. As pointed out by Coulehan and Snyder, this violates an age-old injunction found in the Hippocratic Oath. The discussion should involve an elaboration on the vulnerability of patients, barrier issues, and power differential between patients and physicians. In today's complex world reflection on these issues is extremely important.

In the case considered by Brent and Vidmar in this chapter, the pediatric allergist who gives testimony in an area where he is not competent violates the principle of the primacy of patient welfare and his own commitment to professional competence. He is not upholding the professions commitment to scientific knowledge and he is in conflict of interest, placing his own financial welfare above that of the patient. Several specialties have already issued guidelines indicating that this is wrong and this should serve as the focus of discussion.

Albritton and Hadad reflect on the physician who treats his own family and is ignoring the widely recognized fact that one should not be involved in the care of someone to whom one is emotionally attached. This issue is covered in codes of ethics and the vignette in this chapter nicely illustrates this.

The nursing director who must cope with an abusive surgeon who is critical of other members of the health care team presents an all too familiar problem (discussed by Yeo and Swan in this chapter). The surgeon ignores patient welfare and does not recognize the necessity to function as a member of a team. This certainly will contribute to a decrease in the quality of care and will undoubtedly damage expensive instruments and thus endanger the just distribution of finite resources. Finally, and most importantly, he fails to uphold the collegial nature of medicine. This vignette should lead to a rich discussion of these issues.

Finally, the case involving the orthopedic surgeon who does not wish his patient to be anticoagulated is similar. The discussion should stress the primacy of patient welfare and an individual's commitment to professional competence and scientific knowledge. The obligation to respect one's colleagues on the health care team and to maintain the collegial nature of the profession is covered by Kane and Brigham in this chapter.

Closing Comments

It seems appropriate to close this chapter on professional responsibilities with a quote from an eminent sociologist who believes that professionalism is of fundamental importance, not only to the medical profession itself, but to society. Sullivan has written that "neither economic incentives, nor technology, nor administrative control has proved an effective surrogate to the commitment to integrity evoked in the ideal of professionalism."[79] In attempting to meet their professional responsibility in an exemplary fashion, physicians must constantly strive to maintain this integrity.

Richard L. Cruess, M.D.
Professor of Surgery
Member, Center for Medical Education
Former Dean of Medicine
McGill University, Montreal, Canada

Sylvia R. Cruess, M.D.
Professor of Medicine
Member, Center for Medical Education
McGill University
Former Director of Professional Services
Royal Victoria Hospital, Montreal, Canada

REFERENCES

1. Mancia G, Facchetti R, Bombelli M, Grassi G, Sega R. Long-term risk of mortality associated with selective and combined elevation in office, home, and ambulatory blood pressure. *Hypertension.* 2006;**47**(5):846–853.

2. Ohkubo T, Kikuya M, Metoki H. et al. Prognosis of "masked" hypertension and "white-coat" hypertension detected by 24-h ambulatory blood pressure monitoring 10-year follow-up from the Ohasama study. *J Am Coll Cardiol.* 2005;**46**(3): 508–515.

3. Hippocratic Oath. http://www.pbs.org/wgbh/nova/doctors/oath_classical.html. Accessed January 3, 2007.

4. Perez SG, Gelpi RJ, Rancich AM. Doctor-patient sexual relationships in medical oaths. *J Med Ethics.* 2006;**32**(12):702–705.

5. Council on Ethical and Judicial Affairs. *Code of Medical Ethics. Current Opinions with Annotations.* Chicago: American Medical Association; 1996.

6. American Psychiatric Association. Legal Sanctions for Mental Health Professional–Patient Sex. http://www.psych.org/Departments/EDU/Library/APAOfficialDocumentsandRelated/ResourceDocuments/199302.aspx. Accessed April 25, 2009.

7. Snyder L,Leffler C, Ethics and Human Rights Committee, American College of Physicians. Ethics manual: 5th ed. *Ann Intern Med.* 2005;**142**(7):560–582.

8. ABIM Foundation. American Board of Internal Medicine, ACP-ASIM Foundation. American College of Physicians-American Society of Internal Medicine, European Federation of Internal Medicine. Medical professionalism in the new millennium: A physician charter. *Ann Intern Med.* 2002;**136**(3):243–246.

9. Federation of State Medical Boards. *Addressing Sexual Boundaries: Guidelines for State Medical Boards.* 2006.

10. Sexual misconduct in the practice of medicine. Council on Ethical and Judicial Affairs, American Medical Association. *JAMA.* 1991;**266**(19):2741–2745.

11. General Medical Council. Maintaining boundaries. 2006.

12. Brent RL. Drugs and pregnancy: Are the insert warnings too dire? *Contemporary Obstetrics and Gynecology.* 1982;**20**:42–49.

13. Brent RL. Nongenital malformations following exposure to progestational drugs: The last chapter of an erroneous allegation. *Birth Defects Res A Clin Mol Teratol.* 2005;**73**(11):906–918.

14. Brent R. The Daubert decision. *Pediatrics.* 2006;**118**(5):2222–2225.

15. Brent RL. Litigation-produced pain, disease and suffering: An experience with congenital malformation lawsuits. *Teratology.* 1977;**16**(1):1–13.

16. American College of Obstetrics and Gynecologists. *Professional Liability and Its Effects: Report of a 1987 Survey of ACOG's Membership.* Chicago: ACOG; 1988.

17. Brent RL. The irresponsible expert witness: A failure of biomedical graduate education and professional accountability. *Pediatrics.* 1982;**70**(5):754–762.

18. Lasagna L, Shulman SR. Bendectin and the language of causation. In: Foster KR, Bernstein DE, Huber PW, eds. *Phantom Risk: Scientific Interference and the Law.* Cambridge, MA: MIT Press; 1993:101–122.

19. Brent R. Medical, social, and legal implications of treating nausea and vomiting of pregnancy. *Am J Obstet Gynecol.* 2002;**186**(5 Suppl Understanding): S262–6.

20. Skolnick A. Key witness against morning sickness drug faces scientific fraud charges. *JAMA.* 1990;**263**(11):1468–9, 1473.

21. AMA/Specialty Society Medical Liability Project. A proposed alternative to the civil justice system for resolving medical liability disputes: A fault-based administrative system. 1988.

22. Taragin MI, Willett LR, Wilczek AP, Trout R, Carson JL. The influence of standard of care and severity of injury on the resolution of medical malpractice claims. *Ann Intern Med.* 1992;**117**(9):780–784.

23. Studdert DM, Mello MM, Gawande AA, et al. Claims, errors, and compensation payments in medical malpractice litigation. *N Engl J Med.* 2006;**354**(19):2024–2033.

24. Diamond S, et al. Juror discussions during trials: Studying an Arizona innovation. *Arizona Law Review.* 2003;**45**:1–82.

25. Vidmar N, Hans V. *American Juries: The Verdict*. Amherst NY: Prometheus Books; 2007.

26. Kutnjak-Ivokovic S, Hans VP. Jurors evaluation of expert testimony, judging the messenger and the message. *Law and Social Inquiry*. 2004;**28**:441–482.

27. Shuman D, et al. An empirical examination of the use of expert witnesses in the courts – part 2: A three city study. *Jurimetrics Journal*.;**34**:193–206.

28. Vidmar N, Diamond S. Juries and expert evidence. *Brooklyn Law Review*. 2001;**66**:1121–1180.

29. Geerts WH, Bergqvist D, Pineo GF, et al. Prevention of venous thromboembolism: American College of Chest Physicians evidence-based clinical practice guidelines (8th ed.). *Chest*. 2008;**133**(6 Suppl):381S–453S.

30. Goldhaber SZ. Pulmonary embolism. *N Engl J Med*. 1998;**339**(2):93–104.

31. Simonneau G, Sors H, Charbonnier B, et al. A comparison of low-molecular-weight heparin with unfractionated heparin for acute pulmonary embolism. The THESEE study group. tinzaparine ou heparine standard: Evaluations dans l'embolie pulmonaire. *N Engl J Med*. 1997;**337**(10):663–669.

32. Newman A. Phlegmasia cerulea dolens: A complication of use of the filter in the vena cava. A case report. *J Bone Joint Surg Am*. 1995;**77**(11):1783.

33. Decousus H, Leizorovicz A, Parent F, et al. A clinical trial of vena caval filters in the prevention of pulmonary embolism in patients with proximal deep-vein thrombosis. Prevention du risque d'embolie pulmonaire par interruption cave study group. *N Engl J Med*. 1998;**338**(7):409–415.

34. Merli G, Wetiz H, eds. *Medical Management of the Surgical Patient*. WB Saunders Company; 2007.

35. Wheelan SA, Burchill CN, Tilin F. The link between teamwork and patients' outcomes in intensive care units. *Am J Crit Care*. 2003;**12**(6):527–534.

36. Thomas, Killman. Conflict Management: The Five Conflict Styles. The Collaboration Toolbox Web site. http://web.mit.edu/collaboration/mainsite/modules/module1/1.11.5.html. Updated 2001. Accessed August 26, 2008.

37. Kaplan HI, Sadock BJ. *Comprehensive Textbook of Psychiatry VI*. New York: Williams and Wilkins; 1995.

38. La Puma J, Stocking CB, La Voie D, Darling CA. When physicians treat members of their own families: Practices in a community hospital. *N Engl J Med*. 1991 **325**(18):1290–1294.

39. Aboff BM, Collier VU, Farber NJ, Ehrenthal DB. Residents' prescription writing for nonpatients. *JAMA*. 2002;**288**(3):381–385.

40. American Medical Association. Opinion E-8.19 Self-treatment or treatment of immediate family members. In: *AMA Code of Medical Ethics*. Chicago, IL: American Medical Association; 2006.

41. Carroll R, Tulsky J, Shuchman M, Snyder L. Should doctors treat their relatives? *ACP Observer*. 1999.

42. La Puma J, Priest ER. Is there a doctor in the house? An analysis of the practice of physicians' treating their own families. *JAMA*. 1992;**267**(13):1810–1812.

43. Kenna GA, Wood MD. Prevalence of substance use by pharmacists and other health professionals. *J Am Pharm Assoc (2003)*. 2004;**44**(6):684–693.

44. American Medical Association. *Code of Medical Ethics of the American Medical Association: Current Opinions and Annotations.* 2006–2007 ed. American Medical Association; 2006.

45. Kagle JD, Giebelhausen PN. Dual relationships and professional boundaries. *Soc Work.* 1994;**39**(2):213–220.

46. Thomas Jefferson University. Statement of professional conduct. http://jeffline.jefferson.edu/Professionalism/JMCfaculty.html accessed April 25, 2009.

47. Makary MA, Sexton JB, Freischlag JA, et al. Operating room teamwork among physicians and nurses: Teamwork in the eye of the beholder. *J Am Coll Surg.* 2006;**202**(5):746–752.

48. Rosenstein AH, O'Daniel M. Impact and implications of disruptive behavior in the perioperative arena. *J Am Coll Surg.* 2006;**203**(1):96–105.

49. Arford PH. Nurse-physician communication: An organizational accountability. *Nurs Econ.* 2005;**23**(2):72–7, 55.

50. K Ms, Hallberg LR. The origin of workplace bullying: Experiences from the perspective of bully victims in the public service sector. *J Nurs Manag.* 2007;**15**(3):332–341.

51. Tabak N, Orit K. Relationship between how nurses resolve their conflicts with doctors, their stress and job satisfaction. *J Nurs Manag.* 2007;**15**(3):321–331.

52. Iacono M. Conflict, communication, and collaboration: Improving interactions between nurses and physicians. *J Perianesth Nurs.* 2003;**18**(1):42–46.

53. Tissue plasminogen activator for acute ischemic stroke. The National Institute of Neurological Disorders and Stroke rt-PA Stroke Study Group. *N Engl J Med.* 1995;**333**(24):1581–1587.

54. Baldisseri MR. Impaired healthcare professional. *Crit Care Med.* 2007;**35**(2 Suppl):S106–16.

55. Gastfriend DR. Physician substance abuse and recovery: What does it mean for physicians – and everyone else? *JAMA.* 2005;**293**(12):1513–1515.

56. Shepherd R. Why must you report an impaired colleague? *CMAJ.* 1990;**142**(4):282–283.

57. FASAP. Professional Distress and Impairment: Did You Know?. http://www.jhu.edu/~hrl/fasap/sap/InternalMedicineRetreat.html. Accessed APril 26, 2007.

58. Blumenthal L. The Impaired Medical Professional. Updated 2001. Accessed April 26, 2007.

59. Ethics of Practice. aarogya.com: The Wellness Site Web site. http://www.aarogya.com/Legalities/ethics/ethicspractice.asp. Updated 2004. Accessed April 26, 2007.

60. American Medical Association. Principles of Medical Ethics. http://www.ama-assn.org/ama/pub/category/2512.html. Updated 2006. Accessed April 26, 2007.

61. O'Connor PG, Spickard A, Jr. Physician impairment by substance abuse. *Med Clin North Am.* 1997;**81**(4):1037–1052.

62. Guadagnino C. Treating Pysician Substance Abuse. Physician's News Digest Web site. http://www.physiciansnews.com/spotlight/397wp.html. Accessed April 26, 2007.

63. Alpern F, Correnti CE, Dolan TE, Llufrio MC, Sill A. A survey of recovering Maryland physicians. *Md Med J.* 1992;**41**(4):301–303.

64. Gallegos KV, Lubin BH, Bowers C, Blevins JW, Talbott GD, Wilson PO. Relapse and recovery: Five to ten year follow-up study of chemically dependent physicians – the Georgia experience. *Md Med J.* 1992;**41**(4):315–319.

65. Burton JH. Acute disorders of the joints and bursae. In: Tintinalli JE, Kelen GD, Strapczynski JS, eds. *Emergency Medicine – A Comprehensive Study Guide.* 5th ed. New York: McGraw Hill; 2000:1891–1899.

66. Ezell SL, Kobernick ME, Benjamin GC. Arthrocentesis. In: Roberts J, Hedges J, eds. *Clinical Procedures in Emergency Medicine.* Philadelphia: WB Saunders Company; 1991:847–851.

67. Department of Health and Human Services. Medicare carriers manual. *Centers for Medicaid and Medicare Services.* 2002;**15**:9–12.

68. Association of American Medical Colleges. Background Paper Physicians at Teaching Hospitals (PATH) Initiative. http://www.aamc.org/advocacy/library. Accessed July 30, 2008.

69. See 42 CFR § 415.200 for rules concerning resident billing issues.

70. Corporate Integrity Agreements. http://www.oig.hhs.gov/fraud/cia/agreements. Accessed July 30, 2008.

71. See federal register, vol. **63**, no. 35, February 23, 1998, p. 8987 for the OIG's recommended form of billing compliance plan for hospitals.

72. False claims act, 31 U.S.C. §§3729, et seq.

73. Sarbanes-Oxley Act of 2002, P.L. 107–204.

74. University of Florida College of Medicine. Code of Professional Behavior. University of Florida College of Medicine Web site. Accessed July 30, 2008.

75. Joint Commission on Accreditation of Healthcare Organizations. 2007 Hospital/Critical Access Hospital National Patient Safety Goalss. Joint Commission Web site. http://www.jointcommission.org/patientsafety/nationalpatientsafetygoals/07_hap_cah_npsgs.html. Accessed July 30, 2008.

76. See for example, 49 pa. code § 16.61 regarding complaints for unprofessional and immoral conduct.

77. See, for example, the Balanced Budget Act of 1997, P.L. 105–33 for expanded procedures for suspension or expulsion from the Medicare and Medicaid programs.

78. Relman AS. Medical professionalism in a commercialized health care market. *JAMA.* 2007;**298**(22):2668–2670.

79. Sullivan W. *Work and Integrity: The Crisis and Promise of Professionalism in North America.* 2nd ed. San Francisco, CA: Jossey-Bass; 2005.

80. Cruess SR. Professionalism and medicine's social contract with society. *Clin Orthop Relat Res.* 2006;**449**:170–176.

81. Starr P. *The Social Transformation of American Medicine.* New York: Basic Books; 1984.

82. Krause E. *Death of the Guilds: Professions, States and the Advance of Capitalism, 1930 to the Present.* New Haven, CT: Yale University Press; 1996.

83. Cruess RL, Cruess SR. Teaching medicine as a profession in the service of healing. *Acad Med.* 1997;**72**(11):941–952.

84. Irvine DH. Everyone is entitled to a good doctor. *Med J Aust.* 2007;**186**(5): 256–261.

85. Vogel D. *National Styles of Self-Regulation.* Ithaca, NY: Cornell University Press; 1986.

86. Stacey M. The case for and against self-regulation. *Federation Bulletin.* 1997; **84**:17–25.

87. Collins R. *The Credential Society: An Historical Sociology of Education and Stratification.* New York, NY: Acad Press; 1979.

88. Freidson E. *Professional Dominance: The Social Structure of Medical Care.* Chicago, IL: Aldine; 1970.

89. Larson M. *The Rise of Professionalism: A Sociological Analysis.* Berkeley, CA: University of California Press; 1977.

90. Johnson T. *Professions and Power.* London, UK: Macmillan Press; 1972.

91. Safran DG, Taira DA, Rogers WH, Kosinski M, Ware JE, Tarlov AR. Linking primary care performance to outcomes of care. *J Fam Pract.* 1998;**47**(3):213–220.

92. Patterson SM, Vitello EM. The relationship between credentialing and professionalism: Adversarial or synchronistic. *J Health Ed.* 1994;**25**:201–203.

93. Wolfe J, Cleary H, Stone E. Initiation of voluntary certification program for health education specialists. *Public Health Reports.* 1989;**104**:396–402.

94. Irvine D. *The Doctor's Tale: Professionalism and Public Trust.* Abingdon, UK: Radcliffe Medical Press; 2003.

95. Mechanic D. Physician discontent: Challenges and opportunities. *JAMA.* 2003; **290**(7):941–946.

96. Schlesinger M. A loss of faith: The sources of reduced political legitimacy for the American medical profession. *Milbank Q.* 2002;**80**(2):185–235.

97. Carr-Saunders AM, Wilson PA. *The Professions.* Oxford, UK: Clarendon Press; 1933.

98. Elliot P. *The Sociology of the Professions.* London, UK: Macmillan Press; 1972.

99. Parsons T. The professions and social structure. *Social Forces.* 1939;**17**:457–467.

100. Ihara CK. Collegiality as a professional virtue. In: Flores A, ed. *Professional Ideals.* Belmont, CA: Wadsworth; 1988:56–65.

101. Freidson E. *Professionalism: The Third Logic.* Chicago, IL: University of Chicago Press; 2001.

102. Light DW. The medical profession and organizational change: From professional dominance to countervailing power. In: Bird CE, Conrad P, Fremont AM, eds. *Handbook of Medical Sociology.* 5th ed. Upper Saddle River, NJ: Prentice Hall; 2001:201–216.

103. Cruess R, Cruess S. Professionalism and accreditation – one must accompany the other. *Education for Health.* 1997;**10**:147–152.

104. Irvine D. Standards and revalidation or recertification. *Ann Acad Med Singapore.* 2004;**33**:1–5.

105. Ludmerer KM. Learning to heal: The development of American medical education. 1985.

106. Flexner A. *Medical Education in the United States and Canada: A Report to the Carnegie Foundation for the Advancement of Teaching*. Washington, D.C.: Science and Health Publication; 1910.

107. Kassebaum DS, Culter ER, Eaglen RH. The influence of accreditation on educational change in U.S. medical schools. *Acad Med.* 1997;**72**:1126–33.

108. Bonner TN. *On Becoming a Physician: Medical Education in Great Britain, France, Germany, and the United States*. New York, NY: Basic Books; 1995.

109. Torrance GM. Socio-historical overview. In: Torrance GM, Coburn D, eds. *Health and Canadian Society – Sociological Perspectives*. University of Toronto Press; 1987:6–33.

110. Coburn D. Professional powers in decline: Medicine in a changing Canada. In: Hafferty FW, McKinlay JB, eds. *The Changing Medical Profession: An International Perspective*. New York, NY: Oxford University Press; 1993:92–104.

111. Rosenberg CE. *The Care of Strangers: The Rise of America's Hospital System*. New York, NY: Oxford University Press; 1987.

112. Houle CO. *Continuing Learning in the Professions*. San Francisco: Jossey-Bass; 1980.

113. Stacey M. *Regulating British Medicine: The General Medical Council*. Chichester, UK: John Wiley and Sons; 1992.

114. Dauphinee WD. Revalidation of doctors in Canada. *BMJ.* 1999;**319**(7218):1188–1190.

115. Southgate L, Dauphinee D. Maintaining standards in British and Canadian medicine: The developing role of the regulatory body. *BMJ.* 1998;**316**(7132):697–700.

116. Brennan TA, Horwitz RI, Duffy FD, Cassel CK, Goode LD, Lipner RS. The role of physician specialty board certification status in the quality movement. *JAMA.* 2004;**292**(9):1038–1043.

117. American Board of Medical Specialties. 2003 annual report and revised reference handbook. 2003.

118. Ludmerer KM. *Time to Heal*. Oxford, UK: Oxford University Press; 1999.

119. Choudhry NK, Fletcher RH, Soumerai SB. Systematic review: The relationship between clinical experience and quality of health care. *Ann Intern Med.* 2005;**142**(4):260–273.

120. Salter B. *Medical Regulation and Public Trust*. London, UK: Kings Fund Publishing; 2000.

121. Moran M, Wood B. *States, Regulation, and the Medical Profession*. Buckingham, UK: Open University Press; 1993.

122. Norcini JJ. Recertification in the United States. *BMJ.* 1999;**319**(7218):1183–1185.

123. Shaw GB. *Preface on Doctors. The Doctor's Dilemma*. Penguin Books; 1946.

124. Farber NJ, Gilibert SG, Aboff BM, Collier VU, Weiner J, Boyer EG. Physicians' willingness to report impaired colleagues. *Soc Sci Med.* 2005;**61**(8):1772–1775.

125. Morreim EH. Am I my brother's warden? Responding to the unethical or incompetent colleague. *Hastings Cent Rep.* 1993;**23**(3):19–27.

126. Institute of Medicine (U.S.). *To Err Is Human: Building a Safer Health System.* Washington, D.C.: National Academy Press; 2000.

127. Smith R. All changed, changed utterly: British medicine will be transformed by the Bristol case. *BMJ.* 1998;**316**(7149):1917–1918.

128. Can physicians regulate themselves? *CMAJ.* 2005;**172**(6):717, 719.

129. Secretary of the State for Health. *Trust, Assurance, and Safety- the Regulation of Health Professionals in the 21st Century.* London: Stationery Office; 2007.

130. Sohl P, Bassford R. Codes of medical ethics: Traditional foundations and contemporary medical practice. *Soc Sci Med.* 1980;**22**:1175–1179.

131. Coulehan J, Williams PC, McCrary SV, Belling C. The best lack all conviction: Biomedical ethics, professionalism, and social responsibility. *Camb Q Healthc Ethics.* 2003;**12**(1):21–38.

132. Stevens RA. Public roles for the medical profession in the United States: Beyond theories of decline and fall. *Milbank Q.* 2001;**79**(3):327–53, III.

133. Gruen RL, Campbell EG, Blumenthal D. Public roles of US physicians: Community participation, political involvement, and collective advocacy. *JAMA.* 2006;**296**(20):2467–2475.

134. Whitehead C. The doctor dilemma in interprofessional education and care: How and why will physicians collaborate? *Med Educ.* 2007;**41**(10):1010–1016.

135. Coulter A. Patients' views of the good doctor. *BMJ.* 2002;**325**(7366):668–669.

136. Cruess RL, Cruess SR. Teaching professionalism: General principles. *Med Teach.* 2006;**28**(3):205–208.

137. Cohen JJ. Professionalism in medical education, an American perspective: From evidence to accountability. *Med Educ.* 2006;**40**(7):607–617.

138. Hilton SR, Slotnick HB. Proto-professionalism: How professionalisation occurs across the continuum of medical education. *Med Educ.* 2005;**39**(1):58–65.

139. Boenink AD, de Jonge P, Smal K, Oderwald A, van Tilburg W. The effects of teaching medical professionalism by means of vignettes: An exploratory study. *Med Teach.* 2005;**27**(5):429–432.

Appendix: Cases by Specialty

A. Adult primary care – cases are found in the following chapters: patient welfare, patient autonomy, honesty with patients, managing conflicts of interest, and commitment to professional responsibilities. Cases are also found in Chapter 2 under social justice and improving quality of care.

B. Internal medicine – cases are found in the following chapters: patient autonomy (oncology), patient autonomy (nephrology), social justice (cardiology), patient confidentiality (infectious disease), improving quality of care (gastroenterology, endocrinology, hospital medicine), and professional responsibilities (pulmonary medicine). Cases are also found in Chapter 2 under patient autonomy, maintaining appropriate relations with patients, and commitment to a just distribution of finite resources.

C. Obstetrics and gynecology – cases are found in the following chapters: patient welfare, social justice, patient confidentiality, improving quality of care, managing conflicts of interest. Cases are also found in Chapter 2 under social justice, maintaining appropriate relations with patients, and honesty with patients.

D. Pediatrics – cases are found in the following chapters: patient welfare, patient autonomy, social justice, honesty with patients, patient confidentiality, and professional responsibilities. Cases are also found in Chapter 2 under patient welfare, and patient confidentiality.

E. Psychiatry – cases are found in the following chapters: patient welfare, patient autonomy, social justice, honesty with patients, patient confidentiality, and improving quality of care. Cases are also found in Chapter 2 under patient welfare, managing conflicts of interest, and professional responsibilities.

F. Surgery – cases are found in the following chapters: patient welfare, social justice, honesty with patients, and managing conflicts of interest.

Cases are also found in Chapter 2 under patient autonomy, commitment to scientific knowledge, and professional responsibilities.

G.   Neurology – cases are found in the following chapters – social justice, honesty with patients, patient confidentiality, and professional responsibilities.

H.   Emergency medicine – cases are found in the following chapters: patient welfare, improving quality of care, and professional responsibilities.

Index

CPSIA information can be obtained at www.ICGtesting.com
Printed in the USA
BVOW03s1916280614

357666BV00004B/5/P